Hamid Montakab

with

Solange Montakab-Pont

ACUPUNCTURE FOR TREATING THE HIDDEN ROOTS OF DISEASE

The Mind and the Emotions in Chinese Medicine

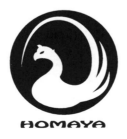

HOMAYA

Editon, design and illustrations: Hamid Montakab
Printed and bound by: Kindle Publishing
Cover design and artwork: Solange Montakab-Pont

ISBN 978-2-9701039-3-6

www.homaya.ch

ACUPUNCTURE FOR TREATING THE HIDDEN ROOTS OF DISEASE

The Mind and the Emotions in Chinese Medicine

Happiness is my nature,
Suffering is my creation

Hamid Montakab MD

Graduated from the Medical School of Paris, did his residency in surgery and completed his acupuncture studies in Paris followed by further clinical training in China. He subsequently explored local healing in the Philippines and India for two years. He practiced for five years in America, obtaining the NCCA certification and a degree in Chinese Herbalism. Later he also studied Osteopathy and Visceral Osteopathy in France.

With his wife Solange they founded the Academy of Chinese Healing Arts in Switzerland in 1986.

Dr. Montakab was commissioned by the Swiss National Science Foundation to conduct a research study on Acupuncture and Insomnia. In 1995 he was the co-founder and president of the Swiss Professional Organization for TCM.

Currently he lectures in Switzerland and in other European countries and the US.

He is the author of Acupuncture for Insomnia (Thieme); Acupuncture Point and Channel Energetics (Kiener); Second Edition (Homaya); Chinese Medicine Revisited (Homaya/ KDP); and Acupuncture for Headaches, Eyes and ENT Pathologies (Singing Dragon). He is also the co-author of Stresskrankheiten (Elsevier) and Bahandlung von Schalfstörungen (MS)

Solange Montakab-Pont

Trained as a Yoga instructor and later studied Naturopathy, Auriculotherapy, Acupuncture and Chinese herbal medicine in Switzerland and in France. She did further trainings in Osteopathy and Visceral Osteopathy in France. She has been practicing *Qi Gong* and meditation, and has been initiated into Tibetan Buddhism. Her particular interest in human psychology led her to the study of a variety of psychotherapeutic methods such as re-birthing, de-hypnotherapy and trans-personal psychotherapy. Inspired by the various Eastern and Western methods, she has developed her own approach for working with patients that she has named "Psycho-Energetics".

Solange Montakab-Pont was the co-founder of the Academy of Chinese Healing Arts and co-author of "Acupuncture for Insomnia" and "Chinese Medicine Revisited". Currently she practices in Saviese- Switzerland.

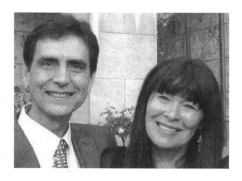

PART- III

EMOTIONS AND THEIR ENERGETIC IMPACT **129**

PART- IV

IMPACT OF TRAUMA **157**

PREFACE

I fell into Chinese medicine without really knowing what I was getting into!

Towards the end of my medical studies, I was becoming more and more disillusioned by our so-called scientific approach, having witnessed how statistical data were collected and manipulated. The medical profession giving the impression of knowing what exactly was the problem and how to treat it, when in fact we were simply applying some protocol based on statistical analysis. Rarely the treatments addressed a patient but rather their diagnosed disease!

At the time, Chinese medicine had offered me the option of getting out of this Western medical "scientific" rut and to look at the concept of health and disease from a different perspective. But rapidly I realised that our Western style of practising Chinese medicine, unfortunately, followed the same pattern of reasoning, which is, to approach the symptom by a cause and effect analysis. Over the years I came to understand that to grasp the full dimensions of a disease nemesis, we as therapists have to change radically our vision of the human, and the world that surrounds us. In this manner, Chinese medicine ceases to be a mere technique and becomes a way of life.

Over 20 centuries ago, the Chinese abandoned the concept of "harmful spirits" at the origin of disease and replaced it with the external and internal causative factors. Emphasising that in the disease aetiology, the internal factors, the mind and the emotions, have predominance over the other, external and combined influences.

In the West, with the separation between church and science in the 16th century, Cartesian science and medicine in particular has been striving to explain the causality of disease, beyond divine will and punishment. Great efforts were made to steer away from the occult and the spiritual, in favour of the visible and material explanations. It even became unavoidable for many scientists to reject totally the notion and the belief in God or in any form of an invisible creating force.

In the 19th century, Pasteur's breakthrough in the germ theory opened the door to understanding and possibly preventing many types of diseases through immunisation. In the 20th century, Fleming developed penicillin and with that the Utopia that if the causative factor was identified and chemically eradicated, then the pathological process could be stopped. Today, after seven decades of using anti-bacterial agents, we are facing a very serious problem, that of antimicrobial resistance, forcing medical science to look in another direction and finally ask the right question when exposed to a pathogen, what makes a particular person develop the disease? Or again, what are the factors influencing the immune system of an individual?

Historically, Chinese medicine had emphasised the continuity of the physical, emotional and spiritual dimensions of the human being. By classifying the causative factors of the disease, into external, internal and mixed, and by delegating the emotions, and mental attitudes to the internal causes, they were emphasising the impact of the psycho-emotional equilibrium of a person. The Chinese premise of "the body holds the mind and the mind contains the body" clearly demonstrates this belief.

Ancient Chinese medicine had already understood the possibility of external infestations, without actually knowing about germs and viruses. *Hoatuo,* in the 2nd century, had even attempted a rudimentary type of vaccination that was to be abandoned later. Chinese medicine explains that the external pathogenic factors (*Xie Qi*) become harmful mainly when the defensive energy (*Wei Qi*) of a person is compromised. The *Wei Qi* is part of the produced energy *Zhong Qi* of the individual and depends on numerous factors such as diet, lifestyle and genetics. All of these factors are directly influenced by the psychology and the temperament of the person.

The Chinese had further emphasised that the *Shen* leads the *Qi*, signifying that the neurophysiology of the body is primarily subject to the mind and the psyche, what is currently broadly classified by allopathic medicine as psychosomatics.

Although Classical Chinese Medicine (CCM) is estimated to be 25 centuries-old, the basic medical and philosophical concepts have been proven to be extremely modern as demonstrated today by the scientific technologies currently available. Despite the prejudice inflicted on to CCM by its contemporary version TCM (Traditional Chinese Medicine; established in the 1940s' and 50s', the Chinese medical theories, in particular, those about subtle energy fields, the psyche, the mind and the emotions are being substantiated by many present-day discoveries.

The powers of the mind are now being extensively researched and have so far demonstrated that not only belief systems and mental training can heal the body ("You are the Placebo" by J. Dispenza), but that the mind actually creates the pathological process in the first place (the causality of accidents and genetics will be discussed later). The works of Dr B. Siegel, amongst many others, on cancer patients, is demonstrating this point (the Nocebo effect). His first question addressed to the cancer patient is "...why do you want to die?"

Such a question would normally scandalise the medical and scientific professions, but then a whole body of research and evidence are supporting the concept that the disease process originates in the psyche.

All life forms have in common the same program: survival and the perpetuation of the species. In humans, this manifests as the "Passion for life" and the "Will to live". When one or the other is lost, the life process is compromised, allowing for various pathological conditions to develop. The New-age concepts and the modern scientific discoveries of the past few decades are joining the ancient Chinese teachings, that the root of all disease is hidden in the mind and that it is through the cultivation of the mind (mental training) that we can treat an individual.

The powers of the mind are boundless, but we are only using, at best 7% of this potential. Not only has the mind the power to generate disease and to heal it but, it is also constantly influencing the outer world, without our conscious knowledge.

Recent discoveries in science are finally confirming the age-old concepts about the importance of "Inner balance" in maintaining health. The role of emotions, the mind and belief systems are now being scientifically evaluated. Just to mention a few:

- The works of C. Pert have demonstrated that the immune system is directly influenced by emotional factors.

- Modern breakthroughs in "Epigenetics" are confirming the impact of the environment (lifestyle and diet) and the psyche on the genes themselves. In fact, only 25% of the transmitted genes are immutable, the majority of the genes could be activated or not depending on a several post-natal influences. Even diet and lifestyle (activity, rest, sleep and sexuality) are all reflecting a person's psychology and temperament. (Biology of belief by B. Lipton)

- The works of E. Kandel on neuroplasticity, confirm that repeated thought patterns and habitual belief systems can change the functioning of the brain, positively or negatively.

- In the 80's several Princeton experiments involving new-born chickens (and rabbits) demonstrated their ability to influence a robot, based on a random event generator, and to change its predefined program. If new-born chicks can change their environment, what can the human mind achieve?

- In quantum physics, Heisenberg proposed the uncertainty principle, applying the "observer effect" to quantum physics, stipulating that the measurements of all wave-like systems cannot be made without affecting and changing the system. In other words, the observer can change the behaviour of the particles at the quantum level. The Chinese paradigm stating that all in existence is a form of Qi was substantiated by Einstein's theories and put into this well know equation ($E=mc^2$). So, it is not anymore, a mystery, that this vibrational world, as well as this vibrational body of ours, is being constantly modified by the "observer" that we are.

Despite all of these findings supporting the New Age claim that the human subconscious is extremely powerful and capable of influencing a person's life and their environment, there is a huge amount of disbelief and scepticism from the hard-line scientific community.

The most common criticism brought to alternative therapies is the lack of a scientific basis, and insufficient evidence to support clinical efficacy. Unfortunately, the methodology that is proposed to study the effects of a given alternative medicine, are un-adapted to the vibrational nature of the alternative method. For instance, a double-blind study is not compatible with acupuncture, manual therapies, energy and vibrational therapies, and many faith healing methods. Furthermore, the main premise in most of the above techniques is to enhance the body's natural healing capacities by changing the mental framework or the belief mechanisms; in other words, to privilege the placebo effect. In scientific studies, the exact opposite is emphasised, that is, to eliminate the placebo. It is quite unfortunate that in an age in which Heisenberg's uncertainty principle has been demonstrated, that we are still relying on older study models that aim at eliminating the observer effect. In the same manner that we cannot use a simple telescope to study the exoplanets, or an old-fashioned microscope to study the molecular structures, the older statistical data collections are obsolete and a new methodology has to be proposed when evaluating the effectiveness of energy healing methods.

It remains that the ancient Chinese had understood some fundamental facts, maybe intuitively, which has taken the West several thousand years to verify and to mathematically quantify. But we are still a long way from applying these concepts to our daily lives. Humanity's collective belief systems have remained Newtonian, and Einstein's contributions have not yet been integrated into what overall humanity believes to be "reality".

Our medical science still relies on the chemical manipulation of the human physiology, as witnessed by well-over 12000 specialities found in most compendiums of pharmaceuticals. The medical belief is that the lack of a certain neurotransmitter is the cause of a person's psychological and emotional state, when in fact Classical Chinese medicine considers the mental state to be the origin of the neuro-physiological dis-balance (dis-ease).

What we see depends primarily upon the belief systems that we use to interpret our observations (see further).

> *...space and time are not conditions in which we live;*
> *they are modes in which we think.*
>
> Albert Einstein

The idea to write this book was not just to add another text on the Psyche in Chinese Medicine, but rather to bring together the discoveries of modern neuropsychiatry with the age-old Chinese concepts, and most pertinently to see to what extent, we practitioners of Chinese medicine, can influence the overall well-being of our patients. Additionally, to explore the impact that our environment has on us and even more important is to discover how our thoughts and belief systems have been influencing our world.

The Chinese concept of the human as a "Microcosm" evolving in the world "Macrocosm", in constant interaction and both submitted to the same laws "*Wu Xing*" the Five Movements, finds a parallel in the modern Lorenz's "Butterfly effect". The Chaos theory proposes the concept of a ripple effect in which small changes may produce great outcomes.

No human is an island….

This book was written in collaboration with my wife Solange.

With her rich background in several Oriental healing arts, Yoga and Buddhist training, and many Western psychotherapeutic methods, she has been able to successfully combine them with the practice of Classical Chinese medicine. Her experience in working with the psychological causes of pathologies in a standard acupuncture setting has been a great contribution to the unravelling and the treatment of the "Hidden Roots of Disease".

Many of the exercises proposed in Annex-IV have been adapted from Eastern and Western methods and refined and applied to the Chinese medical concepts. These methods have proven their clinical efficiency over several decades.

Hamid Montakab
Savièse, Switzerland April 2020

****

I first discovered Chinese Medicine with a feeling of gratitude and relief. Here was finally what I had been searching for, a medicine that understood the human being in its globality and in relation to the world; a holistic approach that tailored the therapy to the individual. A wonderful model to comprehend life. Later as I followed the TCM teachings both in Europe and U.S.A., I became more and more disappointed with the rather mechanical and symptomatic TCM approach, reducing all pathologies to Zang-Fu and Substance disharmony, and geared to the pattern rather than the person. Despite the good results with most of my patients, something essential was missing to truly comprehend the deeper significance and the metaphor of a disease nemesis.

Life being the best teacher, in 1995 after a serious fracture and the following complications I almost lost the use of my right arm, despite the best allopathic and TCM therapies. This challenged me to search in another direction and to seek other alternatives. A year after my recovery I developed new courses combining this difficult experience with techniques that I had learned and practiced previously, some of which is presented in this book.

I must admit that when I was asked to participate in the realisation of this book, there was a great deal of hesitation as it seemed very difficult to transmit the subtility and the complexity of an interpersonal process through the written word. This challenge was further fuelled by the necessity for broadening the scope of Chinese Medicine and to be able to reach a larger group of therapists and patients.

I would like to express my deepest gratitude to my most important teacher, life and all its trials and tribulations; to my parents, and to the many tutors and instructors that I have been fortunate to meet. Special thanks to my beloved Hamid, who believed in me and continuously encouraged me to continue in my search. And finally, I extend my acknowledgments to my patients and students without whom these ideas might not have taken form.

Solange Montakab-Pont
Savièse, Switzerland April 2020

****

The actions and indications of the acupuncture points are based on the Chinese classical texts, the Daoist oral heritage as transmitted by Master. J. Yuen and the European acupuncture traditions, in particular, the French school (Please refer to the Bibliography).

More details and exact references may be found in:

‣ **"Acupuncture Point and Channel Energetics; Bridging the Gap"**. (Kiener Verlag)

or

‣ **"Acupuncture Point and Channel Energetics; Bridging the Gap"**; second edition: **Clinical application of the written and oral traditions of Acupuncture** (Homaya publications / KDP).

INTRODUCTION

- **The "Why of Disease": The ghost in the basement!**

- **The three historical causes of disease in TCM**

- **Emotions and Passions**

- **Life Mandate**

- **Chinese Philosophical traditions**

- **The Three Treasures**

INTRODUCTION:

The "Why of Disease": The ghost in the basement!

The three historical causes of disease in TCM

Health is not only a state of physical or physiological balance but also and maybe even primarily a state of psychological and emotional well-being.

From a Chinese Medical perspective, health is defined as a state of harmony between *Yin* and *Yang*. This equilibrium is relative to each individual. A loss of equilibrium between *Yin* and *Yang* causes disease.

The art of practising Chinese Medicine is primarily to prevent disease; but once pathology has manifested itself, it is to know how to treat its true cause, sometimes its hidden roots.

Since the Song dynasty (circa 10th century AD) the causes of disease have been classified under three headings:

- External Causes: These include climatic variations that are, Cold, Wind, Heat, Dampness and Dryness. The causative factors are the climatic extremes as well as pernicious combinations such as Wind-Cold or Damp-Cold etc. Obviously, besides the most extreme conditions, the outside can only cause disease if the person's inner balance has been compromised.

- Internal Causes: The emotions or rather the psycho-emotional profile and mental states of an individual are the fundamental inner cause of dis-balance. The classical texts have repeatedly emphasised this point:

  > *All diseases are rooted in the Shen*   *Ling Shu* chp. 8

- Half internal - half external, also classified as mixed causes including the constitution, diet, lifestyle, sexual activity, trauma, infections, poisons and radiations, geomagnetic influences and harmful spirits.

Furthermore, the Chinese medical model of the human being stresses two points:

- The human being is a complete "unit"; hence there is no separation between the mind and the body. This implies that our thoughts and emotions are reflections of our energetic and organic physiological functions and vice versa.

- The human being is an integral part of the world in which he or she evolves. The psychological profile of each individual depends not only on the constitutional genetic inheritance but, even more importantly, on the impact of the environment. Our overall health is more often the result of our interaction with the outside world. This interaction is primarily the result of the functioning of the psyche and the "Belief systems". What we consider as reality, truth or fact has a deep impact on how we perceive the world and respond to it.

It is high time for us, practitioners of Chinese medicine, to start applying the outstanding fundamental principles that have been transmitted through the ages:

> *What is most important in the treatment of an individual*
> *is the cultivation of the mind*
>
> Zhang Jiebin (17th c.)

The New-age concepts and the modern scientific discoveries of the past few decades are substantiating the ancient Chinese teachings, that the root of all disease is hidden in the mind and that it is through the Cultivation of the Mind* that we can treat an individual.

* Cultivation of the Mind should be understood as the process through which the habitual mindsets are transformed, allowing for a broader view of reality.

Unfortunately, in modern TCM (Traditional Chinese Medicine), even if we suspect a particular pathology to have its origin in the psycho-emotional profile of the patient, we are still following the Western model of treating the visible cause by simply re-balancing the *Yin* and *Yang* or the *Qi* and Blood to harmonise the psyche. It is so much easier to deal with the "branch" rather than the "root".

Very much like the proverbial character, who has lost his house keys in the basement, but is searching for them in the garden instead, because it is too dark in the basement!!

Then why are we treating the manifestation rather than the origin?

The reasons are quite simple to understand:

- We are lacking the necessary tools to deal with the mind and the belief systems;

- Most often, we, ourselves, have not explored the inner workings of our mind and subconscious; if we have not learnt to swim in the dark waters of the psyche, how can we help save another person from drowning?

Classical Chinese medicine is offering us so many tools to choose from, but often we are just staying with the external approach.

An important Chinese medical paradigm is that *Qi* follows *Shen*. In other terms, the mind and the psyche have an ascendance on the physiological processes and even on exterior phenomena.

Therefore, to understand the "Hidden Roots of Disease", we have to explore primarily:

- The construct of the mind and the psyche that Chinese medicine globally refers to as *Shen*.

- The role and energetic impact of Emotions.

- The importance of the "Belief systems", which are partly the result of the constitution and the temperament of the person, and partly reflect the conditioning by the environment.

Ultimately all disease has its origin in the psyche, according to Daoist or Buddhist beliefs, even external events like accidents, are part of a person's life path. The cultivation of the mind, might not avoid an accident, but it will certainly modify how we live the experience.

Emotions and Passions

The internal causes of disease are defined as the Five Emotions "*Wu Zhi*" 五志 and the Seven Passions "*Qi Qing*" 七情.

One of the originalities of Chinese medicine resides in its holistic understanding of the human being. By indicating the emotions as being the only internal cause, an important emphasis is put on two points:

- Emotions are internal and do not come from the outside, as one often tends to wrongly presume

- Emotional disturbances are the internal root of all disease and suffering

Physical and Psychological Health are interdependent

Emotions are the modifications of the *Shen* (Spirit/ mind) in reaction to changes in the environment. They are necessary for the normal functioning of the organism, thus they are named the "Five emotions" in continuity with the "Five Moving forces". Emotion is considered the driving force behind motivation.

When a particular emotion becomes harmful then it is classified as a "passion". Although Western psychology enumerates numerous types of emotions, the ancient Chinese symbolically classified the harmful emotions as the "Seven passions". The number seven is the symbolic number for the ageing process and for dissolution and destruction.

Modern science is exploring the neuro-humoral factors involved in emotions. Although it is still not clear if a particular chemistry produces an emotion or vice versa, the physiological effects of emotions and their impact on health and disease are indisputable today.

On this point, the ancient Chinese had a very deep understanding by delegating the inner causes of disease to emotional factors and by analysing the physiological impact of each emotion.

Life Mandate

Before going any further, it is imperative to define our personal concepts and beliefs.

The basic Daoist belief considers the human being having a *Ming*, life mandate or curriculum. This concept could be loosely translated as "destiny". In this context many ancient belief systems, Buddhism in particular, agree that human life has a purpose and pre-destination.

We could, very generally, divide the human belief systems into three groups:

- **Human as a creation of God:** A global intelligence or God, creating the universe and human beings, giving them free-will to choose between right and wrong. In this vision, the soul is eternal and would reside for eternity in heaven or in hell based on the actions during this finite life span. Only rare beings may return in physical form, to help guide the humans (avatars or bodhisattvas).

- **Human as part of an evolutionary process:** Each individual spirit is part of a global intelligence, regularly returning and choosing a particular life mandate to complete a specific curriculum or to rectify certain actions. The final realisation (enlightenment, Nirvana) can liberate the soul from this recurring cycle of re-birth.

- **Human as the result of random mutation:** The materialistic and existential belief rejects the notion of a creator. This life is incidental and random and is all that there is, and the soul dies with the physical body. During this very short life, our deeds and actions define the heaven or the hell that we live in.

  Each belief system is supported and substantiated by the socio-cultural environment. An individual may find a confirming proof for one or another of these belief systems. Depending on the observations that we make, our belief systems may change but ultimately, we experience life and the world through the filter of our assumptions and convictions.

The Daoist ideology can easily absorb the first two systems. The ancient Chinese describe conception as the union of three constitutional energies:

- *Yuan Qi* ≈ Source or creative energy; this notion can easily be replaced by the notion of a Universal intelligence or by a creator God. *Yuen Qi* links us with the origin, the source and all in existence.

- *Jing Qi* ≈ Essence, provided by the parental *Jing*. This could be assimilated to the modern concept of chromosomic transmission. The combined essence of the parents will be the foundation of the child's future *Jing*. It was believed that the *Jing* defines the constitution and bestows the vital strength as well as transferring parental life experiences and wisdom. The latter seems to rather indicate the function of *Zong* ≈ Ancestral inheritance.

- *Zong Qi* ≈ Ancestral energy. The *Zong Qi* is considered to be the influence of the environment, the alignment of the stars and the planets (astrology), and the mother's physical and psychological state during the pregnancy. The term "Ancestral" seems to go beyond the simple environmental influences and carries the notion of transmitted parental experiences (both mother and father), and even possibly their beliefs. It is quite logical to equate the *Zong Qi*, to the modern concept of "Epigenetics", according to which the chemo-physical and psychological environment of a child or even an adult may affect the expression of the genetic code through these particular additional segments "Epi", that could block or activate the nucleotides without altering the DNA sequence. This particular modification may be transferred to the offspring, hence the term "Ancestral". (see also section 1.2.8)

It is further believed that *Shen*, the individualised spirit, chooses to appear and inhabit this particular physical residence after conception and that after death, the "Individual" *Shen*, leaves the body and joins the "Universal" *Shen*. Obviously, this belief implies the notion of choice and free will. The choice of taking on a particular physical form, gender, ethnic and religious predilections, is determined by the individual *Shen* before birth, at the very moment of conception.

In this, the three oriental thought systems, Confucianism, Daoism and Buddhism, differ.

Chinese Philosophical traditions

To understand the ancient Chinese vision of the universe, the human being and of medicine, we have to explore the Chinese philosophical beliefs and traditions of that period.

What could be the reason that would explain that the Chinese discovered and developed numerous technologies centuries before the West, to mention just a few:

- Certain agricultural technologies were applied 20 centuries before the West,

- The processing of iron steel, the printing press, and the compass almost 1400 years before the West,

- Discovery of the blood circulation system, 1800 years before Harvey,

- The various concepts about the human physiology and the interactions between the psyche and the soma, and the deep understanding of the origins of disease, prognosis, and treatment,

- Emphasis on prevention, with attempts at vaccination as early as 200 AD

- And most relevantly, the discovery of the binary language 27 centuries before the West invented the computer language.

It is very unlikely that the above discoveries could be explained by simple random chance or some metaphysical genius, but rather a different way of looking at the universe and a different conception of reality.

Historically in the West, the reality was based on facts. A fact is an observed phenomenon in the natural world that is perceived as an elemental principle. It is rarely one that can be subject to personal interpretation. And yet facts such as "the earth is flat" or that "the sun is at the centre of the universe", dominated for centuries man's perceptions and definitions of what is real. Today, the most pertinent of these facts could be said to be the "solid" nature of matter. Even though science has demonstrated that the smallest constituent of matter, the atom, is primarily made of empty space or void, our age-old conditioning does not allow us to perceive it other than solid. And yet, the ancient Chinese had explained the origins of creation very much in the same manner as physicists are doing so today, 25 centuries later!

So, to understand the Chinese concepts, one has to start by understanding the Chinese thought.

Although many schools of thought were the originators of the Chinese religions and philosophies (Hundred Schools of Thought ≈ *Zhuzi Baijia* 諸子百家); between the 6th and 2nd century BC, six schools dominated and influenced the Chinese society, government, lifestyle and medical practices: Confucianism, Legalism, Daoism, Mohism (Universal love), Naturalism (School of Yin-Yang and Five Elements) and Logicians.

There are numerous scholarly books on the above philosophies. The purpose of this text is not to do a historical and sinologic analysis of these thought systems, but rather to realise that each of these thoughts has left its imprints on the Chinese medicine that we are practising today. The following schools of thought may have had the strongest impact on Chinese culture:

- The Confucian school was probably the most influential on the overall Chinese socio-cultural values. The Confucian premise is that human beings are fundamentally good, and may improve and attain perfection through personal and social effort and self-cultivation. For Confucius, the respect of the social order "ethics" was the only effective system of government and social harmony. Interestingly, the concept of emotions being causative factors of a disease, probably stem from this principle. It was believed that emotions, by their disruptive action on social harmony, divert the individual from the path of compassion and social propriety. Furthermore, in medicine, the position of the Heart-Emperor and the ten ministers, as well as the laws regulating the Five Movements (*Sheng* ≈ *Generation/* Production and *Ke* ≈ Control), the concepts of counter-flow Qi and therapeutic technics of *Li* ≈ Rectifying Qi, could be relevant examples of Confucian principles.

- Legalism (法家; *Fajia*; "School of law"), maintained that human nature was incorrigibly selfish; and that the only way to preserve the social order was to impose strict enforcement of laws. Legalism and Confucianism greatly influenced the philosophical basis for the imperial form of government that would remain intact until the late 19th century. The military tendency of the Legalistic thought is reflected in medicine with the concepts of *Wei Qi* ≈ Defensive energy (army), and of *Ying Qi* ≈ Nourishing energy (army camp) and purging therapeutic methods such as sudorification, vomification and purgation.

- Daoism differs from Confucianism by putting more emphasis on physical and spiritual cultivation and less emphasis on political organisation. In many ways, the Daoist philosophy is the opposite of the rigid Confucian morality, focusing on the individual within the universe rather than the individual within society. Hence the life-purpose of each individual is to adjust and adapt oneself to the natural rhythms of the universe, and seek to live in harmony with the world. Naturally, the Daoist teachings advocated an attitude of minimum interference by the government. The Daoist thought deeply influenced the dialectical systems predominant in medical concepts such as the void, chaos, organising principle *Tai Yi*, trinity, etc.; as well as many other medical paradigms. Putting the accent on prevention and living in harmony with the natural rhythms, understanding the psyche and cultivating the mind through contemplation and meditation.

- Although, Buddha, Confucius and Laozi were contemporaries, Buddhism was to integrate the Chinese thought system, much later during the Han dynasty (circa 50 CE), further re-enforced by the teachings of Bodhidharma in the 6th century. Buddhism explores human suffering and relates it to a distorted (illusory) perception of reality (suffering, impermanence and separation) due to faulty mental habits and deeply ingrained beliefs. According to Buddha's teachings, the mind needs to be re-trained through meditation, to be able to truly see the nature of reality and to attain liberation. As Buddhism considers the root of human suffering to be the psyche (belief systems) and the emotions, it seems logical that the inner causes of disease were described to be the "Seven Passions", a typical Buddhist concept.

There are many paintings depicting three men, Buddha, Confucius and Laozi, tasting vinegar; a parable for the leading Chinese philosophical and religious traditions expressing life symbolised by vinegar (▶ Fig. 0.1). Buddha finds the vinegar bitter; Confucius's expression is sour, only Laozi is smiling, stating that life is good as it is. It could also be said that ultimately all teachings are actually one.

Based on these concepts, it becomes quite clear as to why a central role in the disease process is relegated to the psyche and the emotions.

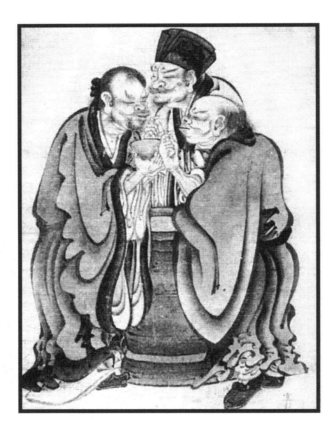

Fig. 01:   The three vinegar tasters

The Three Treasures (*San Bao* 三宝)

In the Chinese art of health maintenance, transformation and search for harmony, the emphasis is put on the "Three Treasures": *Shen - Qi - Jing* (▶Fig. 0.2).

- *Jing* is produced and protected by the Kidneys and is responsible for strength, vitality and the continuation of the species. *Jing*, in turn, depends on the quality "*Jing*" of the air, water and food, and the preservation of the sexual energy.

- *Qi* (refers to True ≈ *Zhen Qi*) is produced by the Spleen and Stomach and maintains life, it clearly depends on the quality of food and water, and the correct lifestyle and the circulation of this *Qi* through appropriate exercises "*Qi Gong*".

- *Shen* is residing in the Heart and enables the evolution and transformation of the human being, mentally as well as spiritually. *Shen* is developed by correct discipline and the cultivation of the mind and the spirit through meditative practices.

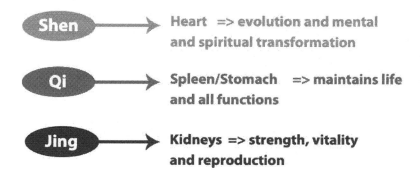

Fig. 02   The three treasures *"San Bao"*: *Shen - Oi - Jing*

PART - I
The Mind and the Psyche

- **The Construct of the Psyche**
  - *Shen*
  - *Hun*
  - *Po*
  - *Yi*
  - *Zhi*

- **Mental Activity and the Brain**
  - The Power of the Mind
  - Consciousness and Sensory Perceptions
  - The Conscious functioning of the Mind
  - The Subconscious
  - Concept of *Gui* ≈ Harmful Spirits
  - Sleep and Dreams (*Shen* and *Hun*)
  - The mind/psyche and the body/soma
  - Pain: the language of the body
  - Memory
  - Intelligence

PART- I

The Mind and the Psyche

1.1 The Construct of the Psyche

The psyche, as seen by the Chinese, follows the Five Element model.

The image is that of each of the five organ-energy systems having a "driving spirit" directing the specific energies of that organ, producing a specific emotion and a mental or spiritual activity. These spirits are subject to the emperor, the Fire Spirit, *Shen*. (▶Fig. 1.1).

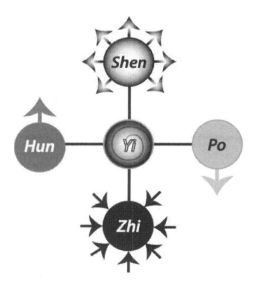

Fig. 1.1: *Shen* ≈ Spirit controlling *Hun, Po, Yi* and *Zhi*

The total manifestation and mental-emotional balance of a person are referred to as their *Shen*.

The closest Western analogy for the concept of the various facets of the *Shen* and its constituents could be found in the Jungian stratification of the human psyche (▶Fig. 1.2):

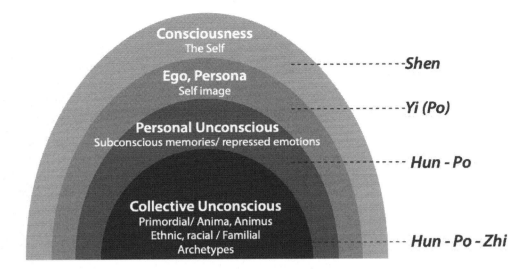

Fig.1.2:   The Jungian image of the stratified human psyche and its parallel with the Chinese concepts of the *Shen* ≈ Spirit-mind

- Consciousness and the concept of the "Self": related to *Shen*

- Ego, Persona, and self-image: related to *Yi*, possibly *Po*

- Personal unconscious/ subconscious: represented by *Hun* and *Po*

- The collective unconscious, ethnical, racial, familial; anima, animus; archetypes: *Hun, Po,* and *Zhi*

The latter concept seems to correspond to the Chinese notion of *Zong* ≈ Ancestral *Qi*

To grasp the concept of the mind and the psyche in Chinese medicine, we first need to explore the notion of the "Five Spirits" that represent the five parts of the mind and the emotions. It is imperative to constantly remember that the human psyche functions as a whole unit and it would be erroneous to consider the five parts separately.

1.1.1 *Shen* ≈ Spirit (神)

The notion of *Shen* in Chinese medicine is quite vast and covers many physical, psycho-emotional and spiritual aspects. As it is often with Chinese terms, it is quite difficult and limiting to translate a word from the ancient philosophical and medical literature into an equivalent concept in Western thinking. *Shen* may have up to twenty different interpretations, which can prove to be quite confusing for the Western practitioner. In most foreign texts *Shen* has been translated as "Spirit" (▶ Fig. 1.3).

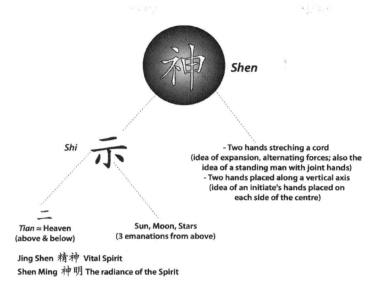

Jing Shen 精神 Vital Spirit
Shen Ming 神明 The radiance of the Spirit

Fig. 1.3: The significance of *Shen*

Historically the concept of *Shen* ≈ Spirit was more developed by the Daoists and transmitted via the oral tradition. The Confucian scholars rather emphasised the notion of "knowing oneself", rather than the attributes of the spirit.

The embodiment of *Shen* is represented by the concept of *Ling* 靈 ≈ Soul. It is believed that *Shen* integrates (incarnates) the original embryo after conception, bringing with it the "desire" to live through a specific experience. The Daoist tradition describes this process as the *Shen* selecting a particular *Jing* ≈ Essence and providing it with a *Ming* ≈ Destiny. It is not exactly clear as to what stage of development the *Shen* integrates the embryo, but it is believed that it provides the 3 *Hun* ≈ Ethereal Souls during the 3rd month and the 7 *Po* ≈ Corporeal Souls during the 4th month.

The notion of "Spirit" primarily includes two outstanding concepts:

➢ The concept of a "Universal *Shen*" which may refer to the notions of:

- Spirit or Spirits*
- Gods
- Creative Instance
- Organising Spirit or Organising Principle
- Subtle influx received from Heaven
- Mysterious cause understood as "Unfathomable" metaphysical principle; Original Mystery (*Suwen* chapter 5)
- Pure action

* C. Larre and E. Rochat translate *Shen* as "Spirits", referring to its multidimensional aspect.

➢   In another context, the references to "*Shen*" seem to describe a more "Individual" dimension:

- Configuring Force: relating to the "Organising" influence actively configuring and transforming the specific characteristics of the "Individual" reflected in "*Ming*", life mandate or destiny. It is even presumed that the *Shen* chooses the physical body that it will inhabit. Once *Shen* has chosen an incarnation it becomes "*Ling*" the "Soul".

- Transforming Force: is the "Creative" force, which enhances growth, elaborates and completes the transformation of an individual and his consciousness of the world.

- *Shen* also represents "Lifeforce" (*Jing Shen* ≈ Vital Spirit). *Shen* is the life principle, represented by the "Passion for Life". When this passion is lost, the motive forces for the perpetuation of life are compromised and the dying process is initiated.

> ....*when Shen departs it is death*   Lingshu chapter 71
>
> ....*losing the Shen is annihilation*   Suwen ch.15

- In post-natal energetics, *Shen* signifies "Vitality": as represented in the concept of "*Shen* being reflected in the eyes". In this context, it is not the spirituality or the intelligence of the person, but simply their vitality, which is evaluated through the eyes. This vitality is seen as a vibrant and sparkling quality, strong in small children and dull and veiled in the elderly. At times, an abnormal intensity can be observed in psychotic patients and referred to as "False *Shen*". Even in tongue diagnosis, when the tongue has normal mobility and moister, it is said that the "Tongue has *Shen*". In this context, a loss of *Shen* signifies a pathological process.

- During one's life, *Shen* represents the consciousness, intelligence, as well as the emotional and the mental functions, all deriving their energies from the Triple Warmer.

  The Daoist beliefs suggest that existence is an unfathomable Spirit or intelligence "Universal *Shen*". Individual life starts by the incarnation of this Spirit into the matter at the moment of conception. At this moment the Individual *Shen* "Little *Shen*" is separated from the "Universal/ Big *Shen*", thus creating the false belief that individuals are separate entities. During one's life span, the "Individual *Shen*" is responsible for maintaining the life force necessary for the person's fulfilment of their individual destiny (*Ming*).

- Chinese medicine delegates the role of the organising principle to the Individual *Shen*, residing in the Heart organ, considered the Emperor. It is symbolically said that the Emperor has two palaces:

- The Earthly palace, is situated in the chest. The chest is part of the trunk, the seat of energy production and human relations. The human body is programmed to grow, evolve and to perpetuate life. Once these basic demands have been completed, the Emperor has to move to its Heavenly palace to fulfil its Heavenly mandate (*Ming*).

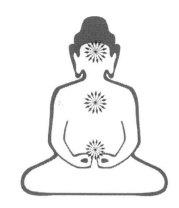

Fig. 1.4: The three *Dan Tian* centres

- The Heavenly palace is symbolically located in the head and behind the third eye. Signifying that the individual should detach from earthly and mundane pursuits and direct their energies towards spiritual matters. The text "Secret of the Golden Flower" describes the necessary steps to transform and ascend the base energies from the lower to the upper "*Dan Tian*" (▶ Fig. 1.4).

It is further underlined that the excessive involvement of *Shen* with Earthly matters is considered a "Passion" and one of the causative factors of disease.

• After death, the "Individual *Shen*" leaves the body to join the global spirit "Universal *Shen*". One of the fundamental premises of oriental spiritual thinking is that the human being, in this separate and dual body, has the opportunity to discover its oneness with existence and with the whole.

This concept of "oneness" with the whole can be represented by the analogy of a cloud made of vaporised water. When the conditions are right, the water vapour freezes and "materialises" to become a snowflake. Each snowflake has its own shape and identity while descending from the sky (▶ Fig. 1.5). But when it reaches the ocean it resumes its water quality once again, losing its physical individuality and dissolving into this vast body of water and at the same time enriching it. By this, it may be implied that the life experiences of the individual (little) *Shen* actually contribute to the growth and evolution of the Universal (big) *Shen*.

It could further be said that during one's lifetime, while separated by the identity of the "Self", the realisation of

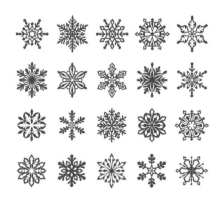

Fig. 1.5: Multitude forms of snowflakes

our true nature and the "oneness" with the rest of existence is what is understood as "enlightenment".

With the body, Unity cannot be realised;

But without the body, the Dao may not be experienced.

At conception, the three "Hereditary" energies of the human being define the body-shape, the constitution, and the temperament, whereas *Shen* defines the destiny of this form.

...Life comes from Jing;

when the male and female Jing unite, Shen is formed...

Each of the five organic systems transform part of the Qi ≈ Energy produced from food and water into a subtle and non-material form that we can call psycho-emotional energy which constitutes one of the five functional energies: Qi, Blood, Fluids, *Shen* and *Jing*.

This concept is symbolically represented by the notion of "*Shen"* that emanates from the "Five Tastes" stored in the Spleen and directed to the Heart. This statement is linking the psycho-emotional energies not only to the Spleen but also to the nature and quality of the food (The five Tastes).

Thus, each organ complex is producing a specific emotion and a mental or spiritual activity, globally represented by the concept of the spirit that resides in that organ: *Suwen* chapter 23 states that *Yi*, resides in the Spleen; *Po* is residing in the Lung; *Hun*, resides in the Liver and *Zhi*, resides in the Kidney. All of these spirits are subject to the emperor, the Fire-spirit "*Shen*" which resides in the Heart. As the Heart-emperor has the charge of the harmony within the state and the empire, *Shen* has the position of coordinator for the other four "Spirits", the *Hun, Po, Yi,* and *Zhi*, maintaining a coherent mental function, manifested in an appropriate connection with the inner and outer worlds, the micro and macrocosm (▶ Fig. 1.1).

Obviously, from a modern Western medical perspective, the notion of a "spirit residing in an organ" is not easy to comprehend. By this symbolic representation, the ancient Chinese have underlined several important points:

- Body and mind are inseparable.

- The mental and emotional manifestations of an individual are the result of the harmonious interaction of organic systems, coordinated by the *Shen*.

- At all times, the inner balance of an individual, the "Microcosm" is dependent on the interaction with the outer world "Macrocosm".

- The overall psychology of a person is represented by the notion of *Shen*

When Qi and blood are complete and harmonised;
when Wei Qi and Ying Qi are complete and unimpeded;
when the 5 Zang are complete and evolved, then the Shen ≈ Spirit
resides in the Heart and Mind ≈ Yi; the Hun and Po contain themselves
within the Zang and Humanity is complete.

Ling Shu Chapter 54

Both in the *I Ching* and the *Suwen* it is stated that:

...the part of Yin and Yang that cannot be measured is "Shen"

Although the psycho-emotional state of a person is referred to as their *Shen*, in fact, this is the sum total of the harmonious interplay of the different attributes of their psyche. *Shen* acts as the Sovereign ruler, directing and orchestrating the other segments of the psyche giving cohesion and coherence to the mental processes, physical functions and harmonising the emotions: coordination, moving into action (Liver - *Hun*), organisation and evaluation (Lung - *Po*), maintenance, concentration, intention (Spleen - *Yi*), advisory aspect, choice, seeing other possibilities (Kidney - *Zhi*).

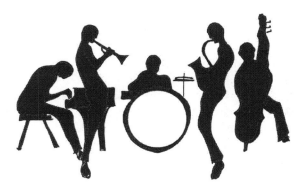

In the image of five musicians who's playing should be coordinated by a band-leader for musical coherence (▶ Fig. 1.6a).

Fig. 1.6a: *Shen* in the image of the band-leader

Or again, the image of the white light that is composed of all the colours of the spectrum (▶ Fig. 1.6b).

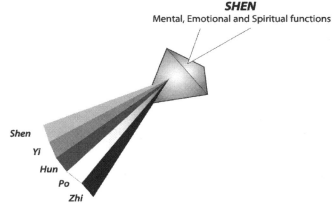

SHEN
Mental, Emotional and Spiritual functions

Shen
Yi
Hun
Po
Zhi

On the human level, the Heart, designated as the Emperor of the state, has the charge of housing the *Shen* ≈ Spirit/ mind. All the other functions attributed to the Heart are actually carried

Fig. 1.6b: *Shen* is the sum of *Shen, Yi, Hun, Po* and *Zhi* out by the Heart's minister, *Xin Bao*. In clinical practice this has two consequences:

- All mental and emotional manifestations will ultimately reflect on the Heart.
- All Heart disharmony patterns will have psycho-emotional expressions.

In Chinese, the word for Heart "*Xin* 心" is the same as for Mind. Thinking, *Si* 思 demonstrates the relation between the Heart and the head as described in the *Ling Shu* chap.10. The ideogram represents the heart bellow and the cranium above.

Shen is reflected in the eyes and manifests through a clear and coherent speech. This statement further refers to the notion that the emperor, envoy of Heaven, receives the virtues of Heaven and Earth and transmits them without alteration. Thus, it is understood that a clear Heart and *Shen*, reflects the world without distorting it. This last statement is fundamental in defining how we perceive the world, interpret reality, and consequently react to the outside. Obviously, a warped mirror can only reflect a distorted image, as a faulty belief system that distorts reality.

On an emotional level, universal love and compassion are the attributes of the Heart. The rather earthly and human relations, love and passion as well as sexuality are the domain of the *Xin Bao* ≈ Heart Envelop/ Protector. Sexuality is an expression of Kidney-Fire that has reached maturity, and through its connection with the *Xin Bao* (Fire-minister), finds an outer expression.

A strong *Shen* manifests with a strong passion for life and a higher degree of intelligence (see further).

A weakened *Shen* presents with the symptoms of loss of vitality and depression. When the *Shen* is unsettled (not rooted in the *Yin* or in Blood), there are manifestations of mental hyperactivity, insomnia and neurotic or even psychotic manic behaviours.

Shen may also be obstructed, usually by Phlegm, causing a progressive loss of contact with the outer world, reduced sensory functions, amnesia, confusion, and may even lead to coma.

Overview of the Functions of Shen

(▶ Fig. 1.7)

- Consciousness: understood as awareness, cognition, and insight
- Thinking: logic, intelligence, memory, ideas, coherence, and wisdom
- Sleep and sleep-quality depend on the quietness of the mind

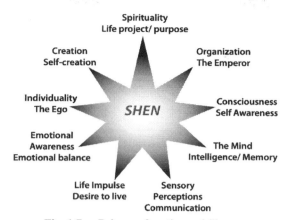

Fig. 1.7:   **Primary functions of** *Shen*

- Integration and comprehension of the five sensory inputs, independent of the sensory organs, the mind has to interpret the information that is received coherently: *Shen Ming* + *Shen Guang* (▶ Fig. 1.8).

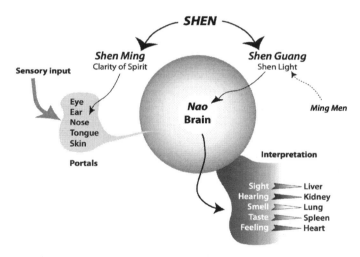

Fig. 1.8:   **Sensory Perceptions:** *Shen Ming* **and** *Shen Guang*

- Spirituality: the capacity to live one's destiny, to comprehend the challenges and lessons, to realise the impermanence of all phenomena, and to accept the illusion of one's separateness from the whole are attributes of *Shen*. In fact, according to Master Yuen, the names of the nine points of the Heart channel, symbolise the nine steps for each person towards redemption (▶ Section A.3.1).

- Mental activity in its capacity of coherence and coordination is an attribute of *Shen* and the Heart, but it also depends on two other organs, the Spleen-Qi, for its functioning, and on Kidney-*Jing* for the production and the maintenance of the brain matter (▶Fig. 1.9).

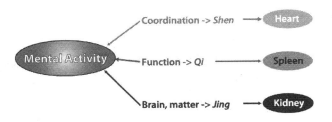

Fig. 1.9:   Mental activity

- Mental clarity ≈ *Shen Ming* is the mind's cognitive capacity; it emanates from Heart-Fire, itself evolving from the original Kidney-Fire ≈ *Ming Men* (▶Fig. 1.10).

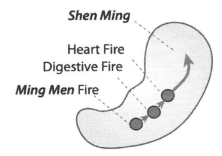

Fig. 1.10: *Shen Ming* and *Ming Men*

Shen disturbances

Shen disturbances are defined by a general loss of control over coordination, organisation, balance, homeostasis and of seeing choices. The mental-emotional disturbances may present in three different ways:

- Weakened *Shen*: associated with depressive states;
- Unsettled *Shen*: manifesting with agitation, anxiety, restlessness, sleep disturbances and manic behaviours;
- Obstructed *Shen*: often involving, Phlegm or Blood stasis, present in conditions such as mental confusion, lack of concentration, reduced sensory functions, hallucinations, disorientation, psychosis, dementia or even coma.

Treatment orientation

- To supplement *Shen*: see under "*Shen*" points (▶Section A.3.2) and Depression (▶Section 6.1)

- To Settle *Shen*:

  – Calming ≈ *An*: for regulating coordination and homeostasis: HE-7 *Shenmen*, ST-40 *Fenglong*, and Spleen channel points

  – Quieting ≈ *Jing*: for a restless mind and agitation: PE-4 *Ximen*, PE-5 *Jianshi*, PE-7 *Daling*. Note that the quieting of *Shen* requires sufficient Liver-Yin and Blood; if the Liver pulse is thin and thready and the Heart pulse is weak, add LR-8 *Ququan*, BL-17 *Geshu*, SP-6 *Sanyinjiao*, and ST-36 *Zusanli*

  – Stabilising ≈ *Ding*: relates to the Lung and Kidney relation, with a tendency to be vulnerable, unpredictable and chaotic. The Heart pulse is scattered and rapid with a weak Lung pulse: PE-5 *Jianshi*; LU-5 *Chize*, ST-45 *Lidui*, SP-1 *Yinbai*; KI-1 *Yongquan*; also, the use of *Ling* ≈ Soul points

- For *Shen* obstruction "Phlegm misting the Heart orifices": PE-5 *Jianshi*; ST-40 *Fenglong*; DM-20 *Baihui*; DM-18 *Qiangjian*; also, the *Jing Bie* ≈ Divergent channel of ST and SP: ST-30 *Qichong*, SP-12 *Chongmen*; RM-12 *Zhongwan*; ST-9 *Renying* and DM-20 *Baihui*

- In general, all *Shen* points may be used for treating *Shen* disturbances (▶Section A.3.2) in particular BL-44 *Shentang* and HE-7 *Shenmen*

- For the loss of desire and the will to live: start with RM-14 *Juque* and ST-23 *Taiyi*; in a second session combine BL-23 *Shenshu* and BL-52 *Zhishi* with BL-15 *Xinshu* and BL-44 *Shentang*

1.1.2 *Hun* ≈ Ethereal (Spiritual) Soul (魂)

Hun is considered the "Reasonable Spirit" and the "Etheric Soul" (▶Fig. 1.11).

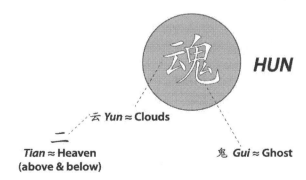

Fig. 1.11: The Significance of *Hun*

It is believed that the *Hun* ≈ Ethereal Soul, becomes activated shortly before birth, initiating the birthing process. Although this idea may be debatable based on the fact that the foetus dreams in the second half of the foetal life, and that dreams are mediated by *Hun*.

Hun is further described as a complement to *Shen* and corresponding to the comings and goings of the mind. This could be understood as the flexibility in thought (imagination) and the capacity to project the mind beyond the physical body; for example, the capacity to imagine oneself lying on a beach while in fact sitting in one's room, or again out of the body experiences. Naturally, dreaming is the domain of the *Hun*.

Hun is the motor force of the mind and yet the mind has to contain, "gather" the *Hun*. Once more, this capacity to imagine needs to be limited otherwise it may lead to delusion, illusion or even hallucination.

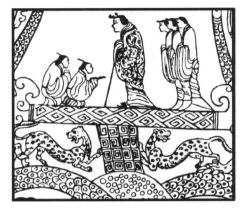

The Chinese tradition states that there are "Three *Hun*". After death, they go back to heaven where they become "glorious ghosts", during life they contribute to imagination, spirituality and dreams, providing they remain rooted in the Yin (▶ Fig.1.12).

Fig. 1.12: The three *Hun* accompany the deceased and become the "Glorious Ghosts"

This underlines the role of the Liver in particular Liver-Blood, considered to be the physical residence of *Hun,* and.

E. Rochat relates the three *Hun,* to the mastery over the three levels of life: emotional, mental and spiritual.

G. Maciocia describes the Three *Hun* as:

- Vegetative Soul: *Shuang Ling* ≈ Clear Spirit
- Animal Soul: *Tai Guang* ≈ Brilliant Spirit
- Human Soul: *You Jing* ≈ Dark Essence

Symbolically "Three" represents the "conditions of creation", and the three constitutional energies, but also the "Three *Hun*" concerning time, corresponds to past, present and future. In fact, by its mobility, *Hun* has the capacity to "visit" various time periods of one's life. This constitutes one aspect of memory. *Hun* is the link between a person's *Ming* ≈ Life Mandate, contained in the *Jing*, and *Shen* the conscious mind, giving a sense of direction and purpose to the individual. *Hun* is said to reside in the Liver, and the Liver channel ends at DM-20 *Baihui*. At birth, the infant's fontanelle is open, hence it is believed that children perceive other realities and dimensions, but as the DM-20 closes there is a loss of memory of previous experiences. The Liver acts as a "time keeper", bringing the deposited *Ming* into the conscious mind *Shen* through life choices, instincts and dreams. (LR-14 *Qimen* and KI-21 *Youmen*).

Choices that we make in life and the directions that we take are greatly influenced by *Hun*. It is even said that "*Hun* has the memory of the future" (*Chen Shi Yuan* 16th c.), again referring to the same concept. As *Hun* is responsible for dreaming, facets of the *Ming* are exposed through dream-imagery (premonitory dreams).

As mentioned above, the movements of *Hun* have to be contained by the mind, that is to say the coordinating role of *Shen* as well as the rooting aspect of Blood, without which *Hun* has a tendency to be dispersed and erratic.

...Hun follows Shen, if the Shen is unconscious

the Hun escapes (is swept away)...

Zhang Jie Bing (16th c.)

A strong *Hun* provides the individual with greater flexibility, imagination and creativity, and the curiosity to explore new ideas, new places and different ways of doing things. *Hun* is in charge of directing and managing the Liver energies. As the Liver is considered the "general of the armies", it is in charge of mobilising the *Wei Qi* ≈ Defensive energy and protecting the boundaries. Disturbances of *Hun* and *Po* are frequently involved in allergic conditions. (see further).

A weak *Hun* causes shyness, hopelessness, and the loss of the sense of direction in life, with a lack of incentive and imagination, as well as difficulty in maintaining personal boundaries.

When the *Hun* is unsettled and erratic, the individual is driven by strong emotional outbursts and even uncontrolled rage. The person becomes overbearing and tends to easily invade another's space.

Hun disturbances

- Weakened *Hun*: lack of imagination, lack of direction in life, aimlessness, lack of clear borders in life with a tendency to attract disrespect and being easily invaded by others; shyness; indecision; anxiety and a vague feeling of fear at night.

- Overactive *Hun*: frustration, irritability, anger; extreme passions; constant need for excitement and risk-taking; impulsive and recklessness; overbearing and insatiable personality.

Treatment orientation

- Supplement or reduce BL-47 *Hunmen*
- To harmonise the relation to others, add BL-23 *Shenshu* and BL-52 *Zhishi*
- Supplement Liver Blood: LR-8 *Ququan*, BL-17 *Geshu*, BL-18 *Ganshu*, SP-6 *Sanyinjiao*, ST-36 *Zusanli*

Overview of the Functions of *Hun*

- Mobilises the mind (wandering of the mind, with *Shen*)

- Intelligence, knowledge, sensitivity, spirituality

- Intuition, inspiration, insight

- Dreaming, imagination

- Assessment, analysis, projects and plans: sense of direction

- Desire, love of life, vital dynamism

- Decision, courage

- Relating to others, balanced expression of emotions

1.1.3   *Po* ≈ Corporeal Soul (魄)

Po is represented as the "Corporeal Soul" or the "Vegetative Spirit" or again the "Receptive Soul" (▶ Fig. 1.13).

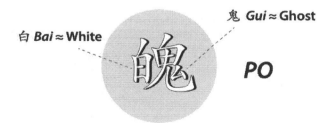

Fig. 1.13:   The significance of *Po*

By its inward momentum, *Po* enables the *Shen* to incarnate into the physical body. *Po* is closely related to the physical body and it oversees the body formation and is in charge of the vital rhythms and regulates the sensations of touch and pain as well as the somatic memory. *Po* defines the outer limits of the physical body, represented by the skin and the mucous membranes. In this manner, the physical separation from the outside, the physical identity and the sense of "self" versus "non-self" are attributes of *Po*. Therefore, it becomes clear as to why the instinct of protection is related to *Po*, defining what is beneficial or harmful to the organism.

It is interesting to note that during the initial stages of the embryonic development, the skin, the brain and the nervous system originate from the same ectodermic structure. In other words, the sensory touch receptors and the brain structures have the same common original cells.

Asides from physical feelings, *Po* is in charge of all sensory perceptions, the concept of "sentiment", defined as sensations, personal experiences and physical feelings, has a Latin origin "sentire", to feel, and in medieval French, "sentment". In French, the verb "sentir", corresponds to feelings, physical sensations, the sense of touch and smell, which are all attributes of *Po,* Metal and Lung.

Together with *Hun*, they manage the defensive mechanisms of the body. The disturbance of *Hun* and *Po* may be at the origin of many allergic reactions (over-reactivity), or even auto-immune conditions (self-destruction).

When the *Hun* corresponds to the comings and goings of *Shen*, the *Po* concerns the entry and exit of *Jing*. This concept of entry and exit should be understood as encompassing all of the vital and instinctive functions of the body concerning survival: starting with birth (entry into the world), breathing, the digestive processes (ingestion, digestion, elimination), the sensory perceptions, and ending with death (exit from the world).

The expression "*Po* mingles with *Jing*" might be a reference to the physiological cycle of *Jing* and the natural ageing process. But it could also be understood as the relation between *Jing Qi* (genetic transmission), and *Zong Qi*, ancestral energy (epigenetic inheritance). As *Po* is in charge of the protection instinct, the necessary protective mechanisms are transmitted to the offspring via the *Zong Qi*. Ultimately, if this protective measure becomes indispensable for the species, it will be registered and transmitted by the genes, the *Jing Qi;* though this process may take numerous generations and thousands of years. For example, the production of skin melatonin which is necessary to darken the skin colour to protect against stronger sun rays is genetically transmitted in those parts of the world where dark skin is necessary for survival. But a certain intolerance to a specific food might only be momentary due to denatured food quality (gluten intolerance), or the presence of certain plant allergens in the environment, necessitating a defensive reaction. This information is transmitted to the offspring not in the genetic code, but in the epi-genetic segment of the DNA (*Zong Qi*), which is only transmitted down to two or three generations as clearly observed in atopic allergic conditions. If the presence of the allergen continues to be a regular aggression threatening survival, then the information passes into the genetic code (*Jing Qi*).

According to classical Chinese texts, there are Seven *Po.*

E. Rochat's describes the Seven *Po* as being in charge of offering the seven earthly essences (*Jing*). After death, the essences return back to the earth from where they had originated from, to be transformed into another life form (▶ Fig. 1.14).

Symbolically, the number seven corresponds to ageing and consequently to the process of dying, therefore the concept of a "Destructive Spirit". But also, seven represents the seven portals of the head, the seat of sensory perceptions. Additionally, seven, in relation to space is represented by the four directions, the above and below and the centre.

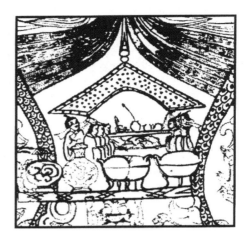

Fig. 1.14: The seven *Po* sit at the banquet of the deceased (Earthly essences)

Po has a downward momentum, it is in charge of eliminating the residue (the anus is called the Door of *Po*), and after death, it is believed to retire into the bones and return to the earth. It is further believed that excessive desires during life may cause the *Po* to become a *Gui* ≈ Ghost: Hungry ghost, sexual ghost or wandering ghost (▶ Section 1.2.5).

At all times this downward movement of *Po* (natural physical decline and ageing) are counter-balanced by the expansive quality of *Shen*. When *Shen's* life-affirming property is lost or obstructed, the momentum of *Po* is accelerated, inevitably leading to the disruption of life.

Po, residing in the Lung, is in charge of life rhythms, breathing, heartbeat, cyclic rhythms, and the ageing process. One of Lung's ministerial functions is to act as "Master of Qi", by circulating the Qi throughout the body, and by preserving the *Zong Qi* ≈ Ancestral/ Gathering Qi in the chest. When the expansion of *Shen* is hampered, as is the case with sadness, grief, or oppression, both *Ying* ≈ Nourishing and *Wei* ≈ Defensive energies are obstructed, exposing the subject to a variety of external pathological conditions.

On the mental and psychological level, *Po* represents correct judgment and evaluation, the sense of correct discernment as to what is right/ good or wrong/ bad for the organism and by extension for a given society. Therefore, fair judgment is an attribute of *Po*; when exaggerated, this quality turns into rigidity, dogmatism and strict morality.

As *Po* is in charge of protecting the body and its environment, it is responsible for planning and foreseeing the future by preparing for any possible upcoming event. Hence, worrying about the future, are attributed to a disturbance of *Po*. On the opposite end, there is a loss of the instinct of protection when the *Po* is weakened or obstructed by sadness and grief.

The function of the Lung has been compared to a fishing net, taking in both the fish and the water, but letting go of the unwanted.

The capacity to "let go" is one of the highest attributes of the *Po*. The loss of this capacity on a physical level may lead to pathologies of asthma or constipation and on a psychological level the incapacity to let go of old habits and ideas, the inability to forgive and a certain mental rigidity. Holding on to unwanted objects and hoarding as seen in the Diogenes syndrome is a good example of this mental condition.

Po disturbances

- Weakened *Po*: loss of the instinct of self-preservation, depression, sadness; inability to evaluate oneself
- Overactive *Po*: rigid beliefs, dogmatism; worrying about the future; holding on to emotions, difficulty to forgive; retained grief

Treatment orientation

- Supplement or reduce BL-42 *Pohu*
- To help release emotions from the chest: add BL-23 *Shenshu* and BL-52 *Zhishi*, LU-7 *Lieque*, PE-6 *Neiguan* and RM-17 *Shanzhong*

Overview of the Functions of *Po*

- Individual ego
- Relating to the self
- Formation of the body
- Sensory perceptions: touch, pain and itching
- Vital functions (rhythms): breath
- Instinct of protection
- Destructive spirit: death

1.1.4 *Yi* ≈ Intellect/ Intent (意)

*Yi is t*he intellectual, reasoning and analytical aspect of the mind (▶ Fig. 1.15).

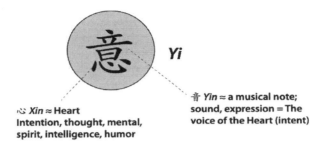

心 *Xin* ≈ Heart
Intention, thought, mental,
spirit, intelligence, humor

音 *Yin* ≈ a musical note;
sound, expression = The
voice of the Heart (intent)

Fig. 1.15: The significance of *Yi*

Yi is said to reside in the Spleen and it represents logic and reasoning. This is the mental capacity to take in information, to break it down (analysis) and store the input by analogy (classification) for future reference (memory). This function is very similar to the digestive process, in which Spleen and Stomach ingest and digest the food by breaking it down into smaller units in order for the nutrients to be assimilated and then transformed into the physical body.

It is the *Yi* that has the charge of giving significance and sense to what has been perceived by comparing the input with previously stored information. Obviously, the *Yi* and the *Shen* have to collaborate intimately in this process. The *Shen* is responsible for the correct reception of outer stimuli through the sensory organs, as well as all the inner information transmitted by the neuro-humoral system. The *Yi* in turn, has to name and give sense to this data, hence the expression "*Yi* is the voice of the Heart", allowing for the *Shen* to verbalise and to express. The *Yi* is the link between the physical body and the mind. When a specific physical sensation is perceived, the *Yi* has the charge of correctly identifying its source before presenting the information to *Shen,* in order for the mind to take action. For example, in a conflicting situation, a person might feel tightness and pain in the solar plexus, signifying an accumulation of Qi. The *Yi* could either correctly identify this feeling as suppressed anger, or erroneously relate it to an organic stomach ache. In this case, the *Shen* not having received accurate information will not be able to respond accordingly. Overtime, this stagnation of Qi (and Blood) will cause an organic pathology, resulting in what is considered a "psychosomatic" disease.

It is therefore not surprising that both the Heart (speech, verbalisation) and the Spleen (identification and discernment of tastes) are related to the tongue.

The capacity to concentrate and to stay focused and maintain attention, are equally attributes of *Yi*. *Yi* is also responsible for some aspects of planning and ideas, although both are attributes of *Hun* as well. Nevertheless, there is a difference between the two; *Hun* represents imagination, intuitive thinking and creation, whereas *Yi* has the potential of materialising and constructing the project. For example, an architect who imagines a building and expresses it in a two-dimensional house layout, but ultimately it needs the engineer or the builder to translate the house-plan into a three-dimensional construction.

A similar process takes place during human conception. The genetic information carried by the parental *Jing* and *Zong Qi* are the potentials of the future being or the original pattern, the actual function of translating this plan into a coherent life form falls on the Extraordinary Vessel *Chong Mai*, intimately connected with the future Spleen channel (SP-4 *Gongsun*).

Yi plays a central role in the memory process. Although each of the five constructs of the psyche have a part in one or another type of memory, *Yi's* function is the most prominent. The actual capacity to retrieve a stored memory depends greatly on how well this information was organised, classified and labelled in the first place by *Yi*.

A strong *Yi* manifests as a strong intellect and logic, the capacity to analyse and synthesise and to construct new concepts from stored ideas. An overactive *Yi* will manifest with a tendency for excessive thinking or thinking in circles, cogitation and obsessive attitudes and worrying about details, and ruminating about the past. A weakened *Yi* will cause difficulties in focusing, logical thought and loss of memory.

Yi disturbances

- Weakened *Yi*: reduced memory, attention and focusing problems
- Overactive *Yi*: obsessions, excessive worry about details, lingering on past events

Treatment orientation

- Supplement or reduce BL-49 *Yishe*
- For thinking in circles: add BL-23 *Shenshu* and BL-52 *Zhishi*

Overview of the Functions of *Yi*

- Memory
- Analysis, synthesis, thinking, classification; discourse, verbalisation
- Concentration, focusing
- Symbolism, abstract thinking, conceptualisation, ideas
- Learning, integration of sensory, mental and emotional input
- Intellect, intention, resolution, opinion
- Physical awareness

1.1.5 *Zhi* ≈ Will (志)

The *Zhi* is represented as the fundamental "Will" or will power (▶Fig. 1.16).

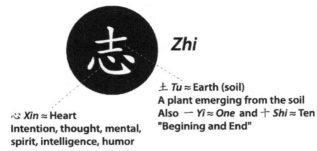

心 *Xin* ≈ Heart
Intention, thought, mental,
spirit, intelligence, humor

土 *Tu* ≈ Earth (soil)
A plant emerging from the soil
Also 一 *Yi* ≈ *One* and 十 *Shi* ≈ Ten
"Begining and End"

Fig. 1.16: Significance of *Zhi*

When *Shen* manifests the "Passion for life", *Zhi* is the "Will to live", hence the terms that designate *Zhi* as the "Creative will", and "Germ of creation".

Will power, resolution, intention, aim and aspiration, are attributes of *Zhi*. For any action to take form and be realised, the will is needed. It is further understood that each organ has its own will. The will of the Liver is to move freely (free flow), the will of the heart is to expand, the will of the Spleen is to transform, the will of the Lung is to gather (condense) and the will of the Kidney is to consolidate.

According to E. Rochat de la Vallée, when the will of an organ is obstructed or hampered, the corresponding emotion manifests. In this context, the Five spirits, *Hun, Shen, Yi, Po* and *Zhi*, are at times referred to as the "Five *Zhi*".

The concept of *Zhi* residing in the Kidney, links *Zhi* to the Kidney *Qi* and *Jing*, therefore the inherited energies, and in a sense, *Zhi* will define the strength of character, of determination and perseverance, hence the notions of courage associated with it.

The Kidney, in its ministerial function, is the imperial councillor, underlining the importance of tempering intelligence (*Shen*) with wisdom (*Zhi*). The wisdom of knowing one's resources and adapting to what one can do is one of the attributes of *Zhi*. This point is symbolically represented by the statement that the "Kidney listens" (is attentive to) the inner reserves", a further analogy between the shape of the ear and the kidney organ.

An aspect of memory is also attributed to *Zhi;* this could represent the stored information and life experiences: memory bank.

A strong *Zhi*, procures a strong character to the individual and a strong will to live, and to survive even against great adversity.

A weak *Zhi* causes fearfulness, especially the fear of change and dreading the future.

The over-activity of *Zhi*, makes the individual overconfident, daring and intrepid.

Zhi disturbances

- Weakened *Zhi*: fearfulness; weak character, "spineless"; loss of the will to live with suicidal tendencies; loss of memory in the elderly

- Overactive *Zhi*: over-dominating, audacious; but also, may retain emotions, fear of change, fear of life, blocked by emotions

Treatment orientation

- Supplement or reduce BL-53 *Zhishi*

- For depression: add BL-23 *Shenshu* also BL-47 *Hunmen*

- To strengthen the character: add *Du Mai* (SI-3 *Houxi*, DM-1*Changqiang*, DM-4 *Mingmen* and DM-20 *Baihui*); BL-11 *Dazhu* and GB-39 *Xuanzhong*.

- For the loss of will to live (suicidal tendency), combine BL-23 *Shenshu* and BL-52 *Zhishi* with BL-15 *Xinshu* and BL-44 *Shentang*

Overview of the Functions of *Zhi*

- Strength of character, courage

- Determination, perseverance

- Drive, capacity to realise

- Will to exist => reservoir of ambitions and desires

- Wisdom

- Memory

1.2   Mental Activity and the Brain

The physical support of the Mind is the Brain ≈ *Nao* (the central nervous system). It is considered one of the six "Extraordinary *Fu*" and is called the "Sea of Marrow" The Brain is formed by Pre-Heaven *Jing* and later maintained by Kidney *Jing*. The Brain is said to be the depository of the "Universal Law" and the "Spiritual Matrix".

On a physical level, the brain matter is supplied and maintained by the Kidney-*Jing*. The necessary Blood and *Qi* are produced by the Spleen, and for its optimum function and coordination, it depends on Heart-*Shen*. Mental activity therefore is closely related to the "Three Treasures: *Shen - Qi - Jing*. (▶ Fig. 1.9)

The brain's function is to coordinate and regulate internally the millions of processes involved in maintaining life, as well as the relation to the outside world, the functions of perception, communication and protection. Only a minute part of these functions is accessible to the conscious mind.

In modern neuroscience, a simple "triune brain" model has been proposed by MacLean (The Triune Brain Evolution; 1990), in which the three brain structures are related to the evolution of the species (▶ Fig. 1.17):

- Brainstem or lower brain: responsible for instinctual behaviours. The brainstem which includes the cerebellum, the medulla and the pons, regulates the heart, lung and the endocrine systems and maintains homeostasis.

- Mid-brain or the limbic system: related to motivation, the emotional, reproductive, feeding and parenting behaviours; it includes the thalamus, hypothalamus, the amygdala and the hippocampus. These brain areas are involved in monitoring and initiating the appropriate behaviour for survival and for socialisation. The mid-brain is commonly referred to as the emotional brain and is further modelled by the pre-frontal cortex, the logical brain.

- Higher brain or neocortex: which confers the ability for logical and abstract thought, language, planning and perception, decision making and moderating the social behaviour. The pre-frontal cortex is often considered the rational brain, while the limbic system is seen as the emotional brain.

The brain stem is developing during the foetal stage, the limbic system develops after birth (till the age of 4-5), and the neocortex completes its maturation during the first seven years. In the brain, the interconnection between neurones, the synapses, are programmed to multiply and to grow for several years, conferring great adaptability and learning potential to children and young adults referred to as "Neuro-plasticity". Later in life, there is a shift

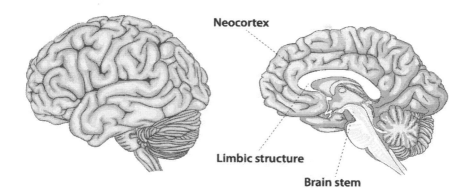

Fig. 1.17: The three brain structures

toward getting rid (pruning) of un-needed or less utilised connections, explaining the reduced mental flexibility, learning and memory functions in the elderly.

As the Heart-emperor has the overall position of overseeing and coordinating the empire, so does *Shen,* residing in the Heart and regulating the activities of the mind. Heart and mind are inseparable, and in Chinese, the word for Heart "*Xin*" is the same as for Mind.

Mental activity is defined as a person's consciousness and thoughts. It could be described as a set of cognitive faculties including consciousness, perception, thinking, judgment, language and memory, further representing imagination, recognition, and appreciation. The mind is responsible for processing feelings and emotions, resulting in attitudes and behaviour.

In Chinese medicine, *Shen* refers to the sum of all the mental functions: consciousness, mental faculties, and intelligence. *Shen* also refers to all the emotional as well as the spiritual phenomena; therefore the Heart is responsible for the overall harmonious mental, emotional and spiritual evolutions; although each mental function and each emotion pertains to its particular spirit, *Hun, Yi, Po,* and *Zhi.*

Shen is on the one hand responsible for being conscious and on the other hand for perceiving and interpreting the sensory input.

Consciousness is defined as a state of being aware of external objects (macrocosm) or something within oneself (microcosm). It can further be qualified as sentience, awareness, subjectivity, the ability to feel, to experience, sensory perception and integration, a sense of self and the control system of the mind.

The conscious part of the mind represents, at best, only 1/10th of our psycho-emotional awareness. The rest is controlled by the unconscious (▶ Fig. 1.18).

The unconscious part of the mind consists of the processes that occur automatically (autonomous nervous system) and are not available to mental processing and introspection, including certain thought processes, memories, interests and motivations, and they exert a strong impact on the behaviour.

These unconscious phenomena include repressed feelings, automatic skills, subliminal perceptions, automatic reactions, hidden phobias and desires.

Human beings naturally relate to and identify with, the conscious part of the mind, which only represents a minute part of the total mental activity.

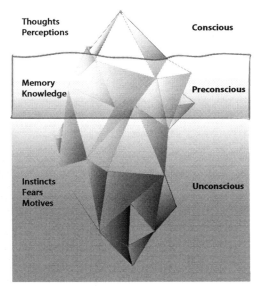

Fig. 1.18 Freud's iceberg model of the psyche

Motivations and desires arising from the unconscious are generally suppressed by the conscious mind due to socio-cultural demands or personal choices. This creates a constant state of separation and strife between the two parts of the mind, and when the conscious part loses the control the condition is labelled as a split personality or schizoid character.

A similar situation is encountered when we understand and mentally decide to stop a harmful attitude or habit, like smoking, drinking, or changing an emotional pattern, and yet we cannot. Aside from a specific chemical dependency, the subconscious has its own needs and reasons for perpetuating a habit; if this need is not understood and satisfied, the conscious mind will invariably lose the battle.

1.2.1 The Power of the Mind

The ancient Chinese had put a lot of emphasis on the "Cultivation of the mind". They had clearly understood the role that human thoughts and emotions play in a given pathological process. Emotions are the responses to outer situations; as one cannot change the outer world, one can only modify one's response to it; in a nutshell, one's mental attitude.

A famous Zen metaphor "blind horse and lame rider" demonstrates the difficulty of taming and channelling the powers of the subconscious. The blind horse represents the subconscious; it is extremely powerful, but cannot see where it is going. The lame rider symbolises the conscious mind and depends on the horse to get to their destination. Only when the conscious part of the mind has learned to master the subconscious may one hope to attain a particular goal.

We are only barely discovering the powers of our minds. The Princeton experiments on new-born chicks (quoted in the preface), demonstrated that even small animal's minds had the power of modulating their environment, then what is the human brain capable of?

Dr Masaru Emoto (Hidden message in Water, 2005 and Miracle of Water 2011), discovered that crystals formed in frozen water reveal changes when specific, concentrated thoughts are directed toward them. He established that water from clear springs and water that has been exposed to loving words show brilliant, complex, and colourful snowflake patterns. In contrast, polluted water, or water exposed to negative thoughts, forms incomplete, asymmetrical patterns with dull colours. These observations demonstrate the impact of our thoughts, not only on our personal health, as we are made of 80% of water, but also the state of the planet.

1.2.2 Consciousness and Sensory Perceptions

All life forms in general and humans in particular, communicate constantly with the outer world. This communication takes place either on a conscious level, involving the sensory perceptions or on the unconscious level, bypassing the conscious and analytical part of the mind (*Shen* and *Yi*) and involving the unconscious parts (*Hun* and *Po*). This universal and unconscious interconnection is one of the main paradigms of Chinese medicine, reflected in the concept of the "microcosm" and the "macrocosm". Many ancient philosophies, Hinduism and Buddhism in particular, have a similar understanding of the human being (microcosm) in inter-relation with the world (macrocosm). In modern times, Sheldrake's theories on "morphic resonance" are very similar to these ancient beliefs. Unfortunately, the scientific world has rejected Sheldrake's concepts as non-scientific and non-verifiable.

For the conscious awareness of the external stimuli in general and the sensory perceptions in particular two aspects of *Shen* are necessary:

- *Shen Guang* (Light): is the faculty of being conscious. *Shen* is considered disconnected in sleep, hypnosis or coma; any state in which there is no conscious awareness of one's participation.

- *Shen Ming* (Clarity): is the capacity of discernment and interpretation of stimuli. All sensory functions depend not only on the related *Zang* organ but equally rely on the acuity of the *Shen,* the "*Shen Ming*". Sensory input may be reduced, misinterpreted, or simply blocked by a dysfunctional *Shen* (▶ Fig. 1.9).

Therefore, any sensory perception involves:

- A functional organic sensory receptor (eye, ear, nose, tongue… related to a *Zang* organ)

- The conscious mind (*Shen Guang*)

- Clear *Shen* (*Shen Ming*)

- Conscious and unconscious memory

The mind interprets the sensory input based on a pre-established program involving conditioning, belief systems, and memory in particular. This could include acquired short term or long-term memory, genetically transmitted unconscious memory, or unconscious conditioning.

In reality, we do not perceive things as they are but as they appear to us. Thus, the perception of the physical world does not necessarily result in a universal reaction amongst observers, for example, a certain colour or smell might evoke a pleasant or unpleasant unconscious memory, resulting in liking or disliking that perception. A sound might be associated with a traumatic experience and be perceived as intolerable etc.

Interestingly Chinese medicine considers the five sensory functions to be:

- Hearing

- Seeing

- Smelling

- Tasting

- Speech

In fact, speech, which is related to the functions of *Shen*, is the conscious response to outer stimuli. It might be actual verbalisation, expressing feelings, like, dislike or pain. Or it could also signify comprehending, interpreting the input and giving it a sense and putting a word or a name on it. In extreme conditions, when the *Shen* is disconnected, overwhelmed or by-passed, the input is perceived by *Hun* and *Po*, hence there are no appropriate words to articulate the experience. As we will explore further, this "naming" process is crucial in therapy when dealing with sub-conscious programs or in post-traumatic disorders.

The tactile sense is not related to a specific organ but is generally managed by *Po*. *Po* is not only responsible for the overall sense of touch and pain, but also several other sensations and emotions. This point is clearly expressed by the meaning of the word "feeling", which in most languages expresses both the capacity to experience the sense of touch and the subjective perception of an emotion. (▶ Section 1.1.3)

As previously mentioned during the initial stages of the embryonic development, the skin, the brain and the nervous system originate from the same ectodermic structure. In other words, the sensory touch receptors and the brain structures have the same common original cells.

It is the conscious awareness of the physical changes that define a particular emotional state.

The *Shen Ming* will interpret and give sense to the tactile stimulus. In certain extreme or potentially dangerous conditions, such as sudden pain or heat, the reflexes bypass the central control of the brain and the body reacts automatically by withdrawing from the harmful stimulus.

1.2.3 The Conscious functioning of the mind

During the conscious state, the outer stimuli are perceived by the sensory organs and integrated and identified by the *Shen* ≈ Mind. The input is then analysed by the *Yi* and compared to pre-existing information, based on which an interpretation and a course of action are proposed (▶ Fig. 1.19).

For example, upon seeing a dog, not only the species is identified, but based on previous interactions with dogs, an evaluation is made as to the attitude to be privileged. In case a dog has bitten one in the past, the recommended course of action would be to select caution and avoid all contact. On the other

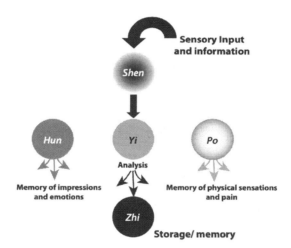

Fig. 1.19 The memory process involving the five Spirits *Shen-Yi-Zhi*, *Po* and *Hun*

hand, when there have been positive memories of having had a pet dog, there is no fear rather the desire to caress or to cuddle the animal.

When the outer situation presents a novelty, the *Yi* would analyse and break down the information and classify each segment by an analogical process. The information is stored by *Zhi* and will constitute the basis for knowledge, to be later retrieved when necessary. Even a traumatic event could be used to enhance a further experience. For example, while running down the stairs, one has lost one's footing, fallen and broken an ankle. As the *Shen*, had not been disconnected, the situation is fully analysed by the *Yi*. The pain and the subjective experience of the fracture will be stored by analogy with other painful episodes, the emotional response, frustration and anger with oneself or with the circumstances, are accordingly classified, as well as the frame of mind in which the person was performing an automatic task, running, without paying full attention in adapting the gait to the stairs. This experience will enable the individual to adopt a different attitude when rushing down a flight of stairs in the future, by either slowing down or by paying full attention to the outer layout to avoid hurting oneself.

During the conscious functioning of the mind, the *Hun* and *Po* have a secondary role.

A good comparison could be made with the computer. When the computer is switched on, it is similar to the state of wakeful consciousness symbolised by *Shen*. The *Yi* represents the RAM (memory) and the software in which the information is introduced. Once this input is complete, it has to be labelled for future reference and then stored on the hard disk, the *Zhi*. In a normal situation when the *Shen* is totally alert and attentive, and that the input has been correctly labelled and stored, all information that has been presented, should be retrievable at all times, unless there is a breakdown in the hard disc. In other words, everything that one has read or learned could be found in the memory banks and remembered. Then how to explain forgetfulness and memory lapses? There are three main categories:

- Lack of full attention, for example, while reading or listening to some information, the mind is drifting elsewhere, and only fragments of the information are effectively absorbed. A similar process occurs when the *Shen* is by-passed as in the case of subliminal stimulation, or if the *Shen* is overwhelmed by the intensity of a given stimulus. In these conditions, although the person is seemingly conscious, the information is handled by the subconscious part of the mind, the *Hun* and the *Po*.

- Incorrect labelling and storage by the *Yi*, in which the information is on the hard disk but the person, simply cannot retrieve it.

- The breakdown of the hard disk, as observed in certain neurological conditions involving the brain such as aphasia, amnesia or dementia.

People, who boast a good memory, are individuals who are capable of maintaining a full concentration during the learning process and possess a good method of tagging, classifying and storing this information.

The greatest part of the human being's interaction with the outer world as well as maintaining the physiological functions is mediated by the subconscious.

1.2.4 The Subconscious/ unconscious functioning of the mind

The unconscious part of the mind is handling and coordinating the thousands or even millions of the physiological processes necessary to maintain life and to adjust to the environment without our conscious realisation. Most of these functions are controlled by the lower brain, constantly modulated by the midbrain, in the form of a reflex (involuntary) action (▶ Fig. 1.20):

- The cerebellum is mainly in charge of motor coordination and balance. It may also be involved in some cognitive functions such as attention and language as well as in regulating fear and pleasure responses.

- The medulla is responsible for autonomic (involuntary) functions such as breathing, heartbeat, blood pressure, sleep-wake cycle, vomiting and sneezing.

- The Pons is in charge of regulating breathing, involuntary actions, hearing, equilibrium, taste, and in facial sensations such as touch and pain, as well as motor roles in eye movement, facial expressions, chewing, swallowing, and the secretion of saliva and tears.

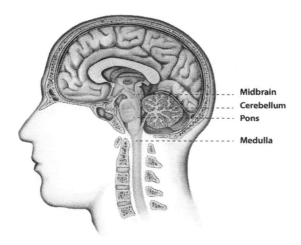

Fig. 1.20: Mid and Lower-brain structures

Besides the numerous physiological functions, many reflex reactions have been previously set in place to safeguard the body and the mind and to shortcut the forebrain and the conscious mind. Some reflexes are genetically transmitted, such as withdrawal from excessive heat or pain, or the blinking reflex to protect the cornea. Very possibly, even some basic fears such as fear of snakes or spiders might have an innate origin as part of the survival instinct.

Some reflexive mechanisms are developed progressively as the infant is growing, the most important being proprioception, the sense of self-movement and body position.

Otherwise, a person might have elaborated a certain protective measure at a certain time, which may later become an unconscious reflex reaction, for example, the ducking of the head in anticipation of being hit in childhood for wrongdoing, could later turn into a habitual neck tension in reaction to any perceived criticism. Similar mechanisms may explain the "conditioned reflex" (Pavlovian conditioning), or even the automatic procedural memory, through which simple daily tasks are performed below the conscious awareness, from tying the shoes to driving a car. The difference being that in the procedural memory, the conscious mind had been present initially, whereas, in the unconscious reflex, the conscious mind was by-passed.

In Chinese medicine, the conscious participation of the mind involves the presence of *Shen* and the logical analysis of *Yi*. Otherwise, any information that has been gathered without the conscious cooperation of *Shen* and *Yi,* is automatically and subconsciously managed by the *Hun* and the *Po*.

In the absence or disconnection of *Shen*, as observed during sleep, anaesthesia, hypnosis, coma, intense physical or psychological shock, or during certain pathological conditions such as high fevers, or even with psychotropic drugs, the outer stimuli is still integrated but without the appropriate scrutiny, analysis and classification of *Yi*. Therefore, the experience is stored in a group "en masse". Consciously the event may not be recalled, but any fragment of the experience, such as an image, a body sensation, a sound or a simple word may trigger the entire incident and have the person re-live the scene as though it was happening in that moment, obviously with intense physical and psychological manifestations, totally unrelated to the present situation. In a sense, the subconscious is re-enacting an experience, and the body is reacting to this with a set of reflex measures such as vasoconstriction, rise in the heart rate and blood pressure, fight or flight instinct, strong emotional outbreak and even coma.

These kinds of un-related manifestations and the alienation from the reality of the moment have been grouped into the concept of *Gui* ≈ Ghost in Chinese medicine. (see below)

1.2.5 Harmful Spirits *Gui* 鬼

The concept of *Gui* was probably a leftover of the earlier beliefs that all diseases were due to harmful spirits. The Chinese notion of *Gui* ≈ Ghost refers to apparently unexplained or inappropriate reactions to outer stimuli without a coherent reason. Today this could be extended to include any unconscious conditioning, hypnosis, phobias, behavioural neurosis, many so-called psychosomatic diseases, and of course in most psychotic manifestations. An appropriate term for *Gui* could be "un-named energy mass", due to unresolved issues causing an energetic disturbance.

Both *Hun* ≈ Ethereal soul 魂 and *Po* ≈ Corporeal soul 魄 contain the radical *Gui* in their respective ideograms.

The Confucian schools replaced the concept of *Gui* by the notion of *Gu* 蛊 ≈ Parasites/ Worms or *Tan* 痰 ≈ Phlegm, as both could be responsible for unexplained symptoms or reactions.

The mechanism of *Gui*:

Normally, mental activity depends on the consciousness of *Shen* ≈ Mind, integrating all inputs, which are then analysed and classified by *Yi* ≈ Intellect to be stored by *Zhi*. When *Shen* is disconnected, as is the case in sleep, hypnosis, coma, or in certain intense traumatic conditions or high fevers, *Hun* ≈ Ethereal soul and *Po* ≈ Corporeal soul, take over and store the memories. Therefore *Yi* ≈ Intellect does not anymore get to evaluate and sort-out the sensory input (▶ Fig. 1.21).

As *Hun* and *Po* do not analyse the experience, the memory is stored in its integrity, and when recalled or re-activated, the person will experience the whole event as though it was occurring right then and there. These unexplained and apparently illogical responses are referred to as *Gui* ≈ Ghost in Chinese medicine.

- *Hun* stores impressions and emotions, producing "Behavioural *Gui*"

- *Po* stores physical sensations and pain, the cause of "Somatic *Gui*"

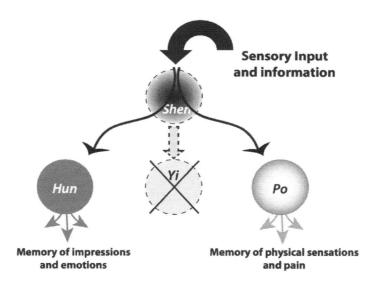

Fig. 1.21: In the absence of *Shen*, *Hun* stores impressions and emotions: "Behavioural *Gui*"; *Po* stores sensations and pain "Somatic *Gui*"

There are three categories of *Gui*:

- Individual *Gui* due to personal un-resolved issues

- Family/ Ancestral transmitted *Gui*

- Collective *Gui*, due to social, ethnic or racial conditioning

During dreaming, the Liver through the offices of *Hun* attempts to release many of the unresolved issues. More serious conditions may be treated with acupuncture, although needles alone without proper psychotherapeutic support seem quite often insufficient.

1.2.6 Sleep and Dreams/ *Shen* and *Hun*

Sleeping is indispensable to health, simply evidenced by the fact that human beings spend in average 25% of their life in sleep. Studies on sleep have demonstrated that two of the sleep phases are the most important:

- N3 or slow-wave sleep (0.5-4 Hz), which represents deep sleep, simply classified as "Delta" sleep and during which the body restores itself and recovers from fatigue.

- Paradoxical sleep (PS), also known as REM (Rapid Eye Movement) sleep or the dreaming phase, during which certain portions of the brain are in full activity while the body is in total inertia. In adults, REM sleep occupies about 20-25% of the total sleeping time. During REM sleep, the brain eliminates many accumulated neuropeptides. Despite numerous neurobiological theories, there is still no consensus as to the reasons for which humans and many mammals and birds dream. Already before birth, the foetus dreams, and after birth, the child is dreaming 50% of their sleeping time.

Studies on total sleep deprivation, or specific dream deprivation, have shown that after 3-4 weeks, the subjects, manifest psychotic behaviour with no apparent physical modification.

In Chinese medicine, dreaming is the domain of the *Hun*. During sleep, the Liver mobilises *Wei Qi* (and Blood) inward, resulting in the relaxation of muscle tone and reduced sensory functions (eyes, nose and ears). This inward movement of *Hun* helps move Qi away from the mind and helps to relax the *Shen*. The internal circulation of *Wei Qi* managed by the Liver (general of the army), first passes through the *Fu* ≈ Bowels before moving to the *Zang* ≈ Organs following the *Ke* ≈ Control cycle: KI ⇨ HE ⇨ LU ⇨ LR ⇨ SP and back to the Kidneys. The purpose of this internal circulation is to expel the residual pathogenic factors as well as the internal pathogens, dietary and emotional. Periodically the *Hun* is released "wanders", producing dreams.

Dreams occur in the last portion of each sleep cycle that usually lasts 90 minutes. Dreams take up from 10 to 40 minutes of the cycle, their length increasing throughout the night. After each dreaming phase, there is a very short waking of a few seconds, which is often not registered by the sleeper. When this waking period is longer, the *Shen* can recall parts of the dream. When the dream-theme has been more intense, the person wakes up with a very clear emotional state and can better remember the details of the dream (▶ Section 4.5.11).

Dreams can be classified into several broad categories:

- Releasing dreams: through which pathogenic factors are being released.

    - Retained external climatic factors or retained dietary factors and the consequent *Zang-Fu* dysfunctions (repletion and vacuity): described in *Suwen* ch. 17 and *Lingshu* ch. 43

    - Emotional processing: releasing unresolved or retained emotions

    - Suppressed emotions: the *Hun* is the link between the unconscious and the conscious mind, helping to move out what has been suppressed.

- Teaching dreams: in which the brain establishes new synaptic connections to enhance performance.

- Healing dreams: the electrochemical changes that occur during dreams directly affect the body (the psychosomatic theories, Shinomya et al 1993; Colic 2007)

- Premonitory dreams: following the idea that *Hun* is in contact with the *Ming* ≈ Life mandate/ curriculum, *Chen Shi Yuan* in *Meng Zhan Yi Zhi* (1562) states that *Hun* has the "memory of the future". This statement refers to the mobility of *Hun*, which can visit all the segments of time, past and future, and therefore reveal in dreams the person's pre-set curriculum. Studies have demonstrated that dream content in patients may actually reveal a future disease location and its seriousness (Kasatkin 1967).

- Lucid dreams: in which the *Shen* ≈ Consciousness is present, with full awareness and participation in the dream, and the capacity to direct the *Hun*. At least half of all adults have experienced episodes of lucid dreaming (Snyder and Gackenbach 1988). Lucid dreaming has been actively pursued in many Eastern traditions, Tibetan Buddhism in particular, by maintaining full consciousness during the dream state (Mullin 1997).

1.2.6 The mind/ psyche and the body/ soma

The impact of the mind on the body has been greatly stressed by Classical Chinese medicine: "Qi follows *Shen*".

Although the concept of "Psychosomatics" seems quite obvious and logical, allopathic medicine still has many reservations concerning the importance of the mind and belief systems on a given pathological process. Nevertheless, the interactions of mind and body are being researched and emphasised by many recent sub-branches of medicine such as Psychosomatic medicine, Neuro-psycho-pharmacology, Psycho-neuro-immunology, and Behavioural medicine etc. The concepts of "Placebo" and "Nocebo" have even been integrated into scientific study projects as having an important impact on the outcome of any statistical evaluation.

The cerebrospinal structures modulate the physiology of the body at all times through neurotransmitters and hormones. The great majority of these automatic regulations are relegated to the subconscious part of the mind.

The neurotransmitters that are produced by various areas of the brain have distal somatic receptors with specific physiological reactions. The release of many of these chemicals is also perceived subjectively as a feeling or an emotion (▶Section 2.3.5).

The mechanism of "Psycho-somatic diseases":

Each emotion manifests with a distinct physical sensation; for example:

- Fear is felt in the lower abdomen, in the "guts"
- Anger and frustration are perceived in the solar plexus area
- Joy produces a distending sensation in the chest
- Sadness and oppression have an opposite effect on the chest
- Worry produces a tightening in various areas: abdomen, chest and head
- Anxiety might be felt in the lower belly and the chest (loss of harmony between the Kidney and Heart)

Therefore, as each emotion has a distinct physiological impact, it will modify the local circulation of Qi and Blood, and in the long run, affect physically the involved organ.

1.2.7 Pain, the language of the body

Pain signifies the stagnation of Blood and Qi in a particular area. Pain is the body's way of focusing the attention on a specific area and to inform us that something is not right.

In Western allopathic medicine a pain may be classified under:

- Organic or structural: for example, pain in the area of the heart due to a coronary obstruction; or pain in an articulation due to osteoarthritis etc.
- Referred pain (pain felt distally from the affected area): for example, pain radiating down the left arm related to a heart attack; or pain radiating down the leg secondary to a discus hernia etc.
- Idiopathic pain: that which has no known cause. Many previously classified idiopathic causes have now found scientific explanations. Today, most idiopathic pains or symptoms are referred to a psychiatrist,

following the general belief that what is not organic must be psychological.

Hence allopathic medicine has three solutions to deal with any pain:

- Remove the organic cause, or in some cases the organ itself
- Pain-killers
- Psycho-pharmaceuticals

Unfortunately, the general trend today in medicine is to rapidly revert to pain-killers. Killing the pain is like killing the messenger that has brought important or even vital information!

When a painful message is ignored repeatedly, the local stagnation of Blood and Qi will result in organic and structural modifications, which will then show up on X-rays, PET-scans or other allopathic exploration methods.

It is paramount for us practitioners of Chinese medicine to understand the importance and significance of pain and to try and transmit this to our patients. In most cases, it is the pain signal that has brought the patient to seek help. Our position as a therapist is not only to relieve this pain but to help the patient discover the hidden roots of their discomfort.

Ancient Chinese medicine makes a clear distinction between pain and suffering. When pain indicates a local modification in the circulation, suffering is how one relates to this pain; the "experience" of the pain. Hence, suffering has a deep psychological foundation.

In Buddhist belief, suffering is the result of the refusal of life experiences. Denial and rejection cause a tightening of the energy points, in particular, the Bladder back Shu points resulting in a protective reaction called "armouring".

1.2.8 Memory and Inherited energies

The operational aspect of the mind and the psyche can be simplified and broken down to two distinct functions:

- The conscious part, which is active during the waking state, and is at all times partly geared to the external world and partly in tune with the internal universe. The sensory perceptions of the outer milieu are constantly analysed and classified based on previously stored information. So, the interpretation of the input from the outside depends mostly on the memorised data. Even if an entirely new situation is presented, it will be analysed and classified by analogy. The conscious mind will then call upon the stored information and decide on the appropriate way to deal with this new event. The other part of the conscious mind is involved in another activity that we call thinking. Most often the thinking mind is disconnected from the outside reality, the "here and now", and involved in past or future reflections. For example, when driving a car, the experienced driver delegates all of the complex procedures to the subconscious, to be free to think and plan about the day's projects or some past event. The automatic pilot can be switched off at any moment if a new, potentially hazardous situation arises on the outside.

- The unconscious mind has the charge of containing the various memories of the species in order to sustain and to conserve life. In humans, the unconscious also has the charge of directing the individual through a pre-established program, *Ming* ≈ Life mandate.

Constitutional energies

Based on the Chinese concept of human creation, there are three constitutional energies involved at the moment of conception:

- *Yuan Qi*: is the "Source" or life principle and the mystery of creation. Here, modern science is lost for an explanation. Creation, starting with the "Big Bang" theory and evolving to the present world, with humans at the top of the evolutionary pyramid, is a fine model, but what about before the Big Bang? Since the beginning of Time, human beliefs and religions have proposed the concept of "God" the creator. Amongst all the various religions, there is no consensus about "God", hence the age-old battle of religions. In Daoism, creation is symbolised by the number "One", the origin of all numbers and containing all of them. Creation is the organisation of the "Void", the original chaos, into two distinct poles, the Yang above, and the Yin below by the appearance of a centre that puts order into the disorder.
Different terms refer to this centre: *Zhong Ji* ≈ Central Ridge 中極 or polar star is the organising centre, also referred to as *Tai Ji* ≈ Supreme Ridge or Great Pole 太極. The passage or way from the original chaos to the manifested order is known as *Dao* 道 (or *Tao*) ≈ Path. It is further said that the Dao has no definition, and if defined it is not the Dao anymore. So, the concept of Yuan Qi, remains a mystery, that may be reflected upon but never defined.
- *Jing Qi*: is the parental essence and can be attributed to the chromosomic transmission. In the fifty's, Watson and Crick discovered the DNA structure and the genetic coding. The genes not only contain parental information, but they also transmit certain structures from the very origins of life. Interestingly only one fourth of the coding genes are expressed "obligatory", the other genes remain apparently dormant, needing to be activated (see further). The information contained in the original cell is half from the mother and half from the father and will be replicated billions of times to constitute the complex human being. The *Jing Qi* may be seen as a memory bank, containing all of the information

concerning not only a particular species but of all life forms from the very beginning. Aside from containing the genetic inheritance, the *Jing Qi* also contains the potential of a person that may or may not be realised during their life.

- *Zong Qi*: is the "Ancestral" energy. The Chinese concept of *Zong Qi* had remained quite confusing for me until recent years. If heredity is transferred by the parental *Jing*, then what would be the "Ancestral" energy? In Chinese medicine, it is believed that the *Zong Qi* is influenced by the planetary configuration at the moment of conception as well as the environment and especially the state of health and well-being of the mother during the gestational period. The breakthrough's in "Epigenetics" seems to have shed light on the ancient Chinese concept of *Zong Qi*. Back in the fifty's, when the DNA structure was unravelled, it was discovered that the genetic code occupied only a section of the DNA helix and that most parts (98%) did not carry any constitutional information. These sections were referred to as "non-coding" segments and considered to have a protective function for the coded section. Epigenetics discovered that these so-called non-coding segments had even greater importance on the genetic code and that they would allow for a gene to manifest or not. In fact, only about 20% of the genetically coded information is "obligatory", this means that the information has to be expressed such as certain racial or organic specificities. 80% of the coded genes may or may not actually materialise and remain dormant, as is the case in certain transmitted diseases that can skip several generations before manifesting. Interestingly the activity of the nucleotides in the coded segment of the DNA is dependent primarily on the environment and life-style; here the modern discoveries of "Epigenetics", joins the ancient Chinese concept of "Ancestral" energy.

Hence the *Zong* ≈ Ancestral Qi relates to family related inheritance. The information transmitted through the parental *Jing* and Ancestral *Zong* constitute the foundation of the racial, ethnic and collective unconscious, and in a sense, is the basis of our memory system. The "Belief" systems are constructed upon these accumulated memories:

- Conscious memories of experiences and events

- In the absence of consciousness or before the full development of the mind (pre and peri-natal period), the memory of a particular experience is contained in the sub-conscious.

- Transmitted and inherited memories

Chinese medicine relegates a different type of memory to each aspect of the mind.

- *Shen* is responsible for the conscious, intentional recollection of information and previous experiences and concepts. This is referred to as "Explicit or Declarative" memory, involving *Yi* for the analysis and classification of previous events, and *Zhi* for the storage (long term memory). Explicit memory is further divided into personal experiences (Episodic memory) and factual information (Semantic memory), concerning accumulated general knowledge and includes concepts, ideas and belief systems.

- *Yi*, represents the analytical aspect of the mind, referred to as "thought". *Yi* analyses (digests) the input and stores the information by analogy with previous events. It is the "Working" memory involved in reasoning and decision-making and behaviour and organisation and manipulation of stored information. In fact, every single input, while the *Shen* is conscious, is analysed and stored by *Yi*. The capacity to retrieve this information depends on the organisational quality of *Yi*. Some consider this to be the short-term memory.

- *Zhi* represents the memory bank or "Long-term" memory. This includes personal experiences (Episodic memory), factual events (Semantic memory), inherited and chromosomic information "*Jing* Qi" (DNA related transmitted information). The latter being further conditioned by the environment, "*Zong* Qi".

- *Po* is the corporeal soul and primarily related to the physical memory of touch and particularly of pain. The common embryonic origin of the skin and the brain cells has been previously underlined. All emotions are first perceived as physical feelings and sensations before the mind has identified them. Therefore, all emotional experiences have a body-based sensation. Before the child's limbic system is fully developed, the body is the depository of all emotional memories. It can be said that the body is the record keeper of all emotional impacts. Even after the full development of the memory centres, during any traumatic event, when the consciousness (*Shen*) is absent, *Po* will register the memory of the incident in the body. Later when this "Body memory" is re-activated, usually by a physical sensation or touch, the person will re-experience the full traumatic episode, physically, physiologically and psychologically. In therapy, the releasing of the body memories is an important stage in the management of psycho-emotional issues.

- *Hun* is responsible for the unconscious memory, perceptions, unconscious learning and language. *Hun* registers impressions and feelings that have not been consciously analysed by the mind. For example, the feeling of shame or rejection when a small child is chastised for having soiled their diaper. This feeling will remain associated with the normal physiological function of elimination throughout the person's life, rejecting the pelvic area as shameful, without any conscious reason. *Hun* is also involved in subliminal programming, in which a certain word or image will trigger a set behaviour. Otherwise, the "Implicit" memory, one of the two main types of long-term memory which is acquired and used unconsciously, and can affect thoughts and behaviours is also the domain of *Hun*. Implicit memory is the counterpart of "Explicit" or conscious memory. One of the common forms of "Implicit" memory is the "Procedural" memory involved in the performance of certain tasks without conscious awareness of the previous experiences. i.e. daily skills (getting dressed, tying the shoes, riding a bicycle, driving a car etc.).

In general, memory is very malleable and can be altered.

Two persons having experienced the same event may remember it quite differently, but ultimately will re-arrange the memory to conform to the majority. Psychologists distinguish two types of memory related to the attempts of an individual to conform to their society: private and social conformity. Private conformity is when the other person's memory is quite similar but with a variance; one can easily accept the difference as one's own memory. In the second instance, the personal memory is very different from the group memory, but the person will conform and accept the public memory as one's own; this is called social conformity. The memory may even be implemented, for example, by replacing an event into a person's early life story, or by changing a traumatic souvenir by a positive and empowering experience. The latter is very useful in the treatment of "Post Traumatic" conditions.

1.2.9 Intelligence

Generally, intelligence is defined as the mental capacity for understanding and retaining information in the form of knowledge, to be later applied in adapting to a given situation, in other words, learning from experience. This could imply, logical reasoning, learning, planning, abstract thinking, problem-solving and attaining goals, self-awareness and emotional insight. The cognitive function of the mind (learning through experience), involves many different mental functions such as attentiveness, analysis and reasoning to deduct information and form knowledge, various types of memory, evaluation, judgment and taking decisions as well as speech. Obviously from a Chinese medical perspective, cognition represents the harmonious collaboration of the five sections of the psyche, *Shen, Yi, Zhi, Po* and *Hun*.

Many of the cognitive factors defining intelligence may also be found in animals as well as in plants.

Based on the above parameters, intelligence was originally measured by a set of standardised tests and scored as IQ (Intelligenzquotient). Since the mid-1960's another aspect of intelligence was identified as Emotional intelligence (EI or EQ), and defined as the ability to recognise one's own and other's emotions. "EI" is the ability to correctly identify different feelings and to use this emotional information to guide thinking and behaviour, to better adapt to the outer circumstances. It seems that people with high EI have superior mental balance, do better in their professions and family lives, and show higher skills as leaders.

The concept of Empathy was associated with this type of intelligence. Empathy is the ability to place oneself in the same framework as another person and to understand or feel what they are experiencing, which could include their emotions (emotional empathy) or their physical conditions (somatic empathy).

Since 1997 several authors have described yet another type of intelligence: Spiritual intelligence (SQ). Although argued and criticised by some, SQ is very broadly defined as the mental capacities based on awareness of non-material and transcendental aspects of the human existence.

D. Zohar defines the 12 principles underlying spiritual intelligence as ($\blacktriangleright$ Fig. 1.22):

- Self-awareness;
- Spontaneity;
- Acting from values and principles;
- Holism (seeing larger patterns);
- Compassion;
- Welcoming diversity;
- Having one's own convictions;
- Humility;
- Seeking the deeper meanings;
- Looking at the bigger picture;
- Positive use of adversity,
- Sense of vocation.

Persons gifted with SQ have a better acceptance of the world and of the others, cope better with difficulties and therefore are better equipped to deal with adversity and disease.

Aside from congenital defects or major traumatic shocks, every human being has access to all three types of intelligence.

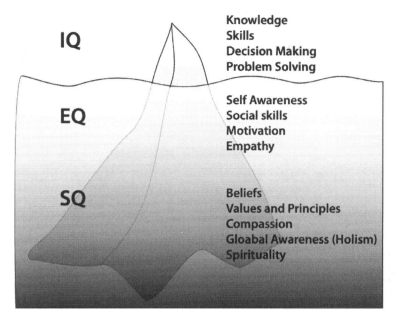

Fig. 1.22:   The iceberg model applied to intelligence

The deficiency of IQ, EQ or SQ is quite often the result of outer social and cultural limitations, in particular, the lack of physical or emotional nourishment in childhood and especially the early mental formatting and the conditioning of faulty belief systems.

Treating the "Hidden Roots of Disease", often implies changing the mind-set and the fixed belief systems of a person. Bringing the person to examine their condition from a different perspective, is the process of helping them get in touch with their Spiritual Intelligence.

PART - II
Belief Systems

- **The Eight Extraordinary Vessels and Psychology**
    - Role of the Extraordinary Vessels in physical and psychological developments
    - Survival Instinct / The Birth Trauma / Bonding Process
    - Compensations / *Gaohuang* Membranes
    - Diagnosis / Psychological profiles
    - Cultivation fo the Mind
    - *Chong Mai* psychological profile
    - *Ren Mai* psychological profile
    - *Du Mai* psychological profile
    - *Dai Mai* psychological profile
    - *Yin and Yang Wei Mai* psychological profile
    - *Yin and Yang Qiao Mai* psychological profile
    - Evaluation Questionnaire

- **Influence of Constitution and Temperaments**
    - *Tai Yang* Temperament
    - *ShaoYin* Temperament
    - *ShaoYang* Temperament
    - *Jue Yin* Temperament
    - *Yang Ming* Temperament
    - *Tai Yin* Temperament
    - Self-assessment questionnaire

- **Influence of the outer world: Psycho-social development**
    - The *Luo* ≈ Connecting vessels in relation to the world
    - Pathology and Diagnosis
    - *Luo* and Personality disorders
    - *Luo* and Mental-Emotional disorders
    - Clinical applications

Part- II

Belief Systems

The belief systems may be defined as the habitual functioning of the mind. This could include a set response mechanism to outer events, well-established value systems (good versus bad), and identification with this primarily fixed mind-set, which constitutes the basis of the individual self-image, the Ego.

Belief systems format and frame the mental functions; when some beliefs are necessary for survival and ultimately the fulfilment of our *Ming* ≈ Life Curriculum/ destiny, other beliefs are self-limiting and may even be self-destructive.

We have previously explored the concept of the small and the big *Shen*. The little *Shen* represents the individualised personality, as separate from the others and the outside. The individual (little) *Shen,* together with *Yi,* the intellect, collaborate to define the "persona", who the individual believes to be and is presenting to the outside. This self-image is the result of various inputs:

- First and foremost, the inherited and constitutional energies that define not only the individual's outer form and body shape but will also greatly influence their behaviour and temperament. The expansive and outgoing energies of Fire and Wood, the more introverted energies of Metal and Water and the centred and balanced position of the Earth element may blend and mix in many combinations to define the variety of human beings on the planet. Many of these psychological traits are genetically (and epigenetically) transmitted and will constitute a great part of the unconscious memories including the collective, ethnic, racial and familial transmissions that are stored in the *Zhi*. These transmitted traits are the basis of the constitution and the archetypal temperaments (▶ Fig. 2.1).

- Culture and conditioning play a fundamental role in the formatting of the belief systems and will further influence the initial constitutional temperament of a person.

- Personal memories and achievements

- Sub-conscious memories registered by the *Hun*
- Sub-conscious physical memories registered by the *Po*

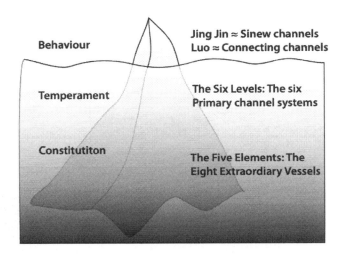

Behaviour

Jing Jin ≈ Sinew channels
Luo ≈ Connecting channels

Temperament

The Six Levels: The six
Primary channel systems

Constitutiton

The Five Elements: The
Eight Extraordiary Vessels

Fig. 2.1:   Foundation of Belief: Constitution- Temperament- Behaviour

How one perceives the outer world and how one reacts to it constitutes the basis of what can be termed as the "Belief system".

Belief always precedes experience

In fact, the mind is formatted to interpret the sensory input based on a pre-established program involving conditioning, belief systems, and memory (conscious or unconscious). The memory system is the sum of our personal experiences, gathered consciously (with the participation of *Yi*) or unconsciously (*Hun* and *Po*) or genetically transmitted (▶ Fig. 2.2).

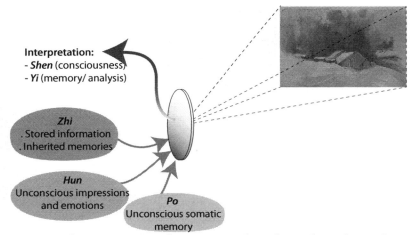

Interpretation:
- ***Shen*** (consciousness)
- ***Yi*** (memory/ analysis)

Zhi
. Stored information
. Inherited memories

Hun
Unconscious impressions
and emotions

Po
Unconscious somatic
memory

Fig. 2.2: The interpretation of sensory input depends on inherited, stored,
and personal subconscious emotional and somatic memories

What we consider to be the consciousness or "Free Will", is actually greatly modelled by the subconscious. Although the conscious functions of the mind constitute merely 1/10th of the brain's activity, it is estimated that only 2 to 4% of our decisions emanate from the conscious mind, 98 to 96% are dictated by the subconscious. Furthermore, the brain does not distinguish between outer or inner input. The outer perceptions or inner imagery (visualisation, dreams), produce the same physiological responses, inducing the same feelings and emotions and the same behaviour (▶ Fig. 2.3).

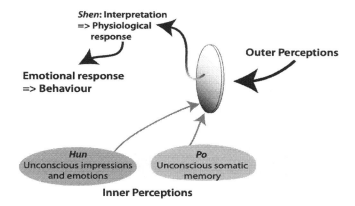

Fig. 2.3: The brain does not distinguish between the inner and outer input; the emotional response is the same.

From early childhood, the mind is conditioned to admit certain perceptions as "real" because others share them equally, and other inputs as "unreal". For example, a small child who is in the process of learning to distinguish between the self and non-self, and the concept of the materiality of objects, has to adapt its visual perceptions in relation to the material limits of the person or object they are experiencing. Now, some small children have been known to perceive forms and colours that surround a person or an object. This is the natural electromagnetic field that surrounds all matter, in particular living organisms. Described as the "aura", it was first evidenced by Kirlian, and now substantiated by modern imagery techniques. The fact that adults do not share the same visual perceptions, will slowly format the child's mind to disregard this type of vision as un-real. But it has been demonstrated that every individual, with a minimum of training, can recover and develop the auric perceptions that were lost in our so-called learning about the outer world.

Belief systems could be defined as the modality by which an individual is learning to conform to their environment. When some belief systems are necessary for protection and survival, for example, the perception of an object or an animal as potentially dangerous, other beliefs may be self-limiting and effectively separating the person from their potential and the full experiencing of the world. In truth, what is considered a "reality" is in fact a filtered and formatted perception of the experience of the environment.

We do not perceive things as they are but as they appear to us

Thus, the perception of the physical world does not necessarily result in a universal reaction amongst observers, for example, a certain colour or smell might evoke a pleasant or unpleasant unconscious memory, resulting in liking or disliking that perception. A sound might be associated with a traumatic experience and be perceived as intolerable etc.

In general, most beliefs are limiting concepts, attempting to maintain a certain social cohesion and mental equilibrium. Most set beliefs narrow down our full experience of the world and of life itself, they inhibit our full potential and are quite often the causes of our suffering and the hidden roots of disease. Learning to identify these hindering beliefs and to change them is the key to psychological and physical health.

Human beings are conditioned to think and to believe in a certain manner. Even when we think that we have free will and free choice, our decisions are quite often rooted in social beliefs.

Some beliefs are leftovers of ancient ideas that do not apply to the modern world anymore.

Here are a few examples:

- Inherited beliefs: collective unconscious:
  - The belief of male superiority: this belief forms the basis of the current "Patriarchal" society, in which women have to fight for their natural rights. Even in the more evolved Western societies, where women have been emancipated, this belief still underlies the subconscious of most people, both male and female.
  - The belief of racial and ethnic differences and the white superiority in Western countries: This belief is at the root of racism and anti-Semitism and has led to the practice of slavery throughout history.
  - Religious beliefs: The deep conviction of following the only "True God", and that the other "Gods" or religions are all in the wrong, has dominated human history since ages and is at the root of religious and sectarian terrorism today.

- Individual conditioning:
  - All of the above beliefs are strongly supported by the family and later social setting during the early formative years
  - The family conditioning: beliefs that are deeply ingrained in the subconscious such as "boys don't cry…"; "be careful…, you will hurt yourself.…"; "eat this if you love mummy…"; "don't touch your genitals, they are filthy…"; "you have to work hard to succeed…";

- Personal beliefs: these are personal experiences and memories, positive or negative, that will condition the manner the psyche will later function and react to the outer world. For example, "love hurts…"; "I am too old to change…"; "my childhood is the cause of my problems…"; "it's bad to show my emotions…";

The relation between "Belief systems" and mental or physical health

Based on the now established certitude that all perceptions produce a physiological response, it is easy to understand that depending on how the sensory input is interpreted, the physiological response will not be the same. For example, upon seeing a dog, based on previous personal experience, the response may be caution or attraction. The same process involves personal feelings, thoughts and concepts that have been previously established as good or bad. A certain belief might have been useful at a certain time in our lives, for example, when we did well in school, we had the teacher's and parent's praise. Later in life, this belief may lead to perfectionism, excessive demands on oneself, and taking on excessive workloads, which will inevitably lead to a "burn-out" condition.

Faulty beliefs are often at the root of the disease process. For example, every time a small child got sick, it got the full attention and care of the parents. Later in life, the same program may reactivate the process in reverse, that is, when the individual feels un-loved or un-cared for, it will get sick. The seriousness of the disease may vary depending on the person or their psychological needs, and may even take the form of a terminal disease, especially if other negative beliefs are associated with the original program, such as "nobody loves me...", "I am not good enough...", "I hate myself...",...

Furthermore, the belief about a particular disease will also greatly influence the outcome of any therapeutic act, for example: "cancer kills...", " I am finished...", "nothing or nobody can help me...", " I don't believe there is any hope...", "chemotherapy is a poison...", etc.

Basis of "Belief Mechanisms"

As the body develops according to a pre-established chronological programme, so does, the mind and the psyche. Outer events and circumstances may alter these developments and manifest on various levels, physical, psychological or mental.

The basic "Constitution" will privilege the activity of a particular set of *Zang-Fu*.

The *Zang-Fu* communicate with the outer world through their superficial channel systems and will define the basic "Temperament" of a person. The secondary channels, *Jing Jin* ≈ Sinew, *Luo Mai* ≈ Connecting/ Network and the *Jing Bie* ≈ Divergent channels, have a more superficial position in relation to the related *Zheng* ≈ Primary channel. In this manner, they complement the functions of the primary channels and protect them against outer influences.

- The *Jing Jin* ≈ Sinew channels are the most superficial channels and carry the *Wei* ≈ Defensive energy. They constitute the main outer line of defence against external aggressions, represented mainly by the six pathogenic factors and physical trauma, but also any other outer stimulus considered too intense by the individual, such as light, sound and even words or emotions. By channelling more *Wei Qi* to a particular area and by tightening up the muscular system, the Sinew channels help to protect the body against these aggressions.

- The *Luo Mai* ≈ Connecting/ Network vessels are deeper and manage and contain the capillary system and Blood. The *Luo* are not that rich in *Wei Qi*, so they attempt to contain the aggressive factor by trapping it in the capillary system.

- The *Jing Bie* ≈ Divergent channels are even deeper. Their defensive role is secondary, but they play an important role in managing the deeper communication between the *Zang-Fu* and the head. Hence, they play an important role in brain physiology and mental functions.

To sum it up, the basic psychological profile of an individual is the result of all of the above influences.

To understand the Belief mechanisms of a person, and to analyse their psycho-emotional responses to the outer world, we need to consider:

- Inheritance: parental, familial, racial and gender (*Jing* and *Zong Qi*)

- Personal *Ming* ≈ Life curriculum (the Eight Extraordinary vessels)

- Basic Constitution and Temperament (Five Elements and the Six channels)

- Socio-cultural developments (the *Luo* ≈ Connecting vessels)

- Personal history of traumatic events (the Eight Extraordinary Vessels and the *Jing Jin* ≈ Sinew channels)

2.1 Eight Extraordinary Vessels and Psychology

The Eight Extraordinary Vessels represent the deepest aspect of one's being. They transmit the constitutional energies and define our genetic make-up and are rooted in the pre-heaven energies. They ensure the perpetuation of the species.

2.1.1 Role of the Extraordinary Vessels in physical and psychological developments

After conception, the primary Extraordinary channels (First Ancestry), *Chong, Ren, Du and Dai Mai*, taking root in the area that will later become *Dong Qi* ≈ Moving Qi between the Kidneys, direct the development of the foetus according to the pre-established programme (plan), defined by *Yuan, Jing* and *Zong* at the moment of conception. After birth, two points communicate directly with the *Dong Qi* area: *Mingmen* ≈ Gate of destiny DM-4, and *Guan Yuan* ≈ Source Gate RM-4 (▶ Fig. 2.4).

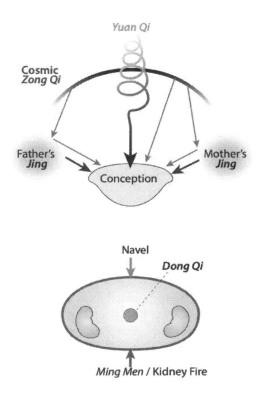

Fig. 2.4: *Yuan, Jing* and *Zong Qi* combine at the moment of conception and become the *Dong Qi* ≈ Moving Qi between the Kidneys

During the foetal stage, the "First Ancestry" comprised of *Chong, Ren, Du* and *Dai Mai*, oversees and coordinates the development of the *Zang-Fu* and of the Primary channels. (▶ Fig. 2.5)

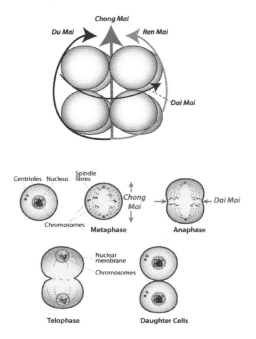

Fig. 2.5: First "Ancestry" and cell division after conception

The original inherited Qi, simply referred to as *Yuan* Qi, is transformed into Kidney Qi and is disseminated from the *Dong Qi* area upward by the *Du Mai* and distributed to the Back *Shu* points, which in turn will direct the *Yuan* Qi towards each *Zang-Fu* ≈ Organ system (▶ Fig. 2.6).

As the primary channels extend from the organs towards the limbs, they will further disseminate the *Yuan* Qi throughout the body. The *Yuan* ≈ Source points located on the distal segments of the channels enhance this movement (▶ Fig. 2.7).

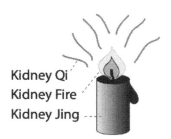

Fig. 2.6: Transformation of *Yuan Qi* into Kidney Qi

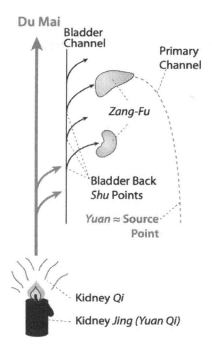

Fig. 2.7: **Distribution of *Yuan Qi* to the *Zang-Fu* and the channels**

The transformation of the original Kidney Yin (*Jing Qi*) into Kidney Qi under the action of Kidney Fire (*Yuan Qi*) is the basis of the *San Jiao* ≈ Triple Warmer system. After birth, the absorbed food and water will constitute the fuel that the digestive Fire will transform into "Qi". The stimulation of a *Yuan* ≈ Source point activates the distribution of this Qi to that particular area.

From a Daoist point of view, the constitutional energies define our fate and destiny.

According to MASTER J. YUEN, the constitutional energies are defined by the *Yuan* ≈ Source Qi, which is reflected by its two components:

- Morphology, the genetic make-up, defined by the parental *Jing* ≈ Essence.

- Destiny*, defined by the *Da* 大 or *Zong* 宗 ≈ Cosmic/ Ancestral Qi at the time of conception.
  * Also referred to as Astrology

After birth, the Extraordinary vessels direct the various developmental stages of the individual, both on the physical as well as on the psychological levels. The activation of the second and third Ancestries, the *Wei Mai* and the *Qiao Mai* coordinate these transformations and define the ageing process, symbolised by the cycles of seven and eight (▶ Fig. 2.8).

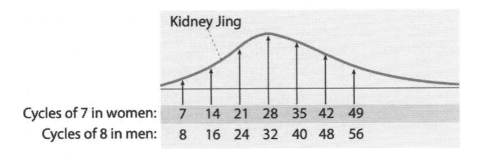

Fig. 2.8:   The cycles of 7 and 8 (The ageing process)

This ageing process does not only concern the ageing of the body but also mental maturity and psychological evolution, hence changes in the person's beliefs, outlooks and value systems.

Normally the pre-defined curriculum "*Ming*" is coordinated and carried out by supporting the Temperament on the one hand, and the physical and physiological evolutions on the other hand, greatly defining the psychology of the person at the various stages of their life.

Aside from transmitted genetic pathologies, Master Yuen relates certain congenital defects to the disturbance of the proper functioning of the Extraordinary vessels without a clear causative factor, for example:

- A consolidation of Yin and the inability of Yang (*Ming Men*-Fire) to disseminate this Yin as observed in Dwarfism, Autism, Down's syndrome and in some types of mental retardation. The most common features in the above pathologies being the shortness of the neck, the webbing of the hands and the clubbing of the feet, and commonly there are tumours or lesions on DM-14 *Dazhui* and DM-4 *Mingmen,* the two primary areas from which Yang needs to disseminate

- An exuberance of Yang with insufficient Yin as seen in seizures and infantile epilepsy, resulting in numbness or paralysis.

- Other, less severe pathologies involving the Extraordinary vessels may cause a separation between the Yin and the Yang due to blockage, stasis or loss. This separation of Yin and Yang may manifest clinically with a disparity between

  - Left and right, treated with *Yin* or *Yang Qiao Mai*

  - Above and below, as seen in *Chong Mai* or *Dai Mai* pathologies

  - Hot and Cold, involving the *Yang Wei Mai*

  - Floating Yang with Yin deficiency, as in menopausal hot flashes, which is dealt with by the *Ren* or *Chong Mai*

  - Sinking Yin with Yang deficiency, as in prolapses, which are classical symptoms of *Dai Mai* or *Chong Mai*

- Some congenital defects, un-related to chromosomal transmission, are due to factors occurring during pregnancy such as exposure to certain medications or chemicals, or certain infectious diseases. The incidence of these defects increases with parental metabolic deficiencies, poorly controlled diabetes, alcohol or tobacco consumption during pregnancy, as well as the mother's age.

- The psychological state of the mother also has a great bearing on the foetus, not only psychologically, but even physically. For example, according to some studies (Archi. Dis. Child. 1978 Jan; 53(1): 66–68) certain physical pathologies, such as pyloric stenosis in the new-born seem to occur with a much higher frequency in mothers who have experienced stressful events during pregnancy. This may also be the case for other congenital but not inherited conditions producing neurological, cardio-vascular or structural defects. Numerous studies have demonstrated the impact of low socioeconomic status on the development of the foetus in utero, growth retardation and premature birth.

- Aside from the above, physical or psychological traumatic events affecting the mother during her pregnancy will also have consequences, not only on the *Jing* but also on the psychology of the child. The mother's stress is experienced as a deep traumatic event for the child. Hence the classical indication of KI-9 *Zhubin*, needled during the third, sixth and ninth month of pregnancy to reduce this impact. Otherwise, the traumatic memory will be buried deep in the unconscious and will constitute an important basis for the person's belief mechanisms. It is recommended to use the *Chong* and *Dai Mai* for clearing out these unconscious events. In general, the Extraordinary Vessels are selected based on the period when a particular shock has occurred.

  - *Chong Mai* is selected for all in utero and peri-natal trauma (see Birth Trauma below);

  - *Ren Mai* involves conditions of lack of, or excessive bonding with the mother, especially in the first year;

  - *Du Mai* is indicated for issues of excessive or absent authority to help shape the individuality of the child, during the second year;

  - The *Wei* and the *Qiao* are involved in transitional periods: puberty, independence age (leaving home), marriage, child-birth, menopause, etc.

  - In all situations *Dai Mai* is the vessel of latency, holding the traumatic event until the person has the necessary means to deal with it.

2.1.2 The Survival Instinct

The instinct to survive is programmed deeply into the genetic structure of all living forms. Any threat to life will automatically set off a reactive response. Shocks affecting the mother, birth, experienced as a major threat, and later the events affecting the infant's life during the first few years will have major effects on the person's psychological traits. Aside from extreme conditions, the impact of a given trauma is not identical for each person. An individual will experience a particular traumatic event very differently based on their constitutional framework. A person having inherited a strong *Jing* will not be affected psychologically by the trauma of birth, whereas a weaker constitution may develop specific psychological traits, such as fearfulness, unexplained anxiety and worry.

For the human being, during these early years, life represents food, water and air, but also touch and care. A lack in any of these may cause certain psychological traits and especially compensation issues.

2.1.3 The Birth Trauma

Master Yuen describes the birthing trauma in the following manner:

> *"If during the birthing process there was a heavy blood loss, this could provoke a constriction in the cervix causing the child to feel a certain degree of suffocation, an unbearable sense of being trapped.*
> *As a result, the child will be high-strung, stressed, hyperactive, with restless sleep and frequent waking, and may later develop attention deficit disorders or infantile epilepsy."*

At birth, the child is adjusting to three basic traumatic events

- The loss of darkness, the child has to adjust to the light, this could later cause fear of darkness, and possible vision disorders.

- The loss of buoyancy, the child is now subjected to gravity, this later manifests in difficulties in walking or walking on the tip of the feet.

- The severing of the umbilical cord, which constitutes the first scar and causes the navel to become a major holding area for a number of unresolved fears and tensions; it also will cause anxiety and worry in the child.

After the severing of the umbilical cord, the child's nourishment comes from the mouth through suckling and also from the nose through breathing. The activation of the Lung Qi and of the mouth Qi "*Qi Ke*" is reflected by LU-9 *Taiyuan* and ST-9 *Renying*. The activation of Lung-Qi activates the Kidney, allowing for the *Jing* ≈ Essence of a new-born to grasp the post-natal Qi of the Lung, regulating the Heart pulsations. As the Qi begins to pulsate the blood; the left side of the Heart (Yang side), develops more pressure. It separates the Heart into left and right differentiated functions and constitutes the Heart barrier.

If the umbilical cord is severed too early, the child is forced to breathe very early and gets into respiratory and circulatory overload, with premature and forceful use of RM-17 *Shanzhong*. This contrived struggle is perceived as a traumatic experience disrupting the *Shen* ≈ Spirit, the child may later tend towards excessive anxiety and worry. This idea is reflected in the name of RM-8 *Shenque* and its function of resuscitating the *Shen* ≈ Spirit.

A caesarean birth has different consequences. The lack of the struggle to pass through the birth canal seems to later affect psychologically the individual who may manifest difficulties with life challenges. Also, the lack of pressure exerted on the skull and consequently on BL-1 *Jingming*, may result in difficulties adapting to day and night rhythms. Additionally, the natural birth exposes the new-born to a large variety of maternal bacteria, which will have a very important role in developing the child's immune system. This bacterial diversity will be missing in the caesarean birth.

2.1.4 Bonding process

Originates in the infant's basic longing to be united back to the maternal nourishment. Exaggerated bonding will engender a relationship of dependency with the mother, which later may transfer to all authority figures, such as parents, teachers, employers, doctors or the partner. This kind of severe dependency on another person is a *Ren Mai* issue.

Conversely, in the absence of an individual to give the infant the required nourishment, may later produce eating and digestive disorders.

During the gestational period and while the child is suckling, the breathing and heartbeat of the mother is a pattern that is embedded in the child (▶ Fig. 2.13).

So, anytime the child looks for nourishment, it will seek the same pattern unconsciously. As an adult, the person will look for relationships that will induce the same kind of breathing patterns and Heartbeat.

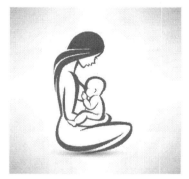

Fig. 2.13: The mother-child bonding; *Ren Mai* connection

These early patterns are further reflected in the manner in which the Sea of Blood – the *Chong Mai* – pulsates the Heart*.

* In this, *Ren* and *Chong* over-lap; in fact, *Ren* is considered the abdominal branch of *Chong*.

In conclusion, for issues with nourishment, both *Ren Mai* and *Chong Mai* should be considered. (see below)

2.1.5 Compensations

A lack of adequate nourishment, air, food, water or care and affection, will produce a sense of deprivation for the infant, who will attempt to compensate this insufficiency, quite often by seeking and retaining Yin. Hence the *Ren Mai*, Sea of Yin is considered the "Compensation Vessel", together with *Chong Mai* "Mother of *Zang-Fu*", they attempt to implement and compensate this sense of deprivation. In fact, both *Ren* and *Chong* are related to the *Gao Huang* membranes, responsible for the nourishment and protection of the *Zang-Fu*.

2.1.6 Gao Huang Protective and Nourishing Membranes

Huang refers to Vitals or Membranes. The points containing the word *Huang* refer to the *Gao Huang*, a term that has been translated by a variety of expressions: vital membranes, or the fatty tissue, etc. Anatomically it seems to refer to the peritoneal folds that surround the abdominal organs and the fatty tissue surrounding the heart. Energetically there is a reference to two concepts (▶ Fig. 2.9):

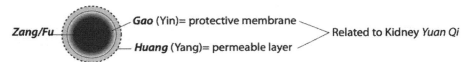

Fig. 2.9: *Gao Huang* ≈ **Protective and Nourishing membranes**

- *Gao*: a protective membrane, Yin
- *Huang*: a permeable membrane, Yang

The latter is referring to "Nourishment" by Blood and Qi of the *Zang-Fu*.

The *Huang* points are:

BL-43 *Gaohuangshu*	Vital Membrane *Shu*
BL-51 *Huangmen*	Vital Membrane Gate
BL-53 *Baohuang*	Womb Vital Membrane
KI-16 *Huangshu*	Vital Membrane *Shu*
RM-6 *Qihai* also called *Huangzhiyuan*	Vital Membrane Source

MACIOCIA adds a sixth point *: *Gaohuang Mu* ≈ Vital Membrane *Mu*

* This point could be RM-15 also named "*Gao Zhi Yuan*"

Clinical Indications

- According to MASTER YUEN, the *Huang* points are related to the *Yuan* ≈ Source Qi and the Kidneys, they activate the *Jingbie* ≈ Divergent channels.

- The French school relates these points to various types and stages of physical and emotional nourishment:

BL-43 *Gaohuangshu*	Relates to affective, self-nourishment (the broken Heart point); it also protects *Yuan Qi* and is a major point in geriatrics (for SUN SI MIAO it is the point of hundred diseases)
BL-51 *Huangmen*	Relates to breast nourishment. A major point for breast diseases
BL-53 *Baohuang*	Relates to sexual nourishment (satisfaction)
KI-16 *Huangshu*	Relates to the maternal (umbilical) nourishment
RM-6 *Qihai*	Considered the gathering point of the Original Qi of the Vital Membranes

According to the above, the *Huang* points may be proposed in a variety of psycho-emotional problems in relation to deficiency of nourishment and its compensation, i.e. anorexia, bulimia, addictions, obesity from affective or sexual frustrations, etc.

2.1.7 Diagnosis

Choosing the appropriate Extraordinary Vessel requires the evaluation of several parameters:

- Chronicity: the pattern has been present since childhood or has started after some major event or life transition

- Organic and energetic dysfunctions and symptoms (▶Appendix-II)

- Particular psychological profiles (see below)

- Palpational diagnosis:

   - Four of the Extraordinary vessels have been described having *Xi*-cleft points; the reactivity of these points may be used to identify the affected vessel: KI-9 *Zhubin* for *Yin Wei*; KI-8 *Jiaoxin* for *Yin Qiao*; BL-59 *Fuyang* for *Yang Qiao* and GB-35 *Yangjiao* for *Yang Wei* (▶ Fig. 2.10)

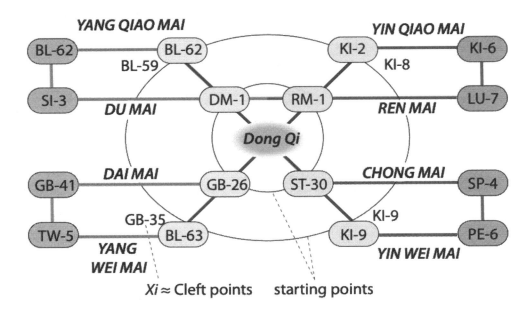

Fig. 2.10: Key, starting, *Xi ≈ Cleft*; and complementary Key points of the Eight Extraordinary Vessels

- Pulses according to Li Shi Zhen or Master J. Yuen (▶Appendix-II)

- Japanese palpational diagnosis based on tension zones according to ITO or MANAKA (▶Appendix-II)

2.1.8 Psychological Profiles

The Psychological profiles for each Extraordinary Vessel will be further analysed under each heading.

As an overview, the main psychological disturbances may be resumed in the following manner:

Chong Mai	Lack of a central axis; lack of connection to the body or emotions; no sense in life; pessimism; idealisation of relations
Ren Mai	Bonding issues: co-dependency, addictions; compensations, eating disorders; issues with control and faith; issues with identity, gender or race
Du Mai	Individuality; over control and rigidity; overachieving; or lack of character; over-dependence; depression

Dai Mai	Holding back and suppression of past violations; disconnection or rejection of the lower body parts; loss of creativity
Yin Wei	Inability to let go of a past event, inability to remain in the present moment; daydreaming; psychosomatic diseases; oppression and panic attacks
Yang Wei	Inability to let go of a past status; self-identification with the social position; over-reactive to external stimuli or criticism
Yin Qiao	Lack of self-acceptance and self-love, lack of self-confidence
Yang Qiao	Non-acceptance or even rejection of the outer conditions, reactivity, political activism, dissatisfaction, indignation

The psychological traits associated with the Eight Extraordinary Vessels will further combine and enhance the constitution and temperament of the person (see under Temperaments).

The resulting "Belief System", will reflect the basic constitution, the temperament as well as the early traumatic events during the gestational period, birth and the first years of infancy.

2.1.9 Cultivation of the Mind

The Eight Extraordinary Vessels are at the core of our belief systems, either through inherited beliefs or through acquired experiences. Hence, the cultivation of the mind requires the cultivation of these constitutional vessels.

According to MASTER YUEN, the Eight Extra Vessels are constitutional channels, reflecting evolutionary and transformational aspects of one's life in relationship to one's gender and ethnic associations or identifications. In some cases, they even represent the evolution of humanity itself. He further indicates their use to help the person in dealing more adequately with their congenital defects, or in situations where the genetic code is being altered post-natally as the DNA and RNA modifications seen in cancer or some acute infectious diseases as in AIDS, tropical diseases and biological warfare.

Furthermore, MASTER YUEN considers the birthing trauma as well as shocks in the early infancy to have certain long-lasting psychological traces on the individual's behaviour for which the Extraordinary Vessels may be effectively utilised.

As the Eight Extra Vessels represent the deepest aspect of one's being, they constitute the deepest form of self-cultivation. The Daoist practice of the "Microcosmic orbit", also called the Small Heavenly cycle, is about re-connecting and opening the *Du* and *Ren Mai* to eventually open up the *Chong Mai*.

The opening of the orbit is achieved by activating the main energy centres through visualisation and breathing (Qigong practice):

- Starting with RM-8 *Shenque*, followed by RM-4 *Guanyuan* for women and RM-2 *Qugu* for men, then followed in order by RM-1 *Huiyin* ⇨ DM-1 *Changqiang* ⇨ DM-4 *Mingmen* ⇨ DM-6 *Jizhong* ⇨ BL-9 *Yuzhen* ⇨ DM-20 *Baihui* ⇨ EP *Yintang*, mouth (tongue touching the palate) ⇨ RM-23 *Lianquan* ⇨ RM-17 *Shanzhong* ⇨ RM-12 *Zhongwan* ⇨ and back to the navel.

- Once this orbit is opened, the practitioner may attempt to open the "Macrocosmic orbit" also called the Large Heavenly Cycle, by activating the *Wei* and the *Qiao* vessels (▶ Fig. 2.11).

Similar results may be obtained through the practice of the Tibetan *Chandali* Meditation, based on the concept of three main channels carrying the life Wind called "*Lung*" (▶ Fig. 2.11).

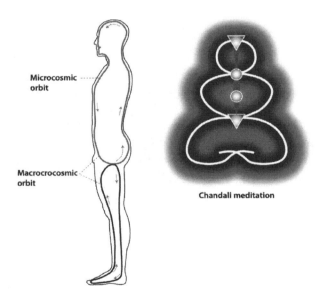

Microcosmic orbit

Macrocrocosmic orbit

Chandali meditation

Fig. 2.11: Micro and Macrocosmic orbit and the Chandali meditation

Normally at conception this life-Wind runs in the two side channels. The *Chandali* Meditation is about manoeuvring this life-Wind into the central channel, which seems quite similar to the concept of the *Chong Mai*.

2.1.10 *Chong Mai* Psychological profile, the "Central Axis"

As *Chong Mai* consolidates the purpose and the reason for one's existence, according to MASTER YUEN, any shock during the gestational period, in the form of disease of the mother, or psychological pressure and stress or the notion of an unwanted child, or birth trauma and early childhood trauma, will manifest later in specific personality traits.

The individual will have an inability to feel connected to the world at a relatively early age, with a deep longing for wholeness and to be united back to the source, the womb. Not feeling complete or whole, not quite incarnated in their bodies or in the world, being quite absent, with difficulty to connect to the Heart and to express feelings and emotions. The desire to find this lost unity, often manifests with a great dependency on the mother, with the image of the mother as a goddess, and is compensated in later life with excessive idealisations of relationships and by projections on to the partner, therapist or teacher. When faced with problems, the individual sees no options or issues, with attitudes of pessimism or even severe states of paranoia or panic attacks.

The *Chong Mai* personality is often depressive, extremely tired, both physically and psychologically, with no desire for anything, sleeping a lot and frequently presenting gynaecological, digestive or lumbar problems, with a tendency to sterility or miscarriage. They frequently experience difficulties in finding meaning in their lives, have difficulties to express their dislikes, and are prone to wheezing or cardiovascular conditions relating to stress.

There are often difficulties in transitional periods of life especially during adolescence with frequent heartbreaks, relationship and marriage difficulties, all reflecting on the *Yin Wei Mai*, which is complementing the *Chong Mai*. As the person does not see any options, they often have no desire to live, although there are very rarely suicidal thoughts during these difficult times.

Chong Mai Treatment protocols

Starting with SP-4 *Gongsun*. PE-6 *Neiguan* is added, especially if there are thoracic or psychological symptoms.

In general, the constituent points are selected according to patterns (please consult Appendix-II for the complete list).

For treating the central axis, manifesting with a lack of centring, feeling disconnected from one's own body and feelings, as well as the outer world and a lack of purpose in life: open *Chong* Mai with SP-4 *Gongsun* and PE-6 *Neiguan*, add according to pattern:

- Due to birth trauma: add KI-16 *Huangshu* and RM-6 *Qihai*
- Due to gestational trauma: add RM-1 *Huiyin*, RM-4 *Guanyuan* and DM-20 *Baihui*

- Due to post-natal trauma: add KI-16 *Huangshu*, BL-43 *Gaohuangshu*, BL-51 *Huangmen*;

- To help release somatic memories treat separately ST-14 *Kufang*, HE-3 *Shaohai* and BL-62 *Shenmai*

- If there is a loss of desire to live (letting oneself die, terminal disease): add RM-14 *Juque* and ST-23 *Taiyi*

- For the loss of will to live (suicidal tendency), combine BL-23 *Shenshu* and BL-52 *Zhishi* with BL-15 *Xinshu* and BL-44 *Shentang*

- For difficulty in moving in the world or taking a stance: add KI-1 *Yongquan* or BL-61 *Pucan* with BL-62 *Shenmai*

- To help accept oneself add KI-6 *Zhaohai* and to help accept the different transitional periods in life add KI-9 *Zhubin*

It should be underlined that just treating with acupuncture or herbs is quite insufficient for influencing the *Jing* ≈ Essence at its deepest levels. To help restore the damage afflicted to the *Jing* and to consolidate the central axis, there is a need to combine psycho-energetic processing and the practice of *Qigong* or martial arts or some other types of meditation (please see under Cultivation).

In this context, MASTER YUEN insists on the concept of *Chong Mai* being about the purpose and the reason for one's existence. In working with *Chong Mai*, we are also harmonising Water and Fire and tapping into the Heart and the *Shen* ≈ Spirit via the great *Luo* of *Shao Yin*. This *Shaoyin* internal link between

the HE and KI is maintained by *Bao Mai* connecting the uterus to the Heart via the Kidney. This connection further involves the *Dai Mai* and the great *Luo* of Spleen: SP-21 *Da Bao*, connecting the *Luo* of *Ren (*RM-15 *Jiuwei)* and *Du Mai* (DM-1 *Changqiang*) (▶ Fig. 2.12).

Besides these points, KI-8 *Jiaoxin* is said to regulate *Chong* and *Ren Mai* and help build trust; especially indicated for children with weak parental *Jing* ≈ Essence, also for adults presenting *Jing* depletion from excessive sex.

For rebellious Qi and "running piglet syndrome" (panic attacks): SP-4 *Gongsun* on the

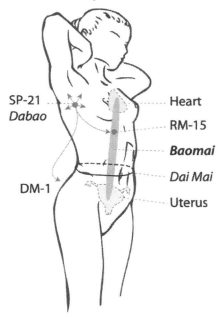

SP-21
Dabao

DM-1

Heart

RM-15

Baomai

Dai Mai

Uterus

Fig. 2.12: *Bao Mai, Dai Mai* and *Dabao*

dominant side followed by PE-6 *Neiguan* on the contralateral side, followed by LR-3 *Taichong* on the opposite side to SP-4 *Gongsun* with contra-lateral PE-7 *Daling* or LI-4 *Hegu*. Other points may be added: KI-14 *Siman*, KI-21 *Youmen*, possibly RM-18 *Yutang*, and in case of rapid and hoarse breathing, RM-17 *Tiantu* and for plum-pit throat ST-5 *Daying*. The abdominal rectus muscle has to be released before actually treating the points along the *Chong*, which could be achieved either with ST-25 *Tianshu*, or by palpating the local points and needling the tight knots, or according to a Japanese method, by needling LR-4 *Zhongfeng* and if not sufficient, followed by LU-5 *Chize*.

2.1.11 Ren Mai Psychological Profile, the "Compensation Vessel"

According to Master Yuen, three main characteristics define the psychology of *Ren Mai*:

- Bonding
- Adaptive behaviour: initial learning of control
- Gender or group consciousness

Bonding

After the initial shock of birth, the bonding process during the first stage of an infant's life is extremely important in helping to establish a balanced psycho-emotional basis for its future development. This bonding concerns the chest-to-chest, mouth-to-nipple and eye-to-eye contact (▶ Fig. 2.13).

In a sense, the *Ren Mai* of the child stays connected with the *Ren* of the mother despite the severance of the umbilical cord (RM-8).

There are two possible situations:

- Excessive protectiveness or over nurturing by a maternal figure, during the first year of its life, causes the child to develop an attitude of over-dependency with feeling easily victimised, never taking full responsibility or commitment, often seeking relationships that involve total dependency on the

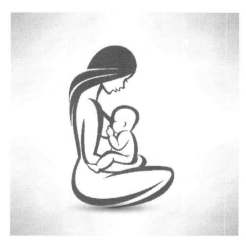

Fig. 2.13: The mother-child bonding; *Ren Mai* connection

other for protection and for decisions, with typical attitudes of co-dependency. The *Ren Mai* personality frequently stays very attached to the mother, living at home for a long time and even after marriage. In the absence of an appropriate replacement for the mother, the person searches for compensations.

- Visual obsessions, daydreaming to compensate for the lack of mother's eye to eye connection;

- Eating disorders, nourishment through Yin type foods (starch) and Damp-Heat producing (sugar), which help to feel contained, heavy and drowsy;

- Addictions, manifesting as food, tobacco and alcohol (oral complex) or drugs (co-dependency).

- On the other hand, an inadequacy of nourishment, due to premature birth, incubator, mother's incapacity, or a working single parent, will result in an insufficiency of Yin. The person never feels contained, content or complete. The condition often involves Yin deficiency with signs and symptoms of Heat and Dryness. The lack of a maternal matrix causes a child to feel that their needs are not being met, that nothing is meaningful or exciting with an underlying feeling of emptiness. There is a further incapacity to feel complete in relationships. This condition reflects the imbalance between *Du* and *Ren Mai* as they are mutually inclusive of each other.

In both cases, over bonding or lack of bonding, may later manifest with compensation issues; either to replace the maternal matrix or because nothing seems to be sufficient. The Chinese concept of "Hungry Ghosts" also referred to as the "Three Worms", relates to these issues:

- Hungry Ghost: concerns unresolved material desires

- Sexual Ghost: resulting from unfulfilled or over indulged sexuality

- Wandering Ghost: relates to frustrated emotional needs

In some ways, these "Worms" are the result of an inability to properly assimilate and be fulfilled and therefore reflect on the digestive process and the post-natal Qi, rendering the *Ren Mai* a veritable vessel of compensation. *Ren Mai* deals with unresolved and unfulfilled issues by a holding pattern, often in the form of Phlegm. Many of the *Ren Mai* points deal with Yin and Phlegm accumulation. (► Appendix-II)

Initial Learning of control

The initial learning how to control and to manipulate the external and internal environment is also developed in the first year, through which the child is learning to adapt to the environment. This could explain some infantile conditions, for example, an early weaning (loss of control of the outside), might result in the infant over controlling their internal environment with manifestations of diaper rash, colic's, reflux, belching, asthma, or later with food sensitivity such as lactose or gluten intolerance or even an irritable bowel syndrome. A child who has difficulties in toilet training (lack of internal control) may develop a need for excessive control of external events manifesting as a need to be first, a leader, having a controlling character.

Gender and group consciousness

Ren Mai as the sea of Yin is also representing "form" and "gender". Issues with physical identity and discomfort about gender or race and colour reflect on the *Ren Mai* development. This may manifest later in the lower abdomen as reproductive, urogenital and intestinal problems.

Ren Mai Treatment protocols

Generally, difficulties with ethnicity and gender involve the lower abdomen; issues with control and digestion, concern the middle abdomen. The chest area deals with the notions of faith and trust in the higher forces. This symbolically can only occur when the individual has relinquished their self-identity (lower Triple Warmer) and control over the environment (middle Triple Warmer) and can now open up to a higher power, God.

Beginning with the key point LU-7 *Lieque*, followed by the complementary key point KI-6 *Zhaohai* and the starting point RM-1 *Huiyin*.

KI-6 *Zhaohai* and RM-1 *Huiyin* are not always used. The treatment could be simplified by choosing LU-7 *Lieque* with the appropriate points along the *Ren Mai* trajectory (please consult the Appendix for the complete list).

For example, points are selected from:

- Lower *Sanjiao* ≈ TW (RM-1 *Huiyin* to RM-8 *Shenque*), for reproductive, uro-genital and intestinal problems; as well as for issues with group or gender identity

- Middle *Sanjiao* (RM-8 *Shenque* to RM-15 *Jiuwei*), for digestive problems, eating dysfunctions and issues pertaining to control and compensation

- Upper *Sanjiao* (RM-15 *Jiuwei* to RM-24 *Chengjiang*), for respiratory and cardio-vascular problems, as well as issues to do with faith and trust

2.1.12   *Du Mai* Psychological Profile, the "Individuality Vessel"

There are two possible psychological profiles:

- An overactivity of *Du Mai*: Maybe due to sensory overstimulation of the child caused either by too many or un-adapted games, or from excessive parental demands, or again by lack of limitations set by the parents. This overstimulation tends to produce hyperactivity and attention deficit in children.

  Or through rebellion against excessive authority and parental rigidity: The person will have a tendency to being overly independent quite early in life, taking risks, having difficulty with commitment, difficulty in being satisfied with their status, becoming overachievers, goal- oriented with an overbearing personality, insensitive to others and over-controlling. They tend to have an over rigid spine as well as rigidity of opinions and ideas.

- A weakness of *Du Mai*: often through over-protectiveness of the mother, smothering the development of *Du Mai* or an overbearing parent crushing the child's identity, which will result in a person with a tendency to be shy and overly dependent, becoming a follower and easily victimised; a depressive type character, with identity and self-affirmation issues, having difficulty in expressing themselves or formulating an opinion. They frequently have a weak back and hold themselves in a hunched (kyphotic) posture. Over-protection from the mother or absence of a father figure is also often the cause of Asthma (Kidney unable to grasp the Lung Qi).

Both types may suffer from vertebral problems.

Note that the psychological profiles for *Du* and *Ren Mai* are complementary, a weakness of *Du Mai* (lack of identity) is accompanied by and repletion of *Ren Mai* (over-dependence), and vice versa.

MASTER YUEN relates the *Ren Mai* to Freudian psychology and the *Du Mai* to behavioural psychology. For him, it is the *Du Mai*, which allows one to interact with people and the world, and is responsible for the behaviour, which can only be measured by action.

Du Mai Treatment protocols

Start with SI-3 *Houxi*, followed by the complementary key point BL-62 *Shenmai*, and the starting point DM-1 *Changqiang*. The *Du Mai* trajectory points may be added according to the symptoms and anatomical correlations

- Lower Curvature (DM-1 to DM-4*)*: In general for intestinal, reproductive and urogenital conditions. In particular DM-4 *Mingmen,* supporting

Kidney-Fire and strengthening the individuality, it is contraindicated for moxibustion until after puberty (this could stimulate the premature unfolding of Kidney Yang, causing premature ageing)

- Middle Curvature (DM-5 to DM-6*)*: Deals with digestive problems
- Upper Curvature (DM-9 to DM-16): indicated for respiratory, cardiovascular, ear, nose, throat and eye conditions as well as for psycho-spiritual issues

  – DM-9 *Zhiyang,* is the gathering point of Yang, supplement for depression

  – DM-10 *Lingtai* and DM-11 *Shendao,* are points that are rarely used in classical acupuncture, it was believed that needling them would scatter the *Shen*≈Spirit and allow for possession

  – DM-12 *Shenzhu,* supports Lungs and *Zhong Qi,* treats Yang type psychological disorders

  – DM-14 *Dazhui,* strengthens Heart-Fire and supports individuality

- Both DM-4 *Mingmen* and DM-9 *Zhiyang* help in making choices
- DM-17 *Naohu,* moves endocranial blood, dispels Wind and Heat
- DM-20 *Baihui,* lifts the mood and stimulates memory
- DM-19 *Houding,* for insomnia and restlessness
- DM-24 *Shenting:* calms the mind, manic behaviour

In general, most *Du Mai* points have psycho-emotional indications. (please refer to *Du Mai* points)

2.1.13 *Dai Mai* Psychological Profile, the "Latency Vessel"

Dai Mai deals with "violations" and deeply held "sentiments", or what can be termed as problems "put under the carpet". The subject holds the issues that have not been dealt with or deeply suppressed, in the form of Dampness and Phlegm in the lower parts.

The original traumas most often involve sexual violations at an early age. The subject is waiting for the right moment to resolve these issues. This holding pattern may also manifest as Phlegm accumulation around the waist, the lower abdomen or the hip areas.

The person has difficulty in finding the necessary energy for creativity or for completing a task, they are often scattered and feel disconnected from their lower abdomen or legs.

Dai Mai, through its connection with the Heart via the *Bao Mai* (▶ Fig. 2.12), is also indicated for chest Blood stasis due to emotions combined with Blood stasis and Dampness in the lower Triple Warmer as observed in vaginal or urinary infections, prostatitis and ulcerative colitis.

Treatment

Begin with the key point: GB-41 *Zulinqi*, coupled with TW-5 *Waiguan*, and the starting point GB-26 *Daimai*.

- To resolve Dampness: GB-41 *Zulingqi* with LR-13 *Zhangmen*, GB-26 *Daimai*
- For Damp-Heat add: GB-27 *Wushu*
- For Damp-Cold add GB-28 *Weidao*

(Please consult the Appendix-II for the complete *Dai Mai* therapeutic applications).

2.1.14　*Yin Wei Mai* Psychological Profile, "Self-identity Vessel"

According to LI SHIZHEN, *Yin Wei Mai* is about self-identification; that is, reflecting and assessing oneself through one's accomplishments. *Yin Wei Mai* is about possessiveness and ownership, the things that make one feel more validated as an individual whereas *Du Mai* represents one's capability and potential. *Yin Wei Mai*, therefore, relates to beliefs and memory, about things that have been accumulated. On this point, it is interesting to recall the Korean study, mentioned previously, on PE-6 *Neiguan* and its effect on the hippocampus area of the brain, related to memory.

Psychologically, the individual is often thinking of the past and may even be stuck in a period of their lives that they don't seem to evolve from such as puberty, a romantic period or a particularly painful episode of physical or emotional shock. Some events or situations in the present might take them back to that particular time and space and have them re-live the traumatic episode again, manifesting as acute episodes of chest oppression, claustrophobia, agoraphobia, panic attacks or even aggression.

Or they may be avoiding the present moment by dreaming about the future, aspiring to become someone important, hoping for the perfect relationship, or dreaming about an ideal living situation. All these attitudes tend to take the person out of the present moment into the past or the future.

Yin Wei Mai is often involved in psycho-somatic diseases, in which there is somatisation of a psychological issue, as seen in patterns such as gastritis, spasmophilia, chest pains and oppressions.

Treatment

Start with PE-6 *Neiguan* coupled with SP-4 *Gongsun*, followed by KI-9 *Zhubin*.

- In general, to calm *Shen* and supplement Blood: add RM-17 *Shanzhong*, LR-14 *Qimen* and Sp-15 *Daheng*

- In case of psychosomatic diseases, or panic attacks and chest oppression, add LR-3 *Taichong,* LR-14 *Qimen*, PE-7 *Daling* or PE-5 *Jianshi* and RM-18 *Yutang*.

- To help talk about a traumatic event; plum-pit: add PE-7 *Daling;* RM-17 *Shanzhong*

- For amnesia; repressed emotions; shyness: add HE-5 Tongli

- Anxiety feeling in the:

  - Stomach add BL-17 Geshu

  - Intestines (holding emotions, constipation): add BL-57 Chengshan

  - Eating to suppress emotions (food compensation): add BL-20 Pishu

- For nine kinds of Heart pain, based on the described type of pain, add the confluent point:

  - Stinging or pinching pain: *Taiyin*; add RM-17 *Shanzhong* and Sp-15 *Daheng*

  - Sharp pains: *Jueyin*; add RM-17 *Shanzhong* and LR-14 *Qimen*

  - Stabbing (transfixing) pains: *Shaoyin*; add RM-17 *Shanzhong* and RM-23 *Lianquan*

- Insomnia: poor sleep quality or superficial sleep: PE-6 *Neiguan*, KI-9 *Zhubin*

  - Difficulty in the first segment of the night: *Taiyin*, add SP-6 *Sanyinjiao* and according to point-sensitivity and other symptoms SP-13 *Fushe* or SP-15 *Daheng* or SP-16 *Fuai*

  - Difficulty in the middle of the night: *Jueyin*, add LR-14 *Qimen*

  - Difficulty in terminal portion of the night: *Shaoyin*, add RM-23 *Lianquan*

2.1.15 *Yang Wei Mai* Psychological Profile, "Reactivity Vessel"

As discussed above, Yin and Yang Wei deal with transitional periods of life, as well as beliefs and aspirations. Having difficulty with these periods, or being stuck in a certain life stage or being too concerned with the future, reflect on these vessels.

For MASTER YUEN, archetypes reflect on *Yin Wei*, whereas social status and social achievements or recognitions are more the domain of the *Yang Wei*.

The *Yang Wei* personality has difficulties with transitions and with adapting to change. They tend to be fixated or even obsessed with their social image of past or future, and material possessions. They tend to be over-reactive to external stimuli and to criticism.

Yang Wei and TW-5 *Waiguan*, are very important for patients facing terminal diseases, to help them embrace death, to feel complete and to let go of possessions and things they are holding-on to; add BL-63 *Jinmen* (starting point) and GB-35 *Yangjiao* (*Xi* ≈ Cleft point).

Treatment

TW-5 *Waiguan* coupled with GB-41 *Zulinqi*, followed by GB-35 *Yangjiao*.

- For chest oppression, with chest knotting: add BL-15 *Xinshu*
- For mania or hysteria: add DM-27 *Duiduan*
- For obsessions with past events or future aspirations: add cupping on GB-29 *Juliao* and SI-10 *Naoshu*
- For helping transitional periods, or the dying process: add BL-63 *Jinmen* and GB-35 *Yangjiao*

2.1.16   *Yin Qiao Mai* Psychological Profile, "Self-image / Self-acceptance Vessel"

The *Qiao* vessels are about rooting the person in the world. The *Yin Qiao* represents the Yin aspect of this rooting, which is the rooting in oneself. It is also about how one sees oneself, about self-acceptance and self-love. The most pertinent question revealing a *Yin Qiao* issue would be: "If you had the choice, who would you choose to be"?

MASTER YUEN also considers the *Yin Qiao* as the first stage of meditation, starting by the rooting of oneself, in the body, which can only take place if there is total self-acceptance and self-love. Maybe this is what ZHANG ZIYANG meant by stating that the *Yin Qiao* is the first vessel?

Treatment

Begin with KI-6 *Zhaohai*, followed by LU-7 *Lieque* and KI-8 *Jiaoxin*

- For lack of self-confidence add KI-8 *Jiaoxin*
- For lack of self-acceptance add LR-8 *Ququan*
- For excessive self-love, narcissism add KI-10 *Yingu*
- For Insomnia: supplement KI-6 *Zhaohai*, reduce BL-62 *Shenmai*, add BL-1 *Jingming*

2.1.17   *Yang Qiao Mai* Psychological Profile, "Rooting Vessel"

As was discussed above, the *Qiao* vessels are about rooting the person in the world. *Yang Qiao* represents the Yang aspect of this rooting and is related to the outer world. Hence a difficulty in accepting the world as it is, a desire to change the world, political or ecological activism, represents a *Yang Qiao* issue. The person is looking for discrepancies and mistakes and becoming rebellious. There is a heightened sensitivity to external stimulation with a tendency to over-react to the outside, and pathologically manifesting as allergies, inflammations and even stirring of internal Wind.

Treatment:

Beginning with the key point: BL-62 *Shenmai,* followed by the complementary key point SI-3 *Houxi,* and the starting point BL-61 *Pucan.* Other confluent points may be added according to the pathology.

- Insomnia: reduce BL-62 *Shenmai,* supplement KI-6 *Zhaohai,* add BL-1 *Jingming*

- To help adjust to external changes, accepting the outer world, add BL-60 *Kunlun*

2.1.18 Life Transitions and the Extraordinary Vessels

The second and third Ancestry, the *Wei* and the *Qiao* vessels are responsible for coordinating the various stages of growth and ageing. This also includes the mental and psychological evolution of the person.

The French school proposes the concept of "Gates" to represent these physical and psychological stages. As *Yang Wei* and the *Yang Qiao* share a several confluent points in certain areas, certain recurrent pathologies may be interpreted as physical manifestations of psychological difficulties with a particular transition (▶ Fig. 2.14).

- Area of the ankles, BL-61 *Pucan*, "Gate of Childhood": representing the notion of standing on one's own feet, letting go of the mother's protective arms, learning to do things on one's own…

- Hip area, GB-29 *Juliao*: "Gate of Adolescence": representing the concept of acceptance of one's gender and sexuality and consequently acknowledging one's role in the reproductive process…

- Shoulder area, SI-10 *Naoshu*: "Gate of Maturity": relating to the acceptance of one's responsibilities in the world; assuming the choices we have made and recognising and coming to terms with the dreams that we have given up...

Clinically, in the presence of a recurrent or resistant physical condition, for example, weak ankles with recurrent ankle sprains, or hip arthrosis, or chronic pathologies of the shoulder, the above "Gate" points should be palpated. If locally the most reactive point is one of the above, the *Xi*-cleft point of the related Extraordinary (BL-59 *Fuyang* and GB-35 *Yangjiao*) will further confirm and orient the diagnosis.

For example, in case of a resistant peri-arthritis of the shoulder in a middle-aged man, with no clear causative factor such as a trauma, or professional over-use; if the most

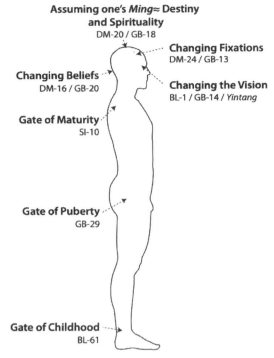

Assuming one's *Ming*≈ Destiny and Spirituality
DM-20 / GB-18

Changing Fixations
DM-24 / GB-13

Changing Beliefs
DM-16 / GB-20

Changing the Vision
BL-1 / GB-14 / *Yintang*

Gate of Maturity
SI-10

Gate of Puberty
GB-29

Gate of Childhood
BL-61

Fig. 2.14: **The Seven Transformational Gates**

reactive point is SI-10, the *Yang Wei* or *Yang Qiao* may be suspected. The palpation of GB-35 and BL-59 (compared to the opposite side) will substantiate the diagnosis. The treatment will select TW-5 *Weiguan* or BL-62 *Shenmai* (or both), together with SI-10. Psychologically it would be important to explore the person's ideas and concepts about their beliefs. These may concern a typical mid-life crisis when the person is examining their life, what they have done or achieved, and what they have left undone…

Similarly, some other meeting areas of the *Wei* and *Qiao Mai* may also symbolically correspond to important landmarks of psychological changes (▶ Fig. 2.14); for example:

- The neck area: GB-20 *Fengchi*, DM-16 *Fengfu* <=> relating to the Sea of marrow; and helping in changing of beliefs. Pathologies in the neck area such as arthrosis, discus hernia (cervicobrachial neuralgia), cervical headaches or certain types of vertigo, maybe expressing issues with rigid belief systems.

- The eye area: BL-1 *Jingming* as well as GB-14 *Yangbai*, and the extra point *Yintang* <=> relate to the changing of vision. Physical pathologies of the eyes or frontal headaches may be relating to difficulties in changing one's outlook in life. The eye area is very complementary to the neck area.

- The forehead area: GB-13 *Benshen*, DM-24 *Shenting* <=> is helping to let go of fixed ideas and assumptions (complements the neck area).

- The apex area: GB-18 *Chengling*, DM-20 *Baihui* <=> assists one in assuming one's spirituality.

2.1.19   Questions for Evaluating the Extraordinary Vessels

Extra-Ordinary Vessel	Questions	Score
Chong Mai	<ul><li>Do you often feel spaced-out?</li><li>Do you find it difficult to be here and now?</li><li>Do you feel disconnected from your roots?</li><li>Do you feel disconnected from your body?</li><li>Do you easily idealise authority figures: teachers, doctors, spiritual leaders, etc.?</li><li>Do you feel uncomfortable in society?</li><li>Do you feel you don't belong...?</li></ul>	
Ren Mai	<ul><li>Do you bond easily?</li><li>Do you frequently need approval before deciding?</li><li>Do you easily feel not respected?</li><li>Do you always agree?</li><li>Do you need to belong to a nation, ethnic or religious group, etc.?</li><li>Are you very attached to familiar surroundings, home etc.?</li><li>Are you attached to your habits?</li></ul>	
Du Mai	<ul><li>Is the notion of independence very important for you?</li><li>Can you easily make choices?</li><li>Can you clearly indicate and realise your needs?</li><li>Are you often overdoing?</li><li>Do you need to explore new horizons?</li><li>Are you easily inflexible?</li><li>Do you tend to be controlling and authoritative?</li></ul>	

Dai Mai	• Is it difficult for you to let go? • Is it difficult for you to forgive? • Are you easily resentful? • Do you often avoid uncomfortable issues? • Do you frequently repress your feelings? • Do you easily put things off for later? • Is it hard for you to be creative?	
Yin Wei Mai	• Are you attached to who you were in the past? • Is it difficult for you to accept the signs of ageing? • Is it hard to for you to let go of past difficult events? • Is it hard for you to accept change? • Is it hard for you to be in the present moment? • Are you often fantasising about the future? • Do you find that your recollection of shared past memories is at odds with others? • Do you have many regrets?	
Yang Wei Mai	• Are you very identified with your social status? • Are you very attached to your material possessions? • Is it hard for you to accept changes in your social status? • Is it very hard for you to accept criticism? • Do you tend to over-react to external change? • Do you dislike wind? • Do you foster many aspirations for the future?	
Yin Qiao Mai	• Do you have a difficult time accepting yourself as who you are? • Do you often wish that you could be someone else? • Is it hard for you to love yourself? • Is it hard for you to trust yourself? • Is it difficult to take a stance and defend your position? • Are you often missing motivation? • Are you easily lacking courage?	
Yang Qiao Mai	• Is it hard for you to accept the world as it is? • Are you often aspiring for a better world? • Do you feel that you have to fight for your place in society? • Do you tend to find mistakes and discrepancies in the system? • Are you easily rebellious? • Are you often involved in activist movements? • Do you have seasonal allergies?	

2.2   Influence of the Constitution and Temperaments on the Belief Systems

To understand the psychology and the mental functions of a person, the analysis of the constitution alone is not sufficient.

The concept of the "Five Elements" describes the basic internal structure and the fundamental energetic and physical profile of a person defined as their "Constitution".

The constitution is transmitted through the parental *Jing* ≈ Essence, which is part of the "Pre-Heaven" energies. This explains the racial similarities found in a particular country or area of the world.

The constitution will further influence the development and activity of the organs *Zang-Fu* and their related "Primary" channels.

The ancestral *Zong Qi* is the cosmic Qi at the moment of conception and defines the *Ming* ≈ Life mandate/ destiny of the person and will therefore, influence the basic "Temperament" of the individual.

According to the Daoist belief, a person's temperament is already defined during the foetal stage:

> *...in the fifth (lunar) month, the five sensory organs are complete,*
> *the temperament is defined and the foetus communicates*
> *with the mother through her dreams...*

This pre-established temperament constitutes the primary basis for the individual's belief systems and emotional responses. The temperament will be modulated after birth by personal experiences and social conditioning.

The "Temperament" will mostly determine how a person communicates and responds to the outer world, defined as their habitual behaviour.

This communication between the inner (microcosm) and the outer world (macrocosm) is carried out partly by the five sensory organs and partly by the outer connections of the *Zang-Fu*, represented by the primary channels and their secondary branches (▶ Fig. 2.15a).

The primary channel systems are expressed as the "Six Great Axis" or "Six Vectors" or simply the "Six Channels" (▶ Fig. 2.15b).

The outermost manifestations of these "Six-Axis" are the twelve "Sinew channels" ≈ *Jing-Jin*, controlling amongst other things, the muscles and the sinews. The interplay of the muscles, their tension or laxity, will define the outer form/ morphology.

The sinew channels also constitute the most superficial defensive layers of the body and therefore will be involved in mostly all physical but also psychological traumatic shocks.

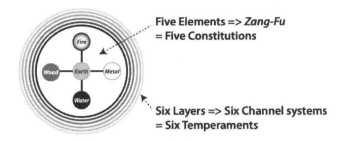

**Five Elements => *Zang-Fu*
= Five Constitutions**

**Six Layers => Six Channel systems
= Six Temperaments**

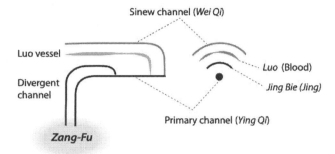

Sinew channel (*Wei Qi*)

Luo vessel

Divergent channel

Luo (Blood)

Jing Bie (*Jing*)

Primary channel (*Ying Qi*)

Zang-Fu

Fig. 2.15a: The Primary and Secondary channel systems

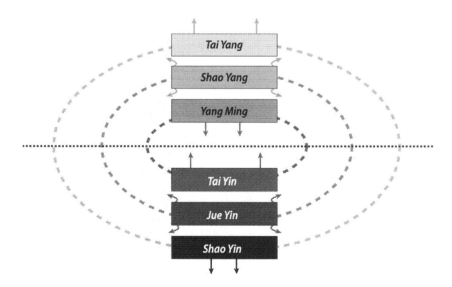

Tai Yang

Shao Yang

Yang Ming

Tai Yin

Jue Yin

Shao Yin

Fig. 2.15b: The Six Levels (Vectors or Axes), connected by the *Luo* system

Another group of secondary channels, the *Luo* ≈ "Connecting vessels", are more in charge of dealing with the human's emotional responses to the outer world. In fact, the *Luo Mai* are described as having two trajectories:

- The transversal trajectory connects two coupled channels: the *Luo-Yuan* point connection maintaining the *Biao-Li* couple (HE and SI or LU and LI etc.). These connections also allow for the emotions produced by the *Zang* organs to be released by the *Luo* of the *Fu* (▶ section 2.3.1)

- The Horizontal trajectory starts at the *Luo* point, follows the primary channel and moves upward and outward: contacts with the outer world and manages the human responses to external changes (▶ Fig. 2.38).

It can be summarised that the "Five Movements" explore the synchronisation of the Microcosm by the Macrocosm; in other words, the Five Movements "*Wu Xing*", explain how the outer world influences the energetics of a person. For example, the rhythmic changes of day and night, or the four seasons, or the sensory input (colour, sound, smell, taste…).

The "Six Channel systems or energy levels" constitute the bridge that communicates the constitution "Microcosm" with the constant changes that occur between Heaven and Earth "Macrocosm". This will further define the person's temperament and habitual behaviour. These habitual responses will manifest as conditions of repletion or vacuity of a particular channel system.

- Repletion (excess) in a channel system may indicate the things to which one is drawn to, for example, a condition of Heart-Heat may result from excessive desires, and seeking excitement; or a Liver-Yang rising reflects on a need to take on too many challenges and to compete...

- Vacuity (deficiency) could underline one's avoidances and inadequacies: for example, the Kidney Qi vacuity would manifest as general fearfulness, lack of motivation and self-trust, and avoiding taking risks.

This explains that a person's physiology as well as their pathology is not only a reflection of their constitution but also of their "Temperament" and "Behaviour".

As long as the temperament is in accordance with the constitution, there is a sense of inner harmony. For example, when a Fire-type constitution has a *Taiyang* (Fire-Water) or *Shaoyin* (Fire-Water) temperament, they will feel generally "at ease". When the temperament is not adapted, there is a feeling of unease, for example, a Fire-type constitution having any other type of temperament, for instance, a *Taiyin* (Earth-Metal) temperament, will manifest a discomfort. This situation often arises from external pressures, such as family, society or conditioning. If this dis-adaptation continues for a longer time it will cause pathology first on the energetic and later on physical levels. In general, each temperament, when not blocked, has the capacity of moving in and out of their preferential level, in order to respond to the needs of the moment, especially to communicate with their complementary Yin or Yang levels.

For example, a *Taiyang* temperament (most extreme Yang), has to be able to withdraw into the *Shaoyin* level (deepest Yin) in order to replenish and harmonise their energies. Otherwise, if the temperament is blocked in a particular level, pathology arises, manifesting at first psychologically, and over time physically as well. It is important to note that with age, as the individual has less Qi, most temperaments tend to either get blocked in their level or in the complementary Yin level, which further enhances the development of the corresponding pathologies. In general, two temperaments get more easily blocked in their levels: the *Taiyin* and the *Shaoyin*.

The "Temperament" is evaluated, based on the outer form as well as the habitual "Behaviour" of the person. With some experience, the constitution and the temperament of a patient are evaluated within minutes of having encountered them. This, not only helps to better understand the pathology of a person but also orients towards the most appropriate selection of therapy and the best choice of channels and points to treat.

Each constitutional element is related to two channels, hence to two possible vibrational levels. For example, a Fire-type constitution may present a *Taiyang* or a *Shaoyin* temperament (▶ Fig. 2.16).

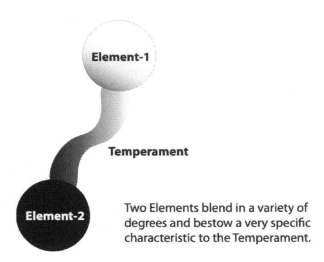

Temperament

Element-1

Element-2

Two Elements blend in a variety of degrees and bestow a very specific characteristic to the Temperament.

Fig. 2.16: The blending of two Elements define the Temperament

Each individual will blend the two elements in their own and very unique manner. Hence two Fire types will have similarities but will not be identical. The same applies to temperaments, for example, a Fire-type might present characteristics of Water or vice versa (▶ Fig. 2.16).

Due to their vibrational affinities, the most common Five Element combinations are:

- Fire and Wood
- Fire and Water
- Earth and Metal

Usually, a person's constitutional element is determined by their most outstanding physical and psychological characteristics. But of course, a third element may influence the above combinations and make it more difficult to define their basic constitution.

It is generally understood that the best combination is the equal combination of the five influences. In practice, this condition is very rarely observed.

Although it is quite easy to determine a typical constitution or temperament, it is much harder when there are mixtures of several influences. Obviously, between the white and black colours there are thousands of shades of grey.

Important note

The six levels or axis are described in their spatial order, that is how they are positioned on the body, from outer to inner:

Taiyang ⇨ *Shaoyang* ⇨ *Yangming* ⇨ *Taiyin* ⇨ *Jueyin* ⇨ *Shaoyin*

Not to be confused with the *Shang Han Lun* description that concerns the progression of disease:

Taiyang ⇨ *Shaoyang* ⇨ *Yangming* ⇨ *Taiyin* ⇨ *Shaoyin* ⇨ *Jueyin*

Pathology of the Temperaments

Ideally, each temperament combines the qualities of their two constitutional elements, providing there is free communication between the two complementary levels. The *Luo* ≈ Network vessels maintain this constant communication.

For example, when *Taiyang* (SI-BL) and *Shaoyin* (HE-KI) are maintained in harmony, the characteristics of Fire and Water are expressed fully (▶ Fig. 2.17). Whereas, when this communication is blocked, certain psychological traits may be exaggerated or distorted, producing faulty and limiting belief systems, resulting in harmful behaviour to the self or to others.

It is very important to underline that the purpose of analysing the temperaments is to better understand the strength and weakness of each individual, and by no means should the following descriptions be taken as a value judgment.

There are three reasons for a specific temperament to get blocked and lose its communication with the complementary level:

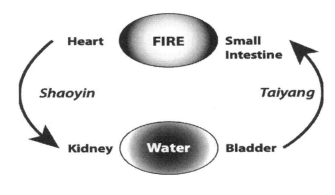

Fig. 2.17:   Fire-Water Constitution

- Conditioning: for example, beliefs that privilege strength and action over softness and contemplation, will enhance the Fire characteristics and discriminate the Water qualities. This condition is very common in the West, where power and action are praised versus meekness and passivity, which are socially condemned.

- Constitutional weakness: for example, a Fire-type person born with a weak Water (Kidney *Jing*), will not have an appropriate complementary level to withdraw to and will be forced to mainly function as *Taiyang* or to compensate in a different Yin level, such as *Taiyin*, which is unnatural for them and will consequently produce psycho-emotional distress, later leading to organic dysfunction. In the image of a person wearing shoes that are one size too small for them, which will cause pain and discomfort at first and later produce callosity and foot deformity.

- Blockage of a *Luo* ≈ Connecting vessel: during the socio-cultural development of an individual, a traumatic event may affect the *Luo* and disrupt its connective function; for example, a lack of parental protection leading to issues concerning limits, or an increased stimulation of the survival instinct, may have an impact on the Bladder *Luo* vessel resulting in the inability of *Taiyang* to interact with *Shaoyin*.

Treatment of Limiting Belief systems

Aside from energetically re-balancing the complementary levels with acupuncture, it is imperative to explore and change the habitual limiting belief systems that have often accompanied the person all their lives and with whom the individual has become identified.

The acupuncture protocols are described for each temperament.

Integrating the psychological work on belief systems is further explored in Part-V with appropriate exercises described in Appendix-IV.

2.1 *Tai-Yang* Temperament

Usually found in Fire or Water-type constitutions combining the expansive nature of Fire with the consolidating aspect of Water and physical and psychological characteristics of both.

The combination of Fire with Water is the combination of extremes and often quite difficult to manage hence it constitutes the least common of the temperaments, combining the qualities of intelligence (*Shen*) and wisdom (*Zhi*), extraversion and introspection, ambition and leadership with humility and detachment. In the Western world, generally, the harder Fire characteristics are more sought after rather than the softer Water qualities; hence this temperament is more frequent in men, especially in the world of business, politics or the army (▶ Fig. 2.18).

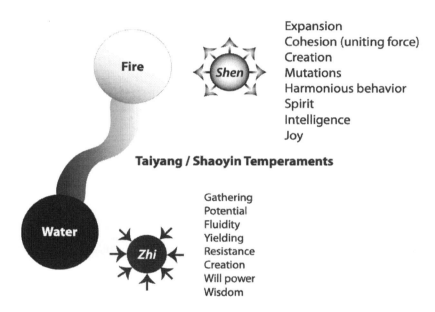

Expansion
Cohesion (uniting force)
Creation
Mutations
Harmonious behavior
Spirit
Intelligence
Joy

Taiyang / Shaoyin Temperaments

Gathering
Potential
Fluidity
Yielding
Resistance
Creation
Will power
Wisdom

Fig. 2.18: Blending of Fire and Water characteristics

The mental and psychological attributes of *Shen* (▶ Section 1.1.1) are quite apparent in the *Taiyang* personality, conferring a superior intelligence and mental cohesion, a harmonious behaviour and the capacity to create and to lead. This intellectual superiority combined with the great ambitions of the *Taiyang* personality often pushes them to lose their connection with their roots, the Water element. This dis-connection is the main causative factor for their physical and psychological issues.

- Physically, the *Taiyang* most often presents the Fire-type body, tall, slender and graceful, with elongated limbs. But they could also have Water-type characteristics, shorter and rounder, or even occasionally dried up and ascetic looking. Even if not tall, the head is carried high, with a certain rigidity of the spine. They usually present an impeccable and precise appearance and clothing, with a preference for uniforms and outer signs of distinction. The complexion may be red or darkish. Eyes are often sparkling (strong *Shen*) and joyful but may also be hard and dominating or even condescending. (▶ Fig. 2.19)

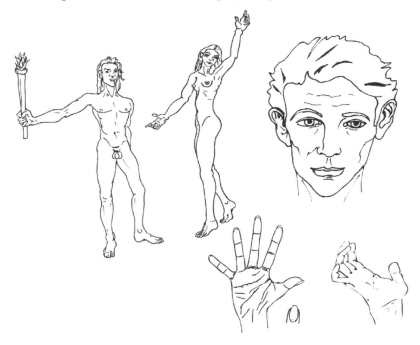

Fig. 2.19 The *Taiyang* physical characteristics

Although the *Taiyang* personalities are quite sensitive, they rarely show their inner feelings, giving an impression of strength or even of hardness.

Their movements are fast or even jerky, they are quite often sportive, liking and needing to win.

Generally, the *Taiyang* dislikes winter but also dislikes excessive heat.

- The strength of *Taiyang* is their extraversion and easy communication with the outside world. When balanced, they radiate a sense of warmth, liveliness and joyfulness that makes them quite charismatic. Their leadership capacities, high ambitions and a good sense of precision, overview and planning, complemented by their capability of directing the action, place them at the head of companies and conglomerates, or as political or army leaders. The *Taiyang* may also be found amongst creators and inventors due to their excellent intellectual and emotional memory, their fast minds and superior intelligence, and their facility in learning, combined with high working capacity.

When the qualities of Fire and Water combine, the *Taiyang* are excellent leaders, good communicators with directness, integrity, sensitivity and vulnerability. They may be generous and devoted, with great self-control, capable of self-sacrifice and austerity to reach an ideal or a pre-set goal.

Issues of family, country and religion are taken very seriously.

- On the negative side, they tend to become easily fanatical, with a fixation on a unique passion. When communication with the *Shaoyin* level is blocked, they tend to have difficulty to integrate with excessive ambition or pretentiousness. Needing to demolish before building. When blocked the *Taiyang* becomes quite intolerable and bossy, dominating, insensitive, commanding, controlling even tyrannical, pushing themselves and others, accepting with difficulty any contradiction; intolerant of mistakes and very impatient. They may at times even

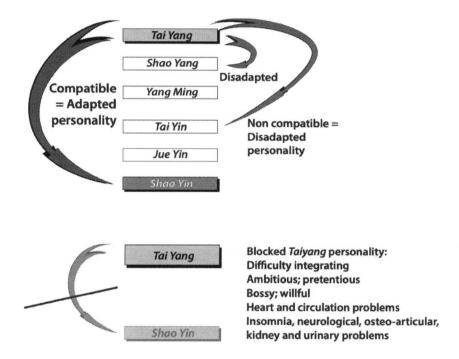

Fig. 2.20: *Tai Yang* dis-adapted or blocked profile

become paranoid (▶ Fig. 2.20).

- Pathologically a blocked *Taiyang* could develop heart and circulation, neurological, osteoarticular or kidney and urinary problems, their sleep is often bad and short.

- *Taiyang* children have an excitable nervous system, especially if there was a difficult birth. They are easily rebellious, opposing authority, especially if they have a *Taiyang* parent.

- The *Taiyang* are quite choosy about their therapists and have to feel a special connection with them. Once a therapist has been accepted, the *Taiyang* types remain quite faithful and will follow the advised treatments and prescriptions dutifully.

- Physically the Fire-type constitution is often present in Scandinavian, Slavic as well as certain East-African races. Examples of *Taiyang* temperament may be observed amongst company directors, army generals, world leaders and presidents.

2.1.1 *Taiyang* Primary Limiting Belief systems

- The superiority complex: I am the best....; I deserve the best....; I have to reach this goal no matter what...;

- Tyranny: just obey me...; I know better what is good for you...;

- Paranoia: I don't trust them...; they don't understand...;

2.1.2 Treatment protocols for *Taiyang*

The treatment strategy consists of helping to re-connect *Taiyang* with *Shaoyin* (▶ Fig. 2.21).

- Re-connecting *Taiyang* with *Shaoyin*: Luo/Yuan: SI-7 *Zhizheng* with HE-7 *Shenmen*; BL-58 *Feiyang* with KI-3 *Taixi*

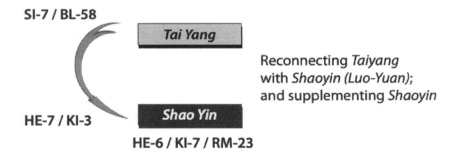

SI-7 / BL-58

Tai Yang

Reconnecting *Taiyang*
with *Shaoyin (Luo-Yuan)*;
and supplementing *Shaoyin*

HE-7 / KI-3   **Shao Yin**

HE-6 / KI-7 / RM-23

Fig. 2.21: Re-connecting *Taiyang* with *Shaoyin*

- Mobilize Taiyang (only if the above treatment was not sufficient): with SI-2 *Qiangu*; SI-6 *Yanglao*; BL-66 *Tonggu* and BL-63 *Jinmen*; also add local Barriers to help move Yang out: BL-10 *Tianzhu*; BL-36 Chengfu, SI-11 *Tianzhong*; and BL-1 *Jingming* (Knot of Taiyang)

- Sedate Taiyang Excess: SI-8 *Xiaohai*; BL-65 *Shugu*; also, TW-10 *Tianjing* (pushing oneself, over-controlling)

- To help relax the excessive wilfulness: supplement BL-44 *Shentang* and BL-23 *Shenshu*; reduce BL-52 *Zhishi*

- Possibly supplement Shaoyin (see below)

The psychological patterns of *Taiyang* reflect on the *Du Mai* or *Yang Wei Mai* psychology (▶ Section. 2.1), hence it is of interest to consider these vessels in the therapeutic strategies.

2.2   *Shao-Yin* Temperament

As discussed above, the *Shaoyin* temperament combines the qualities of Water and Fire elements, but as the Yin energy of Water is pre-dominant, the personality tends to be more yielding and fluid, with more sensitivity and introspection (▶ Fig. 2.18).

- Physically: The Shaoyin types are most often short and rounded; in women, the body could also be quite curvaceous. Often supple but they may have clumsy or choppy movements. Quite rounded features and face, with smooth skin, redness of cheeks, or at times easily blushing, may also have a darkish complexion, especially around the eyes. Swollen and moist eyes with red rims, especially in the mornings. Even if the Fire constitution gives them a tall and slender body, the *Shaoyin* personality makes the individual quite shy and introverted, with a drooping attitude trying not to be noticed. Often self-effacing, looking down or with shifty eyes, speaking slowly, prone to loss of voice. *Shaoyin* type temperaments in general, avoid action and dislike winters and the cold (▶ Fig. 2.22).

- The *Shaoyin*'s capacity for introspection, allows them to recognise their weaknesses and try to change them. Searching for depth and for the essential, which confers great wisdom to the *Shaoyin* types. They are resourceful and creative, self-giving, resigned, modest, vulnerable and detached. In spite of their dislike of action, they are conscientious and serious and will follow through any project that they have initiated; they might even come up with ways of doing things with less effort. The *Shaoyin* tend to be quite artistic and romantic.

- Intellectually, they may have generally a poor memory, having difficulties in learning by heart, but having an excellent emotional memory and great sensitivity and empathy. Although often not good in academic structures, they might excel in certain intellectual aptitudes.

- On the negative side, when blocked they tend to become unsatisfied with life, blaming oneself or the world, shy, introverted, easily discouraged, demoralised, not wanting to live, cautious and fearful, self-effacing and victimised. Ambitious but not daring to move into action; easily considering oneself a looser and even provoking failure. They may also become tricky, sneaky, or even quite clever in business matters. When blocked the Shaoyin can become envious, misanthropic, even rejoicing in other's misfortunes; the tendency for guilt or self-destruction, even masochism; or on the opposite side becoming misanthropic, isolating themselves, seeking contact with nature to get recharged and to find serenity (▶ Fig. 2.23).

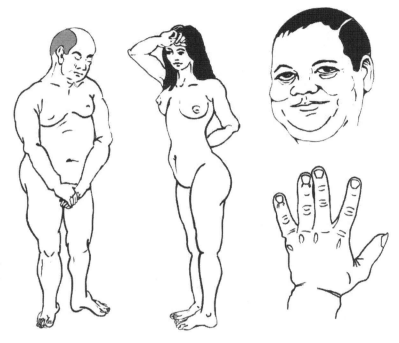

Fig. 2.22 The *Shao Yin* physical characteristics

- As children, they are often fragile, with frequent infections, sore throats, otitis, impetigo, furuncles, rheumatism or even heart problems. In school, other children often pick on them.

- Pathologically, they tend to develop severe infections or chronic diseases, heart and circulation, urinary or osteo-articular diseases. Knowing this and being afraid of death, they will often take good care of their health, consulting early and following prescriptions faithfully.

- The Water-type constitution may be observed in some black races, the inuit, and certain Middle Eastern and Semitic ethnicities. Examples of *Shaoyin* temperament are found amongst philosophers, romantic poets and some unconventional scientists (Einstein).

2.2.1 *Shaoyin* Primary Limiting Belief systems

- The inferiority complex: I am not good enough...; why to bother, I am sure to fail...; this always happens to me...; who could love me...;

- Misanthropic: it is a jungle out there...; I am better off alone...;

- Mistrusting and fearful: I am sure to be cheated...; it is too scary...;
- Self-sacrificing: they need me...; I need to save...

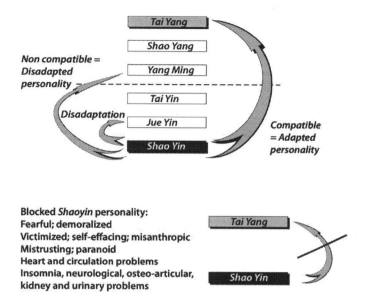

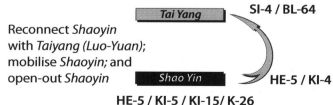

Fig. 2.23: *Shao Yin* **dis-adapted or blocked profile**

2.2.2 Treatment protocols for *Shaoyin*

The treatment aims at supplementing and moving *Shaoyin* and helping it to re-connect with *Taiyang* (▶ Fig. 2.24):

- Luo/Yuan: HE-5 *Tongli* with SI-4 *Wangu*; KI-4 *Dazhong* with BL-64 *Jinggu*

- Mobilise *Shaoyin*: HE-8 *Shaofu*; HE-6 *Yinxi*; KI-2 *Rangu* and KI-5 *Shuiquan*; add RM-23 *Lianquan* (Knot point), and move Yin with RM-4 *Guanyuan* or LR-13 *Zhangmen*

- Help open the *Shaoyin* level with local Barrier points: KI-15 *Zhongzhu*; KI-26 *Yuzhong*

The *Shaoyin* psychology reflects closely the *Ren Mai* or *Yin Qiao Mai* psychological patterns (▶ Section 2.1), which should also be included in the therapeutic strategies.

Reconnect *Shaoyin* with *Taiyang (Luo-Yuan)*; mobilise *Shaoyin;* and open-out *Shaoyin*

HE-5 / KI-5 / KI-15/ K-26

Fig. 2.24: Re-connecting *Shao Yin* with *Tai Yang*

2.3 *Shao-Yang* Temperament

Combines the Wood and Fire characteristics (▶ Fig. 2.25).

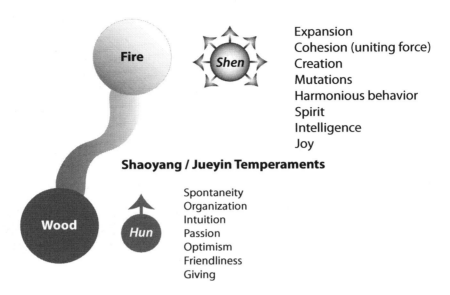

Fire

Shen

Expansion
Cohesion (uniting force)
Creation
Mutations
Harmonious behavior
Spirit
Intelligence
Joy

Shaoyang / Jueyin Temperaments

Wood

Hun

Spontaneity
Organization
Intuition
Passion
Optimism
Friendliness
Giving

Fig. 2.25: Blending of Fire and Wood characteristics

- Physically: average height, proportionate and martial body shape, fearless and may even be reckless at times, agile, restless, nervous or even prone to tics. With open and frank features, large eyes, open eyebrows, warm and penetrating look, extraverted, quite expressive and even seductive. The *Shaoyang* character is most often quite friendly and open, but may also present as an inhibited and shy type with tics, nail-biting, and nervous wrenching of hands; or quite the opposite, the agitated type, talkative, wetting of lips, over excitement, loud or even quarrelsome. The features are tanned or of an olive complexion, but may be pale or blushing. The clothing is often non- conventional or quite coquettish. In general, they seek the cold and dislike wind and heat (▶ Fig. 2.26).

- The *Shaoyang* temperament is spontaneous, intuitive, optimistic, and passionate, living life fully. They are generous, making friends easily, very charming and cordial, they do not like to hurt others and do not keep grudges and in general, dislike conflicts. They are very sportive, and their sense of coordination gives them the ability to be good in sports or artistic performances. The *Shaoyang* is an excellent coordinator and organiser, their flexibility and friendliness and facility in communication puts them often in positions of negotiation or public relations. Their curiosity and interest in the new explain that most explorers and adventures belong to this type. They like work and starting new projects but have difficulty in finishing them.

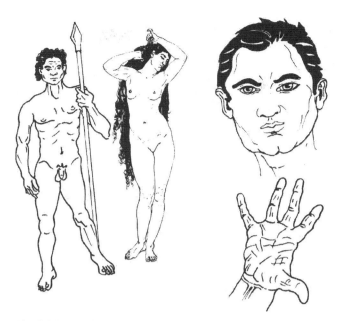

Fig. 2.26: The *Shao Yang and Jue Yin* physical characteristics

- Intellectually they have a good memory that can suddenly decrease with age. Boiling with ideas, imagination, with intense creativity but quite often disorganised intellectually. They are quite active and creative at night but like to sleep late, having difficulty to get going in the morning.

- When blocked the *Shaoyang* has difficulty integrating and becomes insatiable, looking constantly for new adventures or love affairs. Becoming competitive, choleric, reactive, aggressive and vengeful with a tendency to be arrogant, critical, restless and impatient. In some cases, the anger might be interiorised manifesting as anxiety or stress (Liver Qi stagnation). There is a tendency to develop liver and gallbladder problems, hypertension, migraine headaches, stress and tension and various tics or tinnitus (▶ Fig. 2.27).

- In childhood, the *Shaoyang* are often very thin, generally healthy, but sometimes might present with slight liver problems and vomiting (motion sickness) or migraine headaches. In school, they are often the centre of attention, sportive, chief of the band, easily involved in fights.

- Pathologically when blocked the *Shaoyang* might present liver or gallbladder problems, hypertension, migraine headaches, stress and tension, tics, tinnitus and vertigo (Wind). They dislike being sick and usually recover quite fast. In relation to therapy, they might sound very interested and enthusiastic but will follow treatments for a short time only.

- The physical aspect of the Wood constitution is present in the Mediterranean as well as the North American indigenous races.

Examples of *Shaoyang* type temperaments are found amongst explorers and adventurers, in individual sports and extreme sports involving danger, martial arts, visual arts, entertainment and acting.

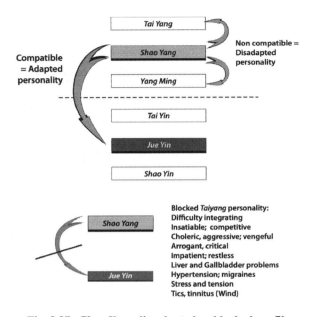

Fig. 2.27: *Shao Yang* **dis-adapted or blocked profile**

2.3.1 *Shaoyang* Primary Limiting Belief systems

- Competitive and comparing: I am better than...; the grass is greener on the other side; they got more...; I'll fight to get what is mine...;

- Insatiable and impatient: I am bored...; it is taking too long...; I am sure I can manage all of this...; I feel trapped...

2.3.2 Treatment protocols for *Shaoyang*

The treatment aims at helping it to re-connect with *Jueyin* (▶ Fig. 2.28):

- *Luo/Yuan*: TW-5 *Waiguan* with PE-7 *Daling*; GB-37 *Guangming* with LR-3 *Taichong*

- Mobilise *Shaoyang*: It is highly recommended to mobilize Shaoyang with great circumspection. This temperament, when blocked, is greatly volatile and may react in unexpected or even a violent manner. TW-2 *Yemen;* TW-6 *Zhigou;* TW-7 *Huizong;* GB-43 *Xiaxi*; GB-41 *Zulinqi*; GB-40 *Qiuxu* and possibly SI-19 *Tinggong* (Knot point).

- Sedate Excess: TW-10 *Tianjing*; GB-38 *Yangfu*

- To help reconnect the above and below: GB-41 *Zulinqi* with TW-5 *Waiguan*

- To harmonize social relations: BL-47 *Hunmen*; BL-23 *Shenshu*; BL-52 *Zhishi*

The *Shaoyang* personality types correspond to *Yang Wei Mai* or in some aspects to *Yang Qiao Mai* psychological patterns (▶ Section 2.1), to be considered in the therapeutic strategies.

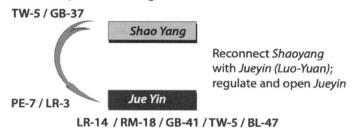

Fig. 2.28: Re-connecting *Shao Yang* with *Jue Yin*

2.4 *Jue-Yin* Temperament

Combines the Wood and Fire characteristics. The *Shaoyang* and *Jueyin* temperaments can easily be confused, both being very extraverted, spontaneous and emotional. The main difference lies in *Shaoyang's* need for action (▶ Fig. 2.25).

- Physically: average height, proportionate body shape, very similar to *Shaoyang* types, but more nervous or even prone to tics, at times difficult to distinguish between the two types. They might either present as a shy type, very nervous, fainting easily, or quite agitated and talkative. Often with open and frank features, large eyes, quite expressive, seductive or mysterious, may be myopic. Often tanned or olive complexion or may be pale. The appearance and clothing attract attention in a provocative or seductive manner, reflecting a passive extraversion. They might be supple and sportive, but get easily exhausted. They dislike wind, heights, aeroplanes, cars, boats and crowds. Liking spring, but sometimes feeling tired at the start of spring (▶ Fig. 2.26).

- The *Jueyin* temperament tends to be spontaneous, intuitive, sensitive, charming, communicative and may be very seductive. They have a great imagination and creativity with a high aesthetical sense, which combined with their non-conformism, gives them many artistic talents. Their natural charm and communicativeness make them good organisers, mediators and public relations. Their mental and emotional flexibility gives them, on the one hand, a facility for acting and on the other hand, the capacity to be quite at ease in the inner and outer worlds, which combined with their strong intuition, confers to them the necessary tools to be excellent psycho-therapists.

- Intellectually they could have a good memory but might become forgetful because of emotions. They have a very lively imagination, high sense of aesthetics, artistic inspirations as well as intuition. They often have very vivid dreams, which could disturb their sleeping patterns.

- When blocked, which means that they are not able to communicate with their complementary Yang level *Shaoyang*, they may become dramatic, hysterical, passionately intense, jealous, pessimistic, with a great tendency to vanity. Emotionally falling in and out of love very quickly. The moods are often inconsistent with swings between anxiety and depression, or dreamy and absent. Their lack of confidence makes them feel conflicts intensely in two possible ways (▶ Fig. 2.29):

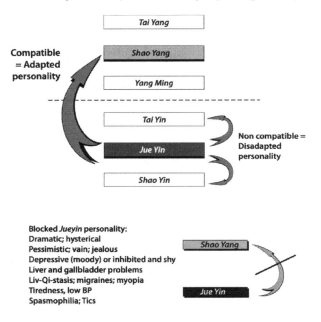

Fig. 2.29: *Jue Yin* dis-adapted or blocked profile

- Inhibition and anxiety "Liver Qi Xu": always on the alert, worrying about small things, having difficulty in giving priority to things, with difficulty moving into action; various kinds of phobia, may even be paralysed by fear. This inhibition can produce great inner tension for even simple daily matters.

- Evasion: often into imagination, closing their eyes to reality, dreaming, creating a false identity, a mask; living often in a world of fantasy and pretence, frequently evading into superficiality, excitements, films, whims, exciting love affairs, with a tendency to addictions, drugs, coffee, alcohol (for which they often have a poor tolerance).

- In childhood, the Jueyin, are quite sensitive, may easily feel unloved, needing a lot of assurance and compliments. They tend to be easily jealous of their siblings. Physically they may suffer from liver problems, eye pathologies and possibly seasonal allergies.

- Pathologically when blocked they can easily develop liver and gallbladder problems; Liver-Qi-stasis; migraines; myopia; tiredness, low blood pressure: various types of spasms (Spasmophilia) and tics. They are difficult patients, as they do not follow through the therapy and the prescriptions, changing often doctors and methods.

- Examples of Jueyin type temperaments are to be found amongst many poets, writers, painters, designers and actors. The Latin races in particular Italians (more Fire) or French (more Wood).

2.4.1 Jueyin Primary Limiting Belief systems

- Insecurity: am I pretty enough...; I wonder how they see me...; I wish I could...; it is so hard to choose...;

- Romanticism, delusions: I am waiting for the perfect one...; I am waiting for the ideal...;

- Intuition, illusions and feelings: I follow my feelings...; I rely on my intuitions...

2.4.2 Treatment protocols for Jueyin

The treatment mainly aims at helping it to mobilise *Jueyin* and to re-connect it with *Shaoyang* (▶ Fig. 2.30).

- *Luo/Yuan*: PE-6 *Neiguan* with TW-4 *Yangchi*; LR-5 *Ligou* with GB-40 *Qiuxu*

- Mobilise *Jueyin*: PE-8 *Laogong;* PE-4 *Ximen*; LR-2 *Xingjiang*; LR-3 *Taichong*; LR-6 *Zhongdu*; also, PE-5 *Jianshi*; LR-14 *Qimen*; and RM-18 *Yutang* (Knot point).

- To help reconnect the above with the below: GB-41 *Zulinqi* with TW-5 *Waiguan*

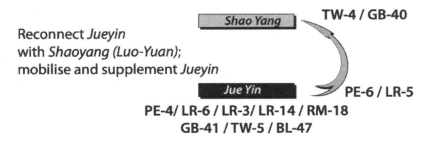

Fig. 2.30: Re-connecting *Jue Yin* with *Shao Yang*

- To harmonise social relations: BL-47 *Hunmen*; BL-23 *Shenshu*; BL-52 *Zhishi*

Many of the *Yin Wei Mai* psychological patterns are found in *Jueyin* personality types and should always be included in the therapeutic strategies. Some other personality traits, in particular relating to "self-image" reflect on *Yin Qiao Mai* patterns (▶ Section 2.1).

2.5   *Yang-Ming* Temperament

Combines the Earth and Metal characteristics (▶ Fig. 2.31). The *Yangming* and especially the *Taiyin* represent the majority of the human race and constitute the backbone and foundation of most societies.

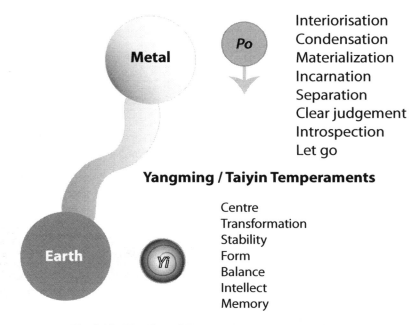

Fig. 2.31: Blending of Earth and Metal characteristics

- Physically: Many combinations of Earth and Metal are possible here.

    - If the Earth element predominates the person has a balanced and centred, earthy look. Large bones, large shoulders and thick thighs with a short neck and a round or large face open and often jovial features, with thick lips, red face or red tip of nose and ears, with soft, reassuring, slightly protruding merry eyes. Not very agile and fast but quite strong, maybe overweight. With age has a tendency to lose hair on the front and top. The general appearance and clothing are often unimportant and might even seem un-kept. They dislike humidity and heat (▶ Fig. 2.32).

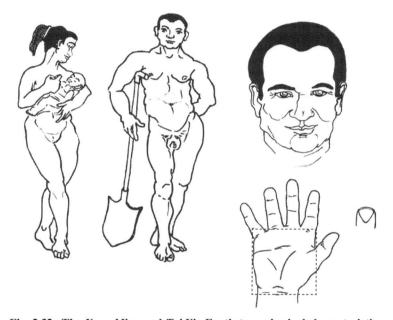

Fig. 2.32: The *Yang Ming* and *Tai Yin* Earth-type physical characteristics

    - When the Metal is dominant the person tends to be taller, with narrow shoulders, a rounded stooping back with a thin, long and pale face, thin lips and eyebrows, high cheekbones. With age the face tends to get deep wrinkles. Dry looking but friendly, calm and patient with slow and precise movements. They are naturally elegant, clean and dress in a very conventional manner. Disliking both heat and cold, preferring the autumn season (▶ Fig. 2.33).

- The *Yangming* temperament is quite calm, non-reactive and non-emotional, with very good objectivity, de-dramatizing situations, seeking harmony, giving support and helping to solve problems in a fair manner. Generally, quite diplomatic, loving human relations and company.

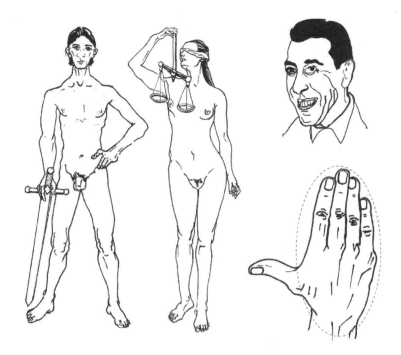

Fig. 2.33: The *Yang Ming* and *Tai Yin* Metal-type physical characteristics

Practical and non-dogmatic, hard-working, tenacious, completing any project. Optimistic, tolerant, liberal, playful with a good sense of humour.

- Intellectually they tend to have a good memory, inventive and clever, having a very good capacity to break down a problem in order to understand and to integrate it. The Metal type *Yangming* has a keen sense of observation, quite comfortable with abstract systems (mathematics). In general, very precise, reliable and punctual, steady and cool, doing a lot with apparent minimum effort.

- When blocked the *Yangming* has difficulty communicating with their counterpart level *Taiyin*. Becoming quite stubborn and obsessive even rigid and intolerant. Lacking comprehension or penetration they deal with their minds rather than with their feelings, they may become quite superficial, ironical, cynical and sceptical. Indulging in all the good things in life, sensual, fun-loving, over-optimistic, tending to overspend or over bet. When angry, they complain rather than explode (▶ Fig. 2.34).

- In childhood, the *Yangming* Earth types are often in quite good health though they tend to overindulge in food, especially sweets. The Metal type is more delicate, often quite skinny with frequent colds and lung problems.

- Pathologically when blocked the *Yangming* Earth types tend to develop digestive problems, with the tendency to obesity, diabetes, gout, excess cholesterol and circulation problems. They are not easy to treat and do not like to follow diets or medical advice. Metal type *Yangming's* present more intestinal problems, sinus infections and teeth decay. They are easy to treat and trust the therapist and follow instructions dutifully.

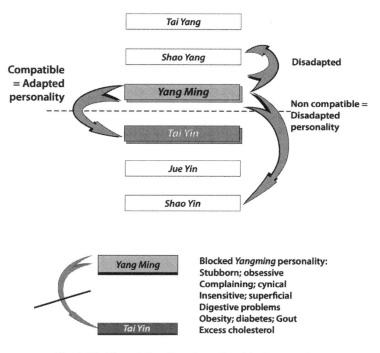

Fig. 2.34: *Yang Ming* dis-adapted or blocked profile

- The Earth-type constitution is predominant world-wide, typically found in native South-Americans and parts of the Middle-East. Examples of *Yangming* Earth-type temperaments are found amongst, farmers, engineers, builders, doctors, nurses, cooks, care-takers and teachers.
  The Metal-type constitution is present amongst large areas of the Eastern populations. The *Yangming* Metal-type temperament is common amongst a number of scholars, mathematicians, doctors and especially surgeons.

2.5.1 *Yangming* Primary Limiting Belief systems

- Over-confidence, lack of empathy: Leave it to me, I will take care of it...; I can concretise this...; don't worry, I can fix this...; let's not get emotional...

- Stubbornness: I have to finish what I start...; this is the way it has always been done...; don't ask me to change, this is who I am...;

- Scepticism: I have to see to believe...

2.5.2 Treatment protocols for *Yangming*

The treatment aims at helping *Yangming* to re-connect with *Jueyin* (▶ Fig. 2.35):

- *Luo/Yuan*: LI-6 *Pianli* with LU-9 *Taiyuan*; ST-40 *Fenglong* with SP-3 *Taibai*

- Mobilise *Yangming*: LI-2 *Erjian*; LI-7 *Wenliu;* ST-44 *Neiting;* ST-34 *Lianqiu* and possibly ST-1 (Knot point).

- Sedate Excess: LI-2 *Erjian*; ST-45 *Lidui*

- To help express feelings RM-17 *Shanzhong*, PE-7 *Daling*

- For repressing feelings with food: BL-20 *Pishu*

- Knotted feeling in the stomach BL-17 *Geshu*

- For obsessions and worry: BL-49 *Yishe*

- Holding emotions in the intestines: BL-57 *Chengshan*

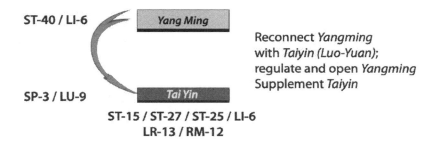

Fig. 2.35: Re-connecting *Yang Ming* with *Tai Yin*

Both *Yangming* and *Taiyin* profiles reflect on *Chong Mai* and *Ren Mai* psychology (▶ Section 2.1).

2.6   *Tai-Yin* Temperament

Combines the Earth and Metal characteristics, and as mentioned above the *Taiyin* temperament constitutes the most frequent of the personality types on earth (▶ Fig. 2.31).

- Physically: The tendency to being large, with a large and fleshy face, quite passive, often "too soft", with thick flesh, very similar to *Yangming* but much calmer, with slow deliberate movements. May also be tall and elastic, or on the contrary quite stiff and dry if the Metal predominates, in this case, the face is long and narrow with a long nose and thin lips.

Facial colour is white or pink with redness of the tip of the nose and ears. They dislike the damp and the cold (▶ Fig. 2.32 and 2.33).

- The *Taiyin* temperament: is very passive, patient, calm, conciliatory and usually a fair referee; often a good listener, non-emotional, capable of consoling with great compassion and insight. Rationalistic, persevering, unattached, deliberate, moving into action only after considering all the options. When the Metal influence predominates, they are very organised, strict and meticulous, paying a lot of importance to detail. Planning for the future, economical. They rather prefer an intimate company to groups.

- Intellectually they tend to be quite rationalistic, dogmatic, analytical, and at times judgmental. In general, they need more sleep, getting easily tired.

- When blocked, this level has difficulty exteriorising towards *Yangming*. May become negligent and lazy, passive, introverted, holding their feelings; indifferent and distracted with bouts of asthenia, depression even melancholia. The Earth type tends to eat to compensate, whereas the Metal type becomes even more rigid and fixed in habits and ideas, obsessed with details, perfectionism, introverted and un-expressive, worrying about the future, holding on to things and even becoming stingy (▶ Fig. 2.36).

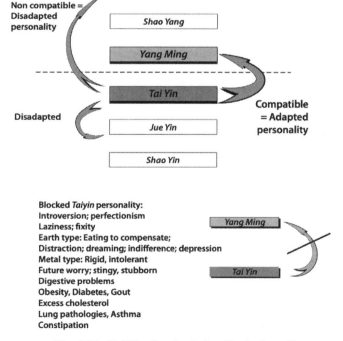

Fig. 2.36: *Tai Yin* dis-adapted or blocked profile

- In childhood: The Earth-types are usually easy children to handle, quite passive, loving to eat. On the opposite the Metal-types are often sickly and fragile, lacking appetite and vitality.

- Pathologically when blocked the *Taiyin* will easily present digestive problems, obesity, diabetes, gout, excess cholesterol as well as lung pathologies, asthma and constipation. The Earth type *Taiyin* often will have difficulty in following diets and treatments, whereas the Metal type *Taiyin* is over-concerned about their health, they will show up at their appointment long before time, will follow the doctor's orders to the letter, will never travel without considering all health risks and having the appropriate medication for it.

- The Metal-type constitution is present in great parts of the Eastern populations as well as in most sedentary and farming societies. Examples *Taiyin*-type temperaments are found amongst precision technicians and factory workers, specialised labourers as well as administration and office employees and service providers.

2.6.1 *Taiyin* Primary Limiting Belief systems

- Passivity: I need rest...; don't ask me to do more...; whatever, I don't mind...;

- Introversion: its demanding to be with people...; leave me alone...;

- Rigidity, prevision: I hate surprises...; I dislike change...; I need to plan for the future...; there is security in repetition...; I will keep this in case...

2.6.2 Treatment protocols for *Taiyin*

The treatment aims at moving *Taiyin* and in helping it to re-connect with *Yangming* (▶ Fig. 2.37):

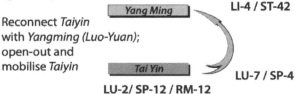

Reconnect *Taiyin* with *Yangming (Luo-Yuan)*; open-out and mobilise *Taiyin*

Yang Ming   LI-4 / ST-42

Tai Yin   LU-7 / SP-4

LU-2/ SP-12 / RM-12

Fig. 2.37: Re-connecting *Tai Yin Yang* with *Yang Ming*

- Mobilise *Taiyin*: LU-10 *Yuji*; LU-6 *Kongzui;* SP-2 *Dadu*; SP-8 *Diji*; a very efficient strategy consists of combining RM-12 (Knot point) with LU-2 *Yunmen* and SP-12 *Chongmen* to help open the *Taiyin* level outward.

- *Luo/Yuan*: LU-7 *Lieque* with LI-4 *Hegu*; SP-4 *Gongsun* with ST-42 *Chongyang*

- Sedate Excess Yin: LU-5 *Chize*; SP-5 *Shangqiu*

- To help express feelings RM-17 *Shanzhong*, PE-7 *Daling*

- For repressing feelings with food: BL-20 *Pishu*

- Knotted feeling in the stomach BL-17 *Geshu*

- For obsessions and worry: BL-49 *Yishe*

- Holding emotions in the intestines: BL-57 *Chengshan*

Both *Yangming* and *Taiyin* profiles reflect on *Chong Mai* and *Ren Mai* psychology, in particular for compensation issues (▶ Section 2.1).

2.7   Self-assessment questionnaire

Temperament	Question	Score
Tai Yang	• Do I need to be the best and on top? • Do I expect things to be perfect? • Am I very confident in my actions and decisions? • Do I have a hard time with contradictions? • Am I very ambitious? • Can I sacrifice to reach a goal? • Am I capable of working long hours to get things done? • Do I see the potential in other people and know what is best for them? • Am I often told that I am bossy?	
Shao Yang	• Do I decide and act quickly? • Do I have fast reflexes? • Am I very competitive? • Am I impatient and restless? • Can I easily show my anger? • Do I constantly need to move and do things? • Do new projects and challenges excite me? • Am I excited by the future? • Am I often bending the rules?	

Yang Ming	<ul><li>Do I rely on my knowledge and analytical capacities?</li><li>Do I enjoy the company and being surrounded by friends?</li><li>Do I feel confident that I can handle things?</li><li>Am I persevering and finish what I have started?</li><li>Do I tend to become stubborn and obsessive?</li><li>Am I optimistic and overspending?</li><li>Do I rely more on my mind rather than my feelings?</li><li>Am I ready to lend a helping hand?</li><li>Am I tolerant and fair?</li></ul>	
Tai Yin	<ul><li>Do I prefer a routine life rather than unexpected events?</li><li>Do I think before saying or acting?</li><li>Do I believe that rules and regulations are important?</li><li>Am I judgemental?</li><li>Am I attached to details?</li><li>Do I have a hard time throwing things away?</li><li>Do I prefer intimate gatherings?</li><li>Do I worry about the future?</li><li>Do I often feel tired and needing rest?</li></ul>	
Jue Yin	<ul><li>Do I have difficulties in deciding and choosing?</li><li>Do I need to be the centre of attention?</li><li>Am I submerged by my emotions at times?</li><li>Do I tend to be overly dramatic?</li><li>Do I like to share my feelings with others?</li><li>Are aesthetics very important to me?</li><li>Do I have a hard time to accomplish what I start?</li><li>Do I spend a lot of time day-dreaming?</li><li>Do I rely on my intuitions?</li></ul>	
Shao Yin	<ul><li>Do I rather blend into the background rather than stand out?</li><li>Do I believe that less effort is the best way?</li><li>Do I frequently doubt my decisions?</li><li>Am I very idealistic and romantic?</li><li>Am I pessimistic and expect the worst?</li><li>Do I often feel that others get more than I do?</li><li>Am I shy and tend to hide my feelings?</li><li>Do I prefer to be alone than with people?</li><li>Am I often fearful?</li></ul>	

2.3 Influence of the outer world: "Psycho-social development and the Luo"

The *Luo Mai* ≈ Connecting/ Network vessels distribute Qi and Blood to all parts of the body, maintain skin, sinews, the five senses and the six portals (orifices). As their name suggests, the *Luo* ≈ Network channels maintain connectivity between the inside and outside, depth with surface and the right with the left.

The *Luo* complement the primary channels and protect them from external aggressions, serving as a reservoir or buffer for external pathogenic factors. This function of a reservoir, which is quite similar to that of the Extraordinary Vessels, could explain the fact that four of the opening points of the Extraordinary Vessels are *Luo* points: SP-4 *Gongsun*, PE-6 *Neiguan*, LU-7 *Lieque* and TW-5 *Waiguan*.

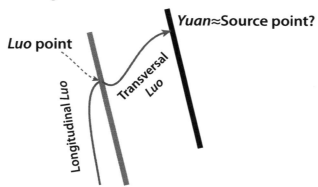

Fig. 2.38: The two *Luo* trajectories

The *Luo* also maintain an inner balance by maintaining the *Biao-Li* connection, thus creating a superficial link between coupled channels. (▶ Fig. 2.38)

In SUWEN, chapter 62 is mentioned:

> *"The five Zang ≈ Viscera along with the Fu ≈ Bowels make an exterior-interior pair with the Jing-Luo vessels as their offshoots. Each of them can manifest emptiness (vacuity) and fullness (repletion)."*

With their relation to the vascular system, the *Luo* also offer a means for the release of internal *Shi* ≈ repletion/excess due to emotional or dietary causes.

The *Luo* are in charge of contact and communication with the outer world. The interaction with the outside implicates:

- The sensory functions, the limbs, movement and contact areas (this concept is more privileged by the French school)
- Emotional responses to outer situations and challenges (emphasised more by the Daoist oral tradition).

2.3.1 The *Luo* in relation to the outer world

The *Luo* are responsible for our contact and communication with the outer world. According to the French school, the *Luo* pathology will also affect all the means and zones of contact and exchange with the outside, including sensory portals and movements.

It is not always clear which of the two branches of the *Luo*, Transversal or Longitudinal, are implicated in the communication with the outer world. In the pathologies of the sensory organs there are two parameters, the sensory function (seeing, hearing etc.), and the sensory orifice or portal (the eye socket, the ear orifice etc.):

The sensory organ itself is maintained by the *Zang* to which it is related; for example, the capacity to see depends on Liver-Blood and reflects more on the harmony between Liver and Gall bladder, hence the role of the Transversal *Luo* to maintain the communication and equilibrium between the two channels of *Zu Jueyin*-LR and *Zu Shaoyang*-GB

The portal or orifice related to the sensory organ represents an area through which the body communicates with the outer world and absorbs the outer influences. This function of "contact" and "protection" implicates also the *Luo* and more specifically the Longitudinal *Luo* (as described by their trajectories). In the above example, when the function of "sight" depends on the Liver, it is the *Luo* of the Heart that maintains the integrity of the eye portal itself. Therefore, visual disturbances such as myopia, night-blindness or optic neuritis address pathologies of the Liver, whereas pathologies of reactivity as in allergic conjunctivitis or again in filtering the outside as in cataract, the notion of protection and contact is implied and would reflect on the Longitudinal Heart *Luo* channel.

Longitudinal Luo and the 9 portals/orifices (▶ Fig. 2.39)

Eyes	HE-5 *Tongli*
Ears	LI-6 *Pianli*
Mouth	LI-6 *Pianli*
Speech	HE-5 *Tongli*, ST-40 *Fenglong*
Nose	BL-58 *Feiyang*
Anus	KI-4 *Dazhong*
Urethra, genitalia	LR-5 *Ligou*

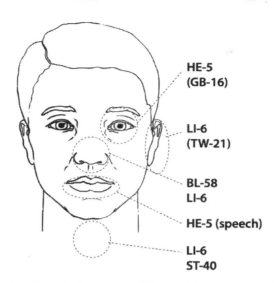

**HE-5
(GB-16)**

**LI-6
(TW-21)**

**BL-58
LI-6**

HE-5 (speech)

**LI-6
ST-40**

Fig. 2.39: **The Longitudinal** *Luo* **and the sensory portals**

Longitudinal Luo and the zones of contact

Skin	SI-7 *Zhizheng*
Throat	ST-40 *Fenglong*
Abdomen	RM-15 *Jiuwei*
Head	DM-1 *Changqiang*, ST-40 *Fenglong*, BL-58 *Feiyang*
Nutrition	SP-4 *Gongsun*
Huang ≈ vitals	HE-5 *Tongli*
Upper TW	PE-6 *Neiguan*
Middle TW	LU-7 *Lieque*
Lower TW	KI-4 *Dazhong*

Longitudinal Luo and movement

All joints	SP-21 *Dabao*
Spine	DM-1 *Changqiang*
Neck	PE-6 *Neiguan*
Lumbar	KI-4 *Dazhong*

Arm	SI-7 *Zhizheng*
Elbow	TW-5 *Waiguan*
Hand	LU-7 *Lieque*
Leg	ST-40 *Fenglong*
Foot	GB-37 *Guangming*

2.3.2 Pathology and Diagnosis

The pathology of the Longitudinal *Luo* is always the result of a *Xie Qi* ≈ External Pathogenic Factor. For each *Luo*, there is a description of symptoms of repletion (excess) and of vacuity (deficiency).

VAN NGHI explains that when the Qi of the channel is deficient, the *Luo* may be invaded by the external pathogens and manifest a state of repletion. When the pathogen has moved into the main channel (most probably via the *Yuan* ≈ Source point), then the *Luo* will manifest symptoms of vacuity.

Luo fullness	*Luo* is replete with *Weiqi* and *Xieqi*
Luo emptiness	*Xieqi* has been emptied into the Primary channel

The fact that most Longitudinal *Luo* move upwards, explains their role of attempting to expel or clear the *Xie* ≈ Pathogenic factor via the head for the Yang *Luo* or the chest and abdomen for the Yin *Luo* (see below "Areas of Concentration").

Aside from the pathological symptoms, there are two main diagnostic elements concerning the state of repletion of the *Luo:*

- The *Luo* become visible when they are replete (excess)
- The *Luo* point becomes painful to palpation and swollen

What is meant by visibility depends on the anatomical layer involved and could manifest as:

On the skin	maculo-papular eruptions
In the sinews	masses, tumours (invisible Phlegm)
Vessels	varicosity

The colour of the varicosity indicates the type of pathogenic factor involved:

Reddish signifies	Heat
Bluish signifies	Cold and pain
Purplish signifies	Blood stasis, which implies an underlying Qi-Xu ≈ Vacuity and the possibility of chronicity and development of a *Bi* ≈ Impediment syndrome

MASTER YUEN recommends taking the moderate pulses (between the surface and the depth) to evaluate the state of repletion or vacuity of the *Luo*.

There are often acute counter-flow Qi patterns:

Sighing, yawning, frequent urine	LU-*Luo*
Frequent bowels, flatulence	LI-*Luo*
Sinking SP-Qi (prolapse), bloating	SP-*Luo*
Nausea, vomiting	ST-*Luo*
Palpitations, angina	HE-*Luo*
Mouth or throat ulcers; reflux	SI-*Luo*
Anuria	BL-*Luo*
Wheezing	KI-*Luo*
Fibrillation, palpitation	PE-*Luo*
Alternating chills and fevers	TW-*Luo*
Alternating symptoms above/below/sides	GB-*Luo*
LR-Yang-rising (high blood pressure)	LR-*Luo*

There are often psycho-emotional issues, but this usually denotes the involvement of the Transversal *Luo*.

2.3.3 Luo and Personality disorders

J. YUEN further relates the development of the mind in relation to the outer world to the *Luo*. According to him the *Luo* are in charge of the various psycho-social phases of life, a disturbance of the *Luo* would have psychological consequences with possible personality disorders. Here he describes the *Luo* in the sequence of the primary channels:

- First unit: cognitive, involving perception, sensation and thought with LU – LI – ST – SP *Luo*

- Second unit: social skills and interaction involve the HE – SI – BL – KI *Luo*

- Third unit: self-preservation and life choices maintained by the PE – TW – GB – LR – Great SP, RM and DM Luo

Luo responsible for the psycho-social phases and personality disorders	
LU-*Luo* repletion out-going towards the world	Communication with the outside: a constant need for stimulation, to touch things and may even cause polymorphic perversity
LU-*Luo* vacuity	Lack of communication: no interest in life; boredom; frequent sighing
LI-*Luo* repletion	Discrimination and assimilation: heightened need to be repetitive; rumination; addictive aspects
LI-*Luo* vacuity	Difficulty to associate and assimilate: lack of concentration and assimilation; cannot chew
ST-*Luo* repletion	Incorporating the world: the process of developing one's emotions: expression and verbalisation of feelings (voice box); difficulty expressing emotions; appearing rational rather than emotional; feelings frequently rooted in fear
ST-*Luo* vacuity	Limited emotional expression: lack of personal satisfaction; frustration (lack of a sense of completion); cogitation; addictive tendency
SP-*Luo* repletion	Absorption and embodiment of the outer world: repeating but unable to understand; habituation; obsessive thinking
SP-*Luo* vacuity	Inability to integrate: desire but no satisfaction; repetitive and obsessive behaviour (repetition relates to Dampness)
HT-*Luo* repletion	Verbal and emotional communication: heart pain: betrayal, broken heart, disappointment; difficulty in interaction and contact with the others; problems with empathy and compassion
HT-*Luo* vacuity	Verbal and emotional communication: loss of speech, linguistic difficulties; inability to name things

SI-*Luo* repletion	Excessive discrimination and feedback: critical; picky; overbearing with obsessions; difficulty sorting out information
SI-*Luo* vacuity	Lack of discrimination: uncertainty, doubting (did I forget to ...?); lack of clarity
BL-*Luo* repletion	Survival instinct: alarm system, survival skills; over-reactiveness; panic attack; post-traumatic stress disorders
BL-*Luo* vacuity	Survival and protection: inability to know limits (enough is enough); addictive aspects
KI-*Luo* repletion	Self-preservation and perpetuation: fearfulness; obsessive-compulsiveness behaviour as a means to control fear
KI-*Luo* vacuity	Self-preservation: paranoia; dreading the end of the world; fear of death
PE-*Luo* repletion	Social interaction: inability to control emotions (stress management); sociopathic
PE-*Luo* vacuity	Social interaction: inability to interact or deal with one's emotions; inability to feel
TW-*Luo* repletion	Adaptability: rigidity, stubbornness; inflexible temperament; antagonistic and persecuting
TW-*Luo* vacuity	Adaptability: indifference; disdain; not caring about other's opinions (I am like this and don't care);
GB-*Luo* repletion	Choices: inability to chose between options; desperate; restless; reckless
GB-*Luo* vacuity	Choices and options: feeling lost; scattered; feeling of "no place to go"; suicidal tendencies
LR-*Luo* repletion	Personality consolidation: split personality; talking to oneself; daydreaming
LR-*Luo* vacuity	Personality consolidation: Multiple personality disorders, loss of *Jing*
SP Great -*Luo* repletion	Connecting all the *Luo*; notion of consciousness: great suffering; pain all over the body
SP Great-*Luo* vacuity	Consciousness: lack of will to live; indicated for coma patients
RM and DM *Luo*	Individuality: accumulation of life experiences; notion of Karma (actions leading to consequences)

Treatment

MASTER YUEN recommends treating the *Luo* over three months in case of personality disorders.

The choice between supplementing and reducing the *Luo* is not always clear from the symptom description; it is better to rely on the local condition of the *Luo* area:

- Reduce (bleeding technique): when the point is painful to palpation, or if there is the presence of local varicosities;

- Supplement (tonify) the *Luo* point: if the point feels empty to touch, and the patient describes the pressure as being agreeable (it feels good when you press there).

Besides the above applications, most Luo are traditionally indicated for the treatment of *Shen* ≈ Spirit or mental-emotional disorders as mentioned in the classical texts.

2.3.4 Luo and Mental-Emotional disorders

The emotional expressions are part of the reactions to the outer events. The *Luo* as connecting vessels, are responsible for managing these emotions.

The Daoist oral tradition describes specific mental and emotional manifestations is relation to *Luo* disorders.

Luo and mental-emotional disorders	
LU-7 *Lieque*	Loss of memory; nervous trembling; manic laughter; dispirited; hallucinations; helps to let go; helps to release and express emotions (sadness)
LI-6 *Pianli*	Manic-depression; talkativeness; anxiety
ST-40 *Fenglong*	Tightness in the solar plexus; anxiety, dizziness; phobia; schizophrenia; *Yangming* type mania (climbing to sing, undressing to run); hallucinations; mind obstruction by Phlegm
SP-4 *Gongsun*	Insomnia; restlessness; manic-depression; epilepsy
HE-5 *Tongli*	emotional over-reactions; stage fright; anxiety and Cold; agitation palpitations; urinary frequency from emotions; fear; hysteria; lack of decisiveness; talking to oneself
SI-7 *Zhizheng*	Anxiety; terror; hysteria; neurasthenia; repressed emotions; incoherent speech; loss of consciousness
BL-58 *Feiyang*	Madness

KI-4 *Dazhong*	Settles the emotions; inferiority complex; lack of authority; disorientation; premenstrual depression; "running piglet syndrome" (panic attacks); hysteria; dementia; anxiety; fear of people; aphasia and somnolence
PE-6 *Neiguan*	Forgetting words; indecision; laziness; stress; anxiety with palpitations; fear and fright; insomnia; hysteria
TW-5 *Waiguan*	Rigidity, stubbornness, inflexible temperament; not caring about other's opinions
LR-5 *Ligou*	Lack of joy; fear, sighing; plum pit when speaking; incoherent speech; excessive worry; panic attacks; fright with palpitations; hysteria; treats three types of "worms" or "ghosts": hungry ghost (food and material desires and obsessions), lusty ghost (sexual desires) and wandering ghost (emotional desires)
GB-37 *Guangming*	Loneliness, hopelessness
RM-15 *Jiuwei*	Insomnia; depression; difficulty finding words; boredom; feeling of doom; absent mindedness; anxiety; mania; hysteria
DM-1 *Changqiang*	Intellectual fatigue; insanity, hysteria

2.3.5 Clinical Applications of the *Luo* in Mental and Emotional disturbances

Each emotion is produced by a specific *Zang* organ, in reaction to a disturbance of its natural movement (see further Part-III).

Each emotion affects the flow of Qi and Blood in a very specific manner; but also, every emotion will affect its corresponding organ by producing Heat. Ultimately all emotions, including Yin type emotions, affect the Heart and produce Heart-Heat. This Heat is referred to as an Internal Pathogenic Factor (IPF). The IPF is transferred to the primary channel, it then passes to the Yang coupled channel via the Transversal *Luo* to be vented or expelled. Therefore, the emotion that is produced by a specific *Zang* ≈ Viscera/organ, is released by the channel of its corresponding coupled *Fu* ≈ Bowel:

- Anger and irritability: are released by the *Zu Shaoyang*-GB channel
- Joy and anxiety: are released by the *Shou Taiyang*-SI Primary channel
- Worry and pensiveness: are released by the *Zu Yangming*-ST channel
- Grief and sadness: are released by the *Shou Yangming*-LI channel
- Fear and shock: are released by the *Zu Taiyang*-BL Primary channel

Treatment

To expel any emotion, the *Luo* system of the Yang channel, is indicated:

- Needling of the *Luo* point
- Bleeding of any varicosity on the pathway of the Longitudinal *Luo*
- Releasing by needling of any accumulations or lumps on the pathway of the Longitudinal *Luo*

According to MASTER YUEN, additionally the Yin *Luo* should also be treated in the following conditions:

- If it is a "mood", in this case the person feels the emotion but cannot explain the reasons: also add LU-7 *Lieque* and LR-5 *Ligou*.
- If the person is aware of the emotion and knows the reason for it, or if it is a suppressed emotion: release with SP-4 *Gongsun* and PE-6 *Neiguan*.
- If it is a habitual emotion (temperament) or even a repression or denial: treat with KI-4 *Dazhong* and TW-5 *Waiguan*.

It is recommended to treat every other day.

Clinical examples for managing the emotions

For a person presenting fear (Water-Kidney):

- Needle and bleed BL-58 *Feiyang*, bleed the varicosities on the BL *Luo* pathway
- If it is a mood, the person is unaware of the reason, add LU-7 *Lieque* and LR-5 *Ligou*
- There is a reason for the fear, add SP-4 *Gongsun* and PE-6 *Neiguan*
- For a fearful personality add KI-4 *Dazhong*, TW-5 *Waiguan*

For a chronically depressed person (Metal-Lung), who is in denial:

- Needle and bleed LI-6 *Pianli*, and the territory of the *Luo*
- Add KI-4 *Dazhong* and TW-5 *Waiguan* as it is a habitual repressed condition

For a patient with suppressed anger (Wood-Liver), who knows the reason but cannot express their anger:

- Needle and bleed GB-37 *Guangming* and bleed the varicosities along the *Luo*
- Needle SP-4 *Gongsun* and PE-6 *Neiguan* to release the suppression.

PART - III
Emotions and their energetic impact

- **Classical description of the "Five Emotions"**
    - Anger
    - Joy / Elation / Excitement
    - Worry / Pensiveness
    - Sadness
    - Fear
    - Oppression
    - Shock / Fright

- **The Seven Passions as "Inner Causes of Disease"**

- **Other common emotions**
    - Love / Romantic love
    - Jealousy / Envy / Craving
    - Hatred / Vengeance / Disgust / Contempt
    - Guilt / Regret / Shame
    - Pride
    - Relief

- **Treatment strategies**
    - *Zang-Fu* disharmonies
    - Impact of Constitution and Temperament

Part- III

Emotions and their energetic impact

Emotion is defined as a strong feeling deriving from one's circumstances, mood, or relationships with others. Strictly speaking, emotions have the role of provoking **an** adaptive behaviour in relation to the outer world.

Originally, the primary emotions, rather defined as instincts, contributed to the basic survival needs and the perpetuation of the species. With the evolution of the species, emotions have become more complex. Although currently there is no scientific consensus on a definition, it is accepted that emotions are mental states associated with the nervous system and due to chemical changes induced by thoughts and feelings as well as behavioural responses to the outside. In other words, emotions are states of feeling producing specific physical and psychological changes that will influence the behaviour of the individual. Hence emotions are closely associated with moods, temperaments and the personality and are considered to be the driving force behind motivation.

According to James and Lange, an emotion would be the subjective feeling of a particular physiological change:

Perception of a stimulus → Physiological response → Feeling of emotion

Embryologically, both the skin and the central nervous system have the same ectodermic origin. It is the conscious awareness of the physical changes that define a particular emotional state.

In fact, all emotional experience is accompanied by changes taking place in the body, it is the awareness of these bodily changes, a particular "feeling", which is interpreted as an emotion. (▶see also 1.1.3 *Po* ≈ Corporeal Soul).

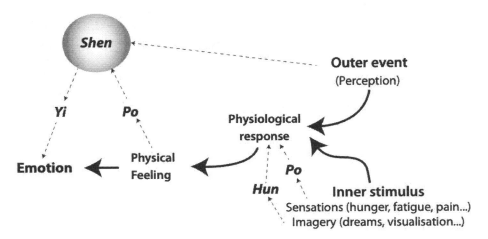

Fig. 3.1:   Production of emotions

The basic emotions may be responses to outer events (anger, joy, fear) or reactions to internal stimuli: pain, hunger, fatigue, pleasure....(▶ Fig. 3.1). In any case, the emotion brings about a physiological change in the form of production of neurotransmitters (dopamine, endorphin, oxytocin, serotonin, noradrenaline etc.), to help preserve and safeguard the individual.

Although the presence of a certain neuropeptide may be associated with a particular emotion, the debate remains as which would the originator of the other. Is it the emotion that releases the transmitter, or is it the presence of the chemical compound that is perceived as an emotion?

The very recent discoveries on the impact of these neuropeptides on distal cells (*Molecules of Emotion* C. Pert), seems to further substantiate the ancient Chinese medical concepts as to the effects of the emotions on movements of Qi, the psyche and the body.

In fact, neurotransmitters or neuropeptides are chemical messengers that transmit a signal across a chemical synapse as from one nerve cell to another cell called a "target" cell, that could be other nerve cells, muscle cells, glands, immune cells etc. These interactions also explain the fact that all emotions are accompanied by specific inner physiological, and outer muscular changes, a kind of "body language".

So far, there are· more than 200 chemical messengers that have been identified, belonging to various types of compounds. Most but not all, are synthesised in the neurones of specific brain structures. Some of these neuropeptides also function as hormones, transported through the circulatory system to target distal organs, regulating the physiology and the behaviour. To mention a few (▶ Fig. 3.2):

- Dopamine: Is synthesised in the brain neurones, the basal ganglia in particular, as well as in the adrenal glands and other distal cells. Although commonly considered to be the chemical component of pleasure, it is in fact, the motivational hormone, regulating the desire-aversion process, modifying the mind and the body towards, or away from achieving a given goal. Any selective action is based on dopamine's role in "initiating action" and the "reward" mechanism (expecting a positive outcome). Several psycho-stimulants and addictive substances (nicotine, cocaine, methamphetamine), act by increasing the brain dopamine levels.

- Endorphin: These are endogenous opioid (morphine-like) hormones produced by the pituitary gland mainly in response to pain, but also by other human activities such as intense aerobic exercises, laughter,

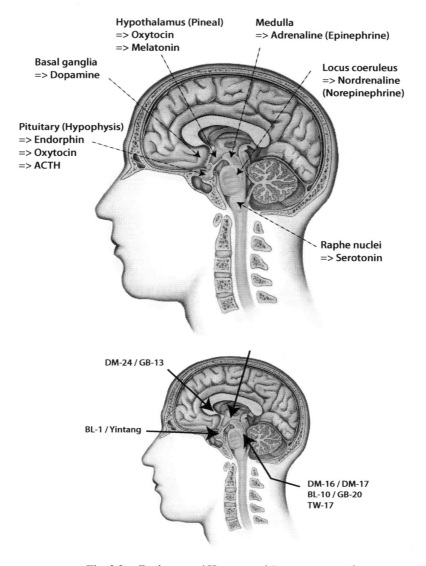

Fig. 3.2: Brain areas / Hormones / Acupuncture points

eating (chocolate in particular), sex and orgasm, or listening to music. It is the hormone that is commonly associated with "happiness".

- Oxytocin: produced by the hypothalamus and released by the pituitary; it plays a role in social and emotional bonding, sexuality (bonding with the partner) and childbirth, and helps with birth, bonding with the child and breast milk production. It is further presumed that oxytocin may have a modulating effect on fear, anxiety and mood.

- Serotonin: primarily produced in the gastrointestinal tract, but also the brain. Although it is generally associated with feelings of well-being and happiness, in fact, it is the modulating hormone, related to cognition, reward, learning and memory.

- Adrenaline (epinephrine) and Noradrenaline (norepinephrine): both are produced by the adrenal glands, whereas the brain equally produces noradrenaline. They are the main activating hormones of the body. Their general role is to stimulate the brain and the body for action (fight or flight), and to inhibit the regenerating and reproductive functions. The emotion related to adrenaline is fear. Fear increases the release of adrenaline; conversely, the presence of higher blood levels of the hormone, induce a propensity to negative feelings and a general state of fearfulness. Usually, the increased adrenergic activity is commonly experienced as "stress". Chronic stress leads to reduced maintenance and regenerative functions, manifesting as the "burn-out" syndrome. In general, adrenergic hormones tend to enhance long-term memory.

- Cortisol: Mostly produced by the adrenals; its release is further increased in response to stress, helping to elevate the blood sugar.

- ACTH (adrenocorticotropic hormone): produced by the pituitary gland in response to stress and fearful stimuli. Its main function is to increase the production and the release of cortisol.

The ancient Chinese medicine described five basic emotions. This might seem very strange today when psychologists are defining almost 80 different variations of emotional behaviour.

Here, it is important to underline that "Five" is not a simple arithmetic number but a numerological symbol. In fact, in the Chinese tradition, "Five" has always represented the structure of the universe, as in the concept of the "Five Elements" in their cosmogenic order (Earth in the centre). Five also represents the relation between the human and the world, the microcosm with the macrocosm, symbolised by the *Wu Xing* ≈ Five moving Forces as expressed by the well-known correspondence system. Therefore, the number "Five" is also representative of emotions, which are the human responses to the outer changes (Microcosm / Macrocosm). (▶ Fig. 3.3)

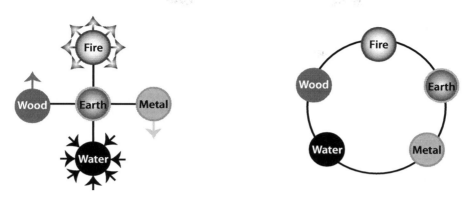

Fig. 3.3: Five Elements and Five Movements ≈ *Wu Xing*

Emotions are mediated by the five sectors of the mind: *Shen, Yi, Po, Zhi* and *Hun*.

Originally, the basic behaviour of any living organism is geared to survival and the perpetuation of the species. This behaviour is mostly instinctual in lower life forms. Any innate, genetically programmed, tendency towards a particular behaviour is defined as an instinct.

The five basic instincts may be represented as:

- *Shen*: Survival instinct; representing the "Passion for Life"

- *Zhi*: Survival and perpetuation instinct; the "Will to Live"

- *Po*: Instinct of protection; helping to develop strategies for protection (den, borrow) and planning ahead (gathering and preserving of food)

- *Hun*: The fight or flight instinct motivated by the circumstance

- *Yi*: Is the caring and nesting instinct, which has greatly developed in the mammalian species and is represented by the need for love and care in humans.

With the evolution of the species and the development of the forebrain and the cortex, emotions have become more adaptive and cognitive. The original instinctive behaviours are progressively adapted to respond to the new threats that a new environment may present. These instinctive behavioural changes may take up to several thousand years before they are actually programmed into the genetic code of the human being or *Jing Qi*. Prior to that the information is epigenetically transmitted as defined in the concept of *Zong Qi* ≈ Ancestral energy (▶ see section 1.2.8).

Although originally all emotions were considered to originate in the limbic area of the brain, recent discoveries made through neural mapping are demonstrating the influence and participation of other areas, for example, the prefrontal cortex. This may suggest the role that the conscious mind may play in adapting and modulating a given emotion (adaptive behaviour). Some neuropeptides associated with distinct emotional expressions are not even produced in the brain but mainly in the body. For example, adrenaline, that is produced by the adrenal glands, or serotonin secreted by the gastrointestinal tract.

In the Chinese concept, the *Zang-Fu* systems as functional units, have three spheres of action: physical, energetic and emotional-mental. This is represented by the notion of the "3 Treasures": *Jing*-essence, *Qi*-energy and *Shen*-spirit. (▶ Fig. 3.3b)

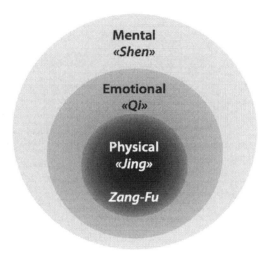

Fig. 3.3b: The three energetic dimensions of the organs: *Jing-Qi-Shen*

The *Jing*-essence of each organ is the base of, not only its physical form but also of its energetic, emotional and mental expressions. The relation between feelings, as body felt experiences, and a particular emotion are clearly emphasised in the tradition.

The basic program of the human body is the "Will to live" in order to fulfil ones "*Ming*" ≈ Life mandate. The specific movement of Qi in each *Zang* is the expression of this "Will". When this strength is used to satisfy the desires (passions) then it becomes an emotion.

Each emotion is produced by a specific *Zang* organ, in reaction to a disturbance of its natural movement. According to E. ROCHAT, the "Will" or modality of the Five *Zang* are:

• The will of the Liver is to mobilise and move forward,

• The will of the Heart is to expand,

• The will of the Spleen is to transform,

• The will of the Lung is to gather,

• The Kidney is to consolidate and give coherence.

When an organ functions according to its will there is no emotion, when this movement is excessive or hampered, there will be an emotion.

Each emotion has been described as affecting the flow of Qi and Blood in a specific manner. Besides this energetic impact, every emotion will affect its corresponding organ by producing Heat. Ultimately all emotions, including Yin type emotions, affect the Heart and produce Heart-Heat.

For example, the ability to move forward is the modality of Liver-Qi

- When it is balanced = There is no emotion

- When excessive = There is "Anger"; this could be explained as: The Liver's potential instead of being expressed through movement and creativity, is rather diverted into passions, irritability and anger.

- When obstructed = There is frustration and depression.

Today, when analysing the complex range of human emotions, it becomes evident that they may not all be conveniently classified into five distinct categories. When it is easy to associate the emotions of anger, rage, irritability and frustration with the movement of Wood, many other emotions overlap and combine the influences of two or more movements, such as guilt, shame or even love, the latter involving the movements of Fire, Earth and Wood.

In Classical Chinese Medicine (CCM), emotions are believed to cause disease if they are not adapted to the external changes:

- Excessive emotion

- Repressed emotion

- In-adapted emotion

Each emotion relates to one of the "5 Moving Forces", and is the non-physical manifestation of the corresponding organ. They are considered Yang as opposed to other organic functions. But in relation to one another, some emotions are classified as Yang, such as anger or elation, as opposed to sadness and fear, which are considered Yin.

The main premises concerning emotions are:

- An excessive emotion harms the corresponding organ and may transform into Fire.

- Disharmony of the *Zang-Fu* may produce an emotional disturbance (*Shi* ≈ Excess/ repletion or *Xu* ≈ Insufficiency/ vacuity). This emotional disturbance may further aggravate the organ disharmony, thus producing a vicious circle.

- All emotions ultimately affect the Heart-emperor, residence of *Shen*

In general Yang type emotions manifest more easily in Yang conditions:

- Yang Excess/ repletion

- Qi or Yang stagnation
- Yin, Blood or *Jin Ye* ≈ Body fluids deficiency/ vacuity

Yin type emotions appear more easily in Yin conditions:

- Qi or Yang deficiency/ vacuity
- Yin Excess/ repletion
- Sometimes in Qi stagnation

In practice three organs are most affected by emotions:

- Heart governs the Spirit "*Shen*", and thus regulates all the other emotions.
- Liver is in charge of defence and of immediate adaptability (adapting the emotional expression to the outer situation), but also draining and de-congesting, in other words releasing the emotional accumulations.
- Spleen is in charge of transforming the essence of food, but also of the processing "digesting" of the emotions and thoughts.

3.1   Classical description of the "Five Emotions"

There has always been a debate as to which are the "Five Emotions".

- *Nei Jing Su Wen* chapter 5 lists five emotional states: anger (LR); joy (HE); pensiveness (SP); worry (LU) and fear (KI); but in later chapters adds sadness (LU and HE) and shock (KI and HE).
- *Chen Wu Ze* (12th c.) describes seven emotions: anger, joy, worry, pensiveness, sadness, fear and shock.
- *Zhang Jie Bing* (16th c.) proposes: anger, joy, worry, pensiveness, sadness, fear, fright and shock.

3.1.1   Anger ≈ *Nu* 怒

Liver produces anger that can be understood as reactivity, or a defensive mechanism, which is also the mobile force behind enthusiasm, passion, competition and decisiveness.

Pathologically anger includes a variety of manifestations: rage, irritability, frustration, annoyance, boredom, repressed anger, hate, contempt, disgust, bitterness etc.

Liver disharmonies produce anger:

- Liver-Qi stagnation or Liver-Yang rising or Liver-Fire produce an explosive anger

- Liver-Blood vacuity produces irritability and frustration
- Liver-Qi stagnation causes repressed anger

On the other hand, excessive anger harms the Liver, producing:

- Liver-Qi stagnation or Liver-Blood stagnation;
- Liver-Yang rising or Liver-Fire.

Effects of Anger

Anger is extremely Yang in nature, and similarly to Wind, causes Qi to rise to the head, producing Heat and Fire symptoms (▶ Fig. 3.4):

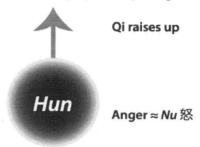

Qi raises up

Hun

Anger ≈ Nu 怒

Fig. 3.4:   The energetics of Anger

- Dizziness, vertigo, tinnitus, which are manifestations of Wind
- Headaches, red face and neck, bitter taste and red tongue, signs of Heat
- Nose bleeds, agitation of the spirit, signifying the transformation in to Fire
- Also produces a greenish complexion, a wiry pulse and red tongue sides

Liver Qi stagnation very often over-controls the Earth (*Ke* cycle) and harms the Spleen and Stomach causing gastritis, diarrhoea and fatigue.

It may also insult Metal (*Wu* cycle), causing Lung counter-flow Qi with asthma and wheezing (▶ Fig. 3.5).

Repressed anger may even manifest as an apparent chronic depression with a red and dry tongue and a tight pulse, versus real depression due to the Lung where the pulse would be weak.

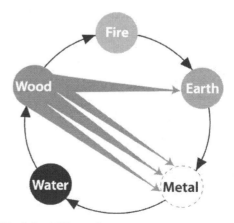

Fig. 3.5:   Effects of anger on Earth and Metal

Management of anger

- Reduce BL-47 *Hunmen*
- Bleed GB-37 *Guangming*
- Harmonise the Liver: LR-3 *Taichong*, LI-4 *Hegu*, LR-14 *Qimen*

Zang-Fu disharmonies and anger

The manifestation of anger may be observed in the following *Zang-fu* disharmony patterns:

- LR-Qi stasis: Anger, nervousness, oppression, depression, burping, sighing; Wiry pulse; treat with He-7 *Shenmen*, LR-3 *Taichong*, PE-6 *Neiguan*, DM-24 *Shenting* and RM-17 *Shanzhong*
- LR and GB-Fire: Anger, agitation, irritability, dysphoria, nightmares, oppression, red eyes, bitter and dry mouth; Wiry-fast pulse, red tongue; treat with PE-5 *Jianshi*, ST-44 *Neiting*, LR-2 *Xingjian* and GB-41*Zulinqi*
- LR and SP disharmony: Anger, agitation, dysphoria, lassitude; treat with SP-4 *Gongsun*, SP-6 *Sanyinjiao*, PE-6 *Neiguan*, LR-3 *Taichong,* LR-2 *Xingjian* and LR-13 *Zhangmen*
- LR and KI-Yin vacuity: Anger, light-headedness, dry throat at night, dry eyes; treat with LR-3 *Taichong*; KI-1 *Yongquan*, KI-3 *Taixi*, KI-7 *Fuliu* and SP-6 *Sanyinjiao*

3.1.2 Joy / Elation ≈ *Lei* 类

The Heart produces Joy and contentment. Joy, ecstasy and serenity are reflections of a harmonious state of Qi, they calm *Shen* and Qi, dilate the vessels, improve the circulation in the brain helping memory and easing the communication with the world. Joy further harmonises *Ying* and *Wei Qi* and protects against illness. Joy is Yang in nature and attached to the expansive movement of the Fire phase.

Obviously, joy is not a cause of disease, but rather excessive excitement ≈ *Shan Xi Xiao,* or excessive interest and vigilance, which may become harmful.

Effects of Excitement

Pathologically too much excitement or pleasure, harms the Heart and disperses the Qi outwards, causing excessive communication (talkativeness; excessive laughter), and may produce (▶ Fig. 3.6):

- Heart-Fire or Pericardium-Fire

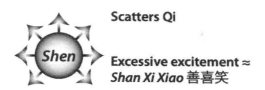

Fig. 3.6: The energetic effects of Excitement

- Heart-Yin or Heart-Blood vacuity

A Heart disharmony can produce excessive or insufficient excitement:

- Heart-Fire produces over-excitement: hysterical laughter
- Heart-Qi or Heart-Yang vacuity produces sadness and crying

Excessive craving or desire produces PE-Fire

Management of Excitement

- Reduce BL-44 *Shentang*
- Bleed SI-7 *Zhizheng*
- Calm, quiet or settle *Shen* (▶ Section 1.1.1).

Zang-Fu disharmonies and Excitement

- HE-Fire: Laughing, incoherent speech, agitation, nightmares; thirst, mouth ulcers; treat with HE-8 *Shaofu*, BL-15 *Xinshu*, BL-44 *Shentang*, PE-7 *Daling*, DM-24 *Shenting*, (EP) *Yin Tang*

- HE-KI not in harmony: Laughing, dreams; weakness of back and knees, empty Heat; Treat with KI-3 *Taixi*, KI-7 *Fuliu*, KI-1 *Yongquan*, KI-10 *Yingu*, HE-7 *Shenmen*, HE-6 *Yinxi*, SP-6 *Sanyinjiao*, BL-52 *Zhishi*; PE-7 *Daling*

- HE-Phlegm-Fire: Laughing, frothing, insomnia, nightmares, amnesia, agitation, jumpiness, bitter taste in the mouth; treat with PE-5 *Jianshi*, HE-7 *Shenmen*, HE-8 *Shaofu*, ST-40 *Fenglong*, ST-44 *Neiting*, DM-24 *Shenting* and DM-20 *Baihui*

- LR-Fire: Abnormal laughter, anger and rage, irritability, dysphoria, nightmares, oppression, bitter taste and a dry mouth; Wiry-fast pulse, red tongue: treat with PE-5 *Jianshi*, HE-8 *Shaofu*, ST-44 *Neiting*, LR-2 *Xingjiang*, GB-41 *Zulinqi*

3.1.3 Worry/ Pensiveness ≈ *Si* 思

The Spleen is responsible for planning and caring, and provides the Heart with accurate information "*Si* ≈ Thought"

A Spleen disharmony produces worry:

- Spleen-Qi vacuity produces mental asthenia with memory and concentration problems.
- A chronic stagnation of Spleen-Qi gives rise to obsessions, worrying and fixed ideas.

Please note that worry and pensiveness have been described separately in the classics (see above), relating pensiveness to Spleen and worry to Spleen and Lung.

Effects of Worry and Obsession

Excessive thinking and worrying harm the Spleen by knotting and depleting its Qi, harming the Lung and the Heart (▶ Fig. 3.7).

- Qi stagnation in the chest and the breasts
- Spleen-Qi stasis, food stasis, Stomach-Heat (ulcers)
- Yellowish-grey colour; slippery or tight pulse
- Worry about the future, also affects the Lung Qi

Knots and depletes Qi

 Worry ≈ *Si* 思

Fig. 3.7: The energetic effects of Worry

Management of Worry

- Reduce BL-49 *Yishe*
- Bleed ST-40 *Fenglong*
- Calm *Shen*: HE-7 *Shenmen* and quiet the mind with KI-23 *Shenfeng*, BL-23 *Shenshu* and BL-52 *Zhishi*

***Zang-Fu* disharmonies and Worry**

- HE and SP-Qi-*Xu*: Obsessions, rumination, insomnia from worry, abundant dreams; treat with BL-15 *Xinshu*, BL-20 *Pishu*, BL-49 *Yishe*, SP-6 *Sanyinjiao*, SP-4 *Gongsun* and DM-20 *Baihui*

- LU-Qi-*Xu*: Worrying about the future, depression, mental rumination; treat with BL-13 *Feishu*, BL-42 *Pohu*, BL-43 *Gaohuangshu*, RM-17 *Shanzhong*, RM-6 *Qihai* and ST-36 *Zusanli*

3.1.4 Sadness ≈ *Bei* 悲

The natural movement of Lung is both downward and upward, to take in and to let go (the image of a fishing net). The natural emotion that is related to the Lung would be a sense of sensitivity, perception, of being in touch (empathy) and the capacity for introspection and to let go (to forgive). This also includes the gentle sadness about the impermanence of life.

When the movement of Lung/ Metal is disturbed, the resulting emotion is sadness; hence the expression: "Lung produces sadness".

Sadness gathers Qi inwards, is Yin in nature and attached to the Metal phase (▶ Fig. 3.8).

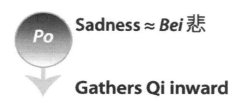

Fig. 3.8: The energetic effects of Sadness

Lung-Qi vacuity produces sadness, melancholia or future worry and a sense of anxiety. Prolonged or intense sadness produces grief.

Effects of Sadness

Excessive or prolonged sadness harms the Lung, preventing its Qi from descending, as well as the Heart, causing loss of communication and joy. Sadness blocks the upper Triple Warmer and the circulation of *Ying* and *Wei* Qi.

Lingshu chapter 28 states: Grief and Worry agitate the Heart and affect the *Zong* ≈ Ancestral Qi, treat with BL-10 *Tianzhu* and GB-3 *Kezhu (Shangguan)*.

The Lung in its function of "Master of Qi", is affected by sadness producing:

- Depression
- Fatigue
- Shortness of breath

- Short and weak pulse in both distal "*Cun*" positions
- In women sadness may cause Liver- Blood-Xu/ vacuity
- Unexpressed sadness (loss of joy) may affect the Kidneys, causing a loss of will to live with suicidal tendencies.

Management of Sadness

- Reduce BL-42 *Pohu*
- Bleed LI-6 *Pianli*
- Help to let go: RM-17 *Shanzhong* and LU-3 *Tianfu*
- Help to forgive: LU-7 *Lieque*, KI-24 *Lingxu*
- Open the chest: BL-17 *Geshu*, BL-43 *Gaohuangshu*, BL-46 *Geguan*
- Support *Zong* Qi: RM-17 *Shanzhong*, PE-1 *Tianchi,* LU-3 *Tianfu*

Zang-Fu disharmonies and Sadness

- HE and LU-Qi-Xu: Sadness and tears, asthenia, spontaneous sweating; treat with LU-7 *Lieque*, PE-5 *Jianshi*, PE-7 *Daling*, BL-42 *Pohu*, BL-15 *Xinshu*, BL-13 *Feishu*, and BL-20 *Pishu*
- HE-Yin or Blood-Xu: Sadness, sudden tears, over sensitivity, dysphoria, absent-mindedness, hysteria, agitation, abnormal behaviour, insomnia; feeling of heat: treat with KI-3 *Taixi*, HE-6 *Yinxi*, PE-6 *Neiguan*, SP-6 *Sanyinjiao*, BL-15 *Xinshu*, BL-23 *Shenshu*; DM-20 *Baihui*
- LR-Fire: Sadness, episodes of tears and anger, chest oppression; introversion, bitter taste and burping; treat with LR-2 *Xingjian*, LU-7 *Lieque*, BL-18 *Ganshu*, BL-13 *Feishu*, BL-42 *Pohu* and BL-47 *Hunmen*

3.1.5 Fear ≈ *Kong* 恐

The Kidneys produce fear, anxiety and apprehension, allowing for the spirit to adjust the true capacities of the person to the will power and drive.

Kidney disharmonies often produce fear:

- Kidney-Qi vacuity produces fearfulness and indecision
- Kidney-Yin vacuity causes an apparent Kidney-Yang repletion with manifestations of temerity and authoritativeness.

Effects of Fear

Fear and chronic anxiety damage the Kidneys (▶ Fig. 3.9):

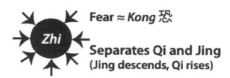

Fig. 3.9: The energetic effects of Fear

- Excessive or sudden fear produce a Kidney-Qi Xu and separate the Qi from the *Jing*, causing the *Jing* to descend to the lower TW, with weakness of the lower orifices; and the Qi to rise to the upper TW producing palpitations and panic attacks.

- Chronic anxiety depletes the Kidney-Yin resulting in Yang rising causing hot flushes, tinnitus, vertigo, night sweating, palpitations and a malar flush.

Management of Fear

- Reduce BL-52 *Zhishi*

- Bleed BL-58 *Feiyang*

- Strengthen the Kidney and the character (▶ A.I.5):

- For lack of self-confidence add KI-8 *Jiaoxin*

Zang-Fu disharmonies and Fear

- KI-*Jing-Xu*: Fearfulness, mental apathy, weak knees and back, tinnitus, agitation, insomnia; treat with BL-15 *Xinshu*, BL-23 *Shenshu*, BL-52 *Zhishi*, KI-3 *Taixi,* SP-6 *Sanyinjiao* and RM-4 *Guanyuan*

- Qi and Blood-*Xu*: Occasional fear, anxiety, palpitations, shortness of breath, paleness, fatigue, spontaneous sweating; treat with HE-7 *Shenmen*, BL-15 *Xinshu*, BL-17 *Geshu*, BL-20 *Pishu*, SP-6 *Sanyinjiao* and ST-36 *Zusanli*

- LR and GB-Qi-*Xu*: Fearfulness, indecisiveness, jumpy, palpitations, blurred vision, insomnia, frequent dreams; treat with LR-13 *Zhangmen*, LR-14 *Qimen*; BL-47 *Hunmen*, BL-48 *Yanggang*, DM-24 *Shenting*, GB-13 *Benshen*; RM-4 *Guanyuan* and GB-35 *Yangjiao*

Classically two other emotional states are added to the above five:

3.1.6 Oppression ≈ *You* 憂

Oppression is linked to grief and represents a condition of lack of circulation, of contraction and immobilisation, causing weakness of Blood and Qi and ultimately producing a Yang-Qi vacuity.

Effects of Oppression

- Oppression is usually related to the Lung, in particular, LU-Qi *Xu* with shortness of breath and a weak cough.
- It may affect the Heart causing HE-Qi *Xu* or HE-Yin *Xu*, with mental tiredness, palpitations, agitation, insomnia and amnesia.
- When it affects the Spleen and Stomach, it disrupts transformation and transportation, causing reduced appetite, bloating, weakness of the four limbs and injury to *Yi* ≈ Mind.
- It can even affect the Liver causing Liver-Qi stasis

Management of Oppression

- Open the chest: BL-17 *Geshu*, BL-43 *Gaohuangshu*, BL-46 *Geguan*
- Supplement LU-Qi: BL-13 *Feishu*, BL-42 *Pohu*, DM-12 *Shenzhu*, LU-7 *Lieque*
- Supplement and harmonise HE-Qi: BL-15 *Xinshu*, BL-44 *Shentang*, KI-3 *Taixi*, KI-7 *Fuliu*, KI-1 *Yongquan*, KI-10 *Yingu*, HE-7 *Shenmen*, HE-6 *Yinxi*, SP-6 *Sanyinjiao*, BL-52 *Zhishi*;
- Supplement and move Qi and harmonise digestion: RM-12 *Zhongwan*, ST-36 *Zusanli*, BL-20 *Pishu*, BL-49 *Yishi*
- Move Liver Qi: LR-3 *Taichong*, LR-14 *Qimen*, LI-4 *Hegu,* PE-6 *Neiguan*

3.1.7 Shock/ Fright ≈ *Jing* 驚（惊）

Shock can be excessive or sudden fear or even sudden joy.

A chronic deficiency of Kidney and Heart-Yin may produce a propensity to be easily startled.

Effects of Shock and Fright

Emotional or mental shock can scatter the Qi, causing a sudden depletion of Kidney essence and Heart Qi:

- Palpitations

- Insomnia

- Other "Empty-Heat" symptoms

- Fast and moving pulse

- White face; or in children, a bluish tinged forehead, or the chin if the shock has been pre-natal.

Management of Shock and Fright

- Settle (stabilise) the *Shen* KI-1 *Yongquan*, PE-5 *Jianshi*

- Bleed BL-58 *Feiyang*

- Harmonise HE and KI: KI-3 *Taixi*, KI-7 *Fuliu*, KI-1 *Yongquan*, KI-10 *Yingu*, HE-7 *Shenmen*, HE-6 *Yinxi*, SP-6 *Sanyinjiao*, BL-52 *Zhishi*; PE-7 *Daling*

- Clear-out the effects of shock: ST-14 *Kufang*, HE-3 *Shaohai*, BL-62 *Shenmai*

Zang-Fu disharmonies and Shock

- HE and GB-Qi-Xu: Chronic fear, jumpiness, mental obsessions, suspicious character, palpitations, disturbing dreams, insomnia, indecision, paleness, shortness of breath, spontaneous sweating: treat with He-7 *Shenmen*, BL-15 *Xinshu*, BL-19 *Danshu*, GB-40 *Qiuxu*, RM-6 *Qihai*

- HE-Yin or Blood-Xu: Fearfulness, sadness, dysphoria, agitation, amnesia, insomnia; paleness or empty heat: treat with KI-3 *Taixi*, HE-6 *Yinxi*, BL-15 *Xinshu*, BL-20 *Pishu*, SP-6 *Sanyinjiao*

- HE-Phlegm-Fire: Fear, jumpiness, palpitations, insomnia with nightmares, agitation, vertigo, amnesia, bitter taste; treat with PE-5 *Jianshi*, PE-8 *Laogong*, HE-8 *Shaofu*, ST-40 *Fenglong*, RM-12 *Zhongwan* and GB-41 *Zulinqi*

- LR-Qi-stasis with Blood-Xu: Anger and fear, nervousness, agitation, dysphoria, oppression, paleness and dizziness treat with LR-3 *Taichong*, LR-8 *Ququan*, LR-14 *Qimen*, PE-6 *Neiguan*, BL-17 *Geshu*, BL-18 *Ganshu*, BL-20 *Pishu*

3.2   The Seven Passions as "Inner Causes of Disease"

The Chinese medical concept of emotions being the roots of disease was previously explored. Certainly, the advent of Buddhist teachings further reinforced this idea. In Buddhism, the source of human suffering is believed to be the ignorance of the "Four Noble Truths"

- *Dukkha*: Identification of suffering: impermanent nature of life; illusory nature of reality; the illusion of being separate…

- *Samudaya*: is the cause of *Dukkha*, which is clinging to things illusory and impermanent and an inclination to the passions, in other words, one's attachments and emotional reactions to the world and to the outer changes;

- *Nirodha*: is the truth that suffering may end and peace of mind may be attained by ceasing the craving and clinging

- *Magga*: Is the path to reach this goal, through self-cultivation and mindfulness.

In simple terms, we humans suffer because of our misconceptions about life and reality, or in other terms, because of our belief systems.

Chinese medicine proposes the concept of the "Seven Passions" as the inner causative factors of disease. It is customary to add two more emotional states to the above five, usually oppression and shock, thus leaving a lot of material for debate as to which are the seven pathological emotional states.

Once again, the symbolism of the number has to be understood. "Seven" is a number associated with "Time" and with the lunar cycle, which in the earlier days represented an accurate reference for time (4X7). The lunar cycle was also used to subdivide the solar year. The human creation and the gestational period is described by (4X7X10), and the ageing process is symbolised by multiples of 7 (puberty 2X7; wisdom 3X7; full strength 4X7; end of fertility 7X7 …). "Seven", not only represents the process of psychological maturity (Seven challenges), but also the process of dissolution and progression towards death (Seven *Po*).

Hence the "Seven Passions" should be understood symbolically and not purely mathematically.

Today the myriad emotions could be analysed in terms of their subjective perception (pleasant and unpleasant) and their physiological response (activating or deactivating/ calming).

Generally, people suffer from unpleasant emotions and seek pleasant feelings. But the emotional response to an outer situation is not identical in two different persons. Hence in therapy, we must not simply rely on the emotional identification proposed by the patient, but we have to do our own assessment and establish the energetic impact that a given emotion may have on the patient.

For example, a patient consulting for a state of depression might actually be suffering from a lack of joy (Fire), lack of motivation (Qi), sadness and grief (Metal), chronic anxiety (Water), or even a suppressed anger (Wood).

In general, each emotional state perceived as pleasant has an unpleasant counterpart that may be related to the same *Zang-Fu* organic system and its psycho-emotional manifestations. For example:

- Joy and sadness reflect on the Fire-Heart and *Shen*

- Friendliness and it's opposite aggressivity relate to Wood-Liver and *Hun*

- Fear and courage both stem from Water-Kidney and *Zhi*

- Tolerance and rejection involve the Metal-Lung and *Po*

- Love and nurturing or lack of caring are both expressions of Earth-Spleen and *Yi*

As to why a particular emotion manifests in its pleasant or unpleasant feeling, depends on several factors:

- The energetic state of a *Zang* organ: for example, the lack of joy that results from a condition of Heart-Qi vacuity

- The harmony within a particular movement, maintained by the equilibrium between the *Zang* and the *Fu*, and in particular their respective channels. This equilibrium is reflected in the "Temperament" of the person: for example, when the *Taiyang* temperament is in harmony with its complementary level *Shaoyin*, the noble emotions of unconditional love and compassion and altruism may be manifested, whereas when the connection between *Taiyang* and *Shaoyin* is blocked, the person may become self-centred, insensitive, contemptuous or even dehumanising.

- Previously established and ingrained "Beliefs", from personal experiences or social conditioning, for example, phobic attitudes towards certain animals or insects, contempt or hatred towards racial differences, fear of change and novelty, or disgust for certain tastes or smells etc.

- Traumatic experiences during the foetal phase, birth or the early years, greatly contribute to the emotional response patterns (▶ Section 2.1: The Extraordinary Vessels and Psychology)

3.3   Other common emotions

3.3.1 Love / Romantic love

Love is probably the most misunderstood of all the human emotions. It is defined as a strong emotional and mental state, ranging from universal love to the feelings of pleasure.

In Chinese two terms express love:

- *Ren* 仁 which denotes a rather benevolent love. As a Confucian concept, love is rather focusing on duty and evaluated through action, such as the veneration of ancestors, love of parents, children and the concept of loyalty to clan and king.

- *Ai* 愛 is a concept developed by *Mozi* (Mohism), emphasising universal love. This term evolved later to represent passionate love and desire.

  In Buddhism *Ai* could be considered either selfish (a passion) or selfless (compassionate) love.

The ancient Greek distinguished five types of love:

- Kinship, friendship and platonic love: "Philia"

- Romantic love and desire: "Eros"

- Parental love and affection: "Storge"

- Hospitality: "Xenia"

- Divine love, pure love or ideal love: "Agape"

In Chinese medicine, different types of love are expressions of different movements:

- Universal and unconditional love, are attributes of Fire-Heart and *Shen*.

- Parental love and caring originates from the Earth-Spleen and *Yi* and enhances the caring instinct. The psychological disturbances brought about by the lack or excess of this caring (bonding process), have been explored under the *Ren Mai*.

- Romantic and passionate love as well as sexuality, involve the Wood-Liver and *Hun*. The driving and outgoing force of Wood enables the expression of this desire and provides the necessary means to attain it; quite often symbolised by Cupid's arrow transfixing the heart of the beloved! Hence it becomes clear as to why this passionate love may easily turn into envy, jealousy, aggression and even hatred.

Emotions that arise from human interactions and relationships, in particular, those concerning passion, desire and romantic love, all reflect on the Fire minister-PE. Actually, Heart minister ≈ *Xin Bao*, is also considered the envoy of the Kidney-Fire. At puberty the Kidney Fire reaches maturity, enhancing the development of the outer and inner genitalia, and at the same time through the Fire-minister it modifies the psychological behaviour of the individual towards the outer world and in particular the interpersonal relations. Therefore, the Fire-minister will be managing the emotional issues relative to relationships, desire, passion, excitement, jealousy, rejection and a broken heart; hence the importance of PE-7 *Da Ling*; PE-6 *Nei Guan* and BL-43 *Gao Huang Shu*. Together with the Liver (the *Jue Yin*), they also regulate sexuality (LR-5 *Li Gou*; LR-3 *Tai Chong*; LR-4 *Zhong Feng;* LR-12 *Ji Mai*). On the other hand, excessive attachment and co-dependency reflect on the *Ren Mai*, the bonding vessel (LU-7 *Lie Que;* RM-17 *Shan Zhong*; RM-12 *Zhong Wan*).

3.3.2 Jealousy; Envy; Craving

Jealousy has several components:

- Desire (Fire): wanting what the other person has, envy and craving scatter Heart Qi and produce Heart-Fire: HE-7 *Shen Men*; PE-7 *Da Ling*; for excessive sexual desire: LR-4 *Zhong Feng;* BL-10 *Tian Zhu*

- Lack of self-worth and self-confidence, Fire minister (see above): BL-43 *Gao Huang Shu*; KI-8 *Jiao Xin*; LR-8 *Ququan* (self-acceptance)

- Fear of losing a relation or a situation, fear of change: BL-52 *Zhi Shi*

- Anger towards the person responsible for provoking this feeling: BL-47 *Hun Men,* GB-37 *Guang Ming;* further re-enforced by lack of self-love and the feeling of abandonment (add LR-8 *Ququan*).

- Resentment: BL-47 *Hunmen*

3.3.3 Hatred; Vengeance; Disgust; Contempt

- Hatred and vengeance are like anger and aggressivity but they also affect the Heart, producing Heart-Fire. Chronic hatred may involve the Spleen with obsessive thinking about a particular situation. Hatred tends to stagnate the Qi in the solar plexus area causing Liver Qi stagnation, with the possibility of Liver Yang rising or even Liver Fire (rage).

- Disgust and contempt are rooted in non-acceptance and contain elements of rejection, hence the Wood movement, but also of evaluation and judgment (Metal/ *Po*).

- Contempt: SP-14 *Fujie*, KI-14 *Siman*

- Hating life: KI-17 *Shangqu*

- Hating light: KI-18 *Shiguan*

3.3.4 Guilt; Regret; Shame

Both the feelings of guilt and shame are rooted in social morality and social values (Earth-Spleen-*Yi*) as well as social judgments (Metal-Lung-*Po*).

Although guilt is one of the primary emotions in the West and constitutes the core premise of the Judeo-Christian and Islamic religions, it seems to be missing in the Chinese culture and the three primary philosophies of Confucianism, Daoism and Buddhism.

One of the strongest constituents of the collective unconscious and the foundation of the Western belief systems is the concept of the "original sin", at the root of the feelings of guilt and shame.

Both guilt and shame may cause Qi stagnation in particular in the chest area, affecting the Heart and Lung, and further causing Blood stasis. Shame may also cause the Qi to sink affecting the Kidney and the lower TW, with the production of Dampness and Phlegm. Very frequently, the feeling of shame is related to early toilet training, genitalia and sexuality. These early traumas involving the pelvic area are retained by the *Dai Mai*: GB-41 *Zu Lin* Qi; GB-26 *Dai Mai,* GB 27 *Wu Shu* and GB-28 *Wei Dao*, to help release these un-processed issues.

- Guilt is more self-directed, with feelings of inadequacy, low self-esteem, self-value and self-trust. In a sense, of how we see ourselves (*Yin Qiao Mai*; KI-6 *Zao Hai*; KI-8 *Jiao Xin*), and lack of self-love and self-esteem (BL-43 *Gao Huang Shu*).

- Shame is in relation to the outside and to how one appears to the others. Actually, the feeling of shame has been re-enforced in Confucian morality as a means for self-regulating the social order. It requires "Rectification" and "Letting go" as well as re-enforcing self-value.

- Social judgment and values reflect on the Spleen; emotions stemming from these require the "Rectification of Qi": *Chong Mai; SP*-4 *Gong Sun*; SP-12 *Chong Men*; SP-14 *Fu Jie*; SP-17 *Shi Dou*. Letting go of these feelings with LU-7 *Lie Que*, and enhancing self-esteem and self-confidence with BL-43 *Gao Huang Shu* and KI-8 *Jiao Xin*.

- To help let go of a shameful or guilty feeling: LU-7 *Lie Que;* KI-24 *Ling Xu;* HE-4 *Ling Dao*

- To help let go of retained emotions, sorrow and regret: PE-6 *Neiguan*; KI-9 *Zhubin*; RM-17 *Shanzhong*

- Regrets: HE-1 *Jiquan;* GB-35 *Yangjiao;* DM-11 *Shendao*

- Feeling vulnerable or embarrassed by guilt: LU-9 *Taiyuan*

3.3.5 Deception; Disappointment

Expecting a certain outcome and not getting it produces a strong feeling of disappointment.

- Deception may be the result of excessive or unrealistic desires (HE-7 *Shen Men,* PE-7 *Da* Ling)

- This feeling may be oriented towards oneself: "I am not good enough", with feelings of lack of confidence, low self-esteem, even guilt or shame (*Yin Qiao Mai*; KI-8 *Jiao Xin,* BL-43 *Gao Huang Shu*; LR-8 *Ququan*).

- Or oriented towards the outside: "...it is the fault of....", or "I am not appreciated" with feelings of rejection (*Yang Qiao Mai*)

3.3.6 Pride

Pride is generally a positive, pleasant and activating type of emotion and can be seen as the opposite of the feelings of guilt and shame. LI SHIZHEN considered *Yin Wei Mai* to be in charge of self-identification and self-assessment through one's accomplishments. Therefore, the sense of pride would be about owning the things that make one feel more validated in life. Although, excessive pride may become counterproductive and harmful:

Maintaining a person in past personal or social achievements (*Yin* and *Yang Wei Mai*): use TW-5 *Waiguan* and cupping on GB-29 *Juliao* and SI-10 *Naoshu* (to help let go of past images) or BL-63

- Disconnection from one's true resources (HE-KI not in harmony; blocked *Tai Yang* level with a loss of connection with the *Shao Yin): *SI-7 *Zhizheng* with HE-7 *Shenmen* and BL-57 *Feiyang* with KI-3 *Taixi* also RM-23 *Lianquan* also RM-4 *Guanyuan* and RM-17 *Shanzhong*

- Lack of discernment and self-evaluation (Metal-Lung and Po): LU-1 *Zhongfu*; ST-25 *Tianshu* and BL-42 *Pohu*

- Excessive self-love (narcissism): add KI-10 *Yingu*

- Excessive pride: SP-14 *Fujie*, KI-14 *Siman*

3.3.7 Relief

Relief is another powerful and pleasant feeling, stemming from the cessation of emotions causing stasis, such as anticipation, worry, anxiety or fear. Very similar to joy, it relaxes the stagnation of Qi and helps it circulate. Although a feeling of relief may not be directly enhanced, in therapy by moving the Qi stagnation and a change in the patient's perspective can often produce this feeling.

3.4   Treatment strategies

In the management of emotions, several questions have to be clarified:

- Is it a *Zang-Fu* disharmony causing the particular emotion, or is it the habitual emotion that is affecting the *Zang-Fu*?

- Is a particular emotion a reflection of the person's constitution, temperament and belief systems?

- Is the emotion part of a reflex defence mechanism, helping to protect the individual?

In most cases the roots of a particular emotion may involve all three, hence several therapeutic strategies have to be implemented.

Some general considerations:

- Mood disorders: when the subject cannot determine a causative factor. This involves the *Weiqi* ≈ Defensive Qi. Master Yuen indicates the *Jing* ≈ Well points and points around the upper portals (eyes, nose, ears…).

- Emotion: in relation to the outside, with a clear cause; involving the *Xue* ≈ Blood and the *Luo* ≈ Connecting channels

- Temperament: habitual tendency to a particular behaviour and the overall personality involve the *Yuan* ≈ Source Qi and the *Yuan* points.

3.4.1 *Zang-Fu* disharmonies causing emotions

The treatment strategy includes:

- Treating the *Zang-Fu* disharmony (▶Appendix-I)

- Releasing the emotion with the *Luo* ≈ Connecting channels (▶ Section 2.3.5: Clinical Applications of the *Luo*)

- Releasing the emotion with the *Zhi* ≈ Will (Five Spirit) points. Their palpation may reveal a state of repletion/excess or vacuity/deficiency. In general, a retained emotion causes a state of excess in which the point feels full to the touch and is painful when pressed. This has great importance in the accurate evaluation of an emotional state, based on the reactivity of the point:

  - BL-42 *Pohu*: retained sadness and grief
  - BL-43 *Gaohuangshu*: rejection, deception, shame, broken heart
  - BL-44 *Shentang*: excessive excitement, desires, anticipation
  - BL-47 *Hunmen*: retained anger, rage, revenge, frustration, irritability
  - BL-49 *Yishe*: excessive worry and pensiveness; obsessions
  - BL-52 *Zhishi*: fear of the future, fear of change, fear of life

3.4.2 Impact of constitution and Temperament

The impact of constitution and temperaments was explored in section 2.2. In normal conditions when a temperament is balanced with its complementary level, there is a flexibility in feeling and expressing all emotions. When a temperament is blocked and unable to freely communicate, there is a tendency to specific emotional patterns:

- Blocked *Taiyang*: tendency to excitement, pride, contempt, anger, intolerance, lack of sensitivity…

- Blocked *Shaoyang*: tendency to anger, rage, hatred, vengeance, disgust…

- Blocked *Yangming*: obsessiveness and worry; complaining; avidity; stubbornness…

- Blocked *Taiyin*: worry, sadness, melancholia, shyness, introversion; rigidity…

- Blocked *Jueyin*: irritability and frustration, anxiety, jealousy, envy, shame and regret…

- Blocked *Shaoyin*: fear, anxiety, insecurity, guilt, shame, deception…

PART - IV
Impact of Trauma

- **"*Po*": Body memories and sensations**
    - Concept of "Body Armours"
    - Clinical application of Body Armours
    - Treatment strategies

- **Description of the segments**
    - Ocular and Crown segments
    - Oral segment
    - Cervical segment
    - Thoracic segment
    - Diaphragmatic segment
    - Abdominal segment
    - Pelvic segment
    - Body Armour self-test
    - Body Armours and EFT
    - Adapted PAT exercises for releasing Body Armours
    - Changing the Mind-set

- **"*Hun*": Psychological trauma (images, words, sentiments)**

- **"*Gui*": the wrench in the gears**

- **Emotions and Dreams**
    - Emotions as Internal pathogenic Factors (IPF)
    - Dreams of fear; loss; control; vulnerability…
    - Excessive dreaming
    - Nightmares / Night-fright
    - Dreams of flying; falling; sexual
    - Working with dreams

Part- IV

Impact of trauma

Trauma is often the result of an overwhelming amount of external input that goes beyond the individual's ability to cope with or to integrate (understand).

Humans have in common with all other life forms, the instinct for survival; although compared to most animals, humans are the least equipped to survive individually.

It can, therefore, be presumed that any event that involves a menace of death or serious injury, or any threat to the physical or psychological integrity of a person, maybe perceived as a traumatic experience.

Individuals react to a similar traumatic event very differently depending on their constitutions, temperaments, conditioning and personal subjective experiences.

A traumatic experience may be caused by a variety of events involving:

- Extreme sensory input, particularly sight and sound
- Physical sensations, primarily pain
- Psycho-emotional causes, involving either extreme emotions or situations in which the person's core beliefs are being challenged causing a state of confusion and insecurity

Traumatic events may even involve all of the above causes. Furthermore, trauma may result from either a single distressing experience or be the consequence of recurring and repeated overwhelming situations. Therefore, the effects of the trauma need to be treated physically as well as psychologically. The body can store and recreate emotional trauma in much the same way the mind can store and recreate physical trauma.

The conscious functioning of the mind has been explored in Part-I.

When faced with a potentially threatening situation, the *Shen* calling upon previous experiences that have been analysed and classified by *Yi* will react in most appropriately: expression, fight, flight or withdrawal (disconnection or shut down of *Shen*).

Withdrawal occurs when the threat is too strong, or the physical and the psychological inputs are too intense, in this event, the *Shen* may disconnect in an attempt to maintain the sanity, very similar to an electrical fuse or a circuit breaker that acts as a safety device and disconnects the current to safeguard the whole mechanism. The shut-down of *Shen* can be considered as a loss of communication between the fore-brain and the limbic structures, as well as a disruption between the hemispheres of the brain. The restoration of this connection constitutes an important phase in the management of post-traumatic conditions.

In the absence of *Shen*, *Hun* and *Po* (emotional brain) take over to deal with the traumatic event.

In the absence of *Shen*, *Yi* (logical brain) cannot analyse and store this information in the conscious part of the mind therefore other sectors of the psyche take over:

- *Po* stores the trauma in the body, in particular in the muscles managed by the *Jinjin* ≈ Sinew channels;

- *Hun* will register the event in the subconscious memories, in the form of feelings and emotions or words.

The traumatic experiences, when stored by *Hun* and *Po*, have not been properly analysed, processed and integrated, hence they remain "un-digested". The sensory input becomes muddled; sight, sound, touch and emotion blend into one. Each time that any aspect of the traumatic event is reactivated, be it a touch, a word, a sound or even a smell, the whole initial episode is re-experienced. The person will re-live the whole trauma as though it was happening at that moment. In Chinese medicine, this condition of "alienation" is referred to as "*Gui*" ghost, or in more modern terms the concept of "Energy Mass".

It is important to note that before the full development of the limbic system, responsible for the storage of emotional memory, in infants and small children, most traumatic experiences are stored in the body by *Po*, contributing to the formation of the "Body Armours".

In fact, during the first developmental months of their life, the infant's brain is unable to clearly distinguish the source of a specific sensory input; vision, hearing, and touch blend into a unitary perceptual experience (D. Levitin; McGill University; Monreal).

4.1 *Po*, body memories and sensations

Our bodies are both a source and a storage site for our emotions. This is frequently the case after a trauma, be it physical or psychological.

4.1.1 Concept of "Body Armours"

The *Jingjin* ≈ Sinew channels, which constitute the most superficial defensive layers of the body, are primarily responsible for mobility (sinews and muscles) and protection (*Wei* ≈ Defensive energy). Hence in case of intense or repeated trauma to a particular area of the body, the Sinew channels may develop a protective territory, similar to the ancient armours.

The "Body Armours" are defined as organised defence mechanisms involving *Wei Qi* accumulation in a group of *Jingjin* ≈ Sinew channels, in a particular area of the body.

Although this terminology was never used in the Chinese texts, it comes very close to the Mongolian massage known as *Chua-Ka* (*Chuoka*). The Mongolian warriors believed that fear was trapped in the body in the muscles and sinews and that it was important to release this fear before confronting the enemy. They would utilise a smooth piece of wood to dig into and release the trapped pain or tension. According to the Mongolian belief, memories of pain, be it physical or emotional, get deposited in the muscles. With this deep tissue massage, the trapped pains and tensions, as well as the corresponding fears and memories, are released.

As we have seen previously, the *Jingjin*, acting as the first organised line of defence, react to all external aggressions, not only climatic but also emotional or mental. When a particular aggression is repeated it causes a meshing and binding of the *Taiyang*-BL Sinew channel, the main protective layer of the body, which will, in turn, affect the back *Shu* ≈ Transport points, and often cause the abnormal development of the muscles in a particular area, producing not only mechanical malfunctions but also energetic disturbance of the related *Zang-Fu*. With time, this abnormal muscular tension results in postural and even facial modifications, as analysed in Chinese face diagnosis.

It takes a great deal of energy, *Wei Qi,* in this case, to maintain a constant state of protection, this results in Qi and Blood accumulation in that part of the body, often leading to organic diseases.

With the interconnection and crossing over of the Sinew channels, slowly there results a defensive band, around that particular area, involving all the six Sinew channels, rather than the customary linear Sinew channel involvement.

The concept of muscular defence, in response to repeated or unresolved psychological aggression, led psychiatrist WILHELM REICH (1897–1957) to describe the seven segments of body Armouring (▶ Fig. 4.1). Based on these concepts, ALEXANDER LOWEN developed a type of body-psychotherapy named Bioenergetic Analysis.

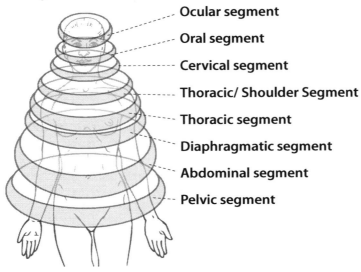

- Ocular segment
- Oral segment
- Cervical segment
- Thoracic/ Shoulder Segment
- Thoracic segment
- Diaphragmatic segment
- Abdominal segment
- Pelvic segment

Fig. 4.1:   The Body Armours

It is important to underline that although the "Body Armours" are implicating the protective instincts of *Po* and the surface layers, the muscles and sinews, their activation does not only concern physical trauma and pain but any type of psycho-emotional aggression as well.

4.1.2 Clinical application of the Body Armours

The concept of "Body Armours" and its application in Chinese medicine is relatively recent and quite unknown to the general acupuncture public. Although the basic concept of releasing an "Energy mass" trapped in the muscles and sinews, has been developed in many of the modern "new age" therapy methods, the contribution of acupuncture has not been much explored.

Body Armours may prove to be extremely valuable in the following conditions:

- Chronic muscular tensions or pains
- Correcting body postures
- Recurrent and resistant organic pathologies
- Psychosomatic diseases
- Fixed psychological habits and attitudes
- Releasing long-standing traumatic memories

4.1.3 Treatment strategy

The treatment is based on releasing the trapped energy by shallow needling of the main local *Guo* ≈ Binding points. The points are selected based on palpational sensitivity. The *Jing* ≈ Well and the convergent Sinew channel points are not used in this case.

It is very important to point out that just needling a given set of points is not enough to release long standing defence mechanisms, especially if the latter have been installed at a very early age. Birth or early childhood traumas might require the use of the Extraordinary Vessels, especially the *Chong Mai*. Working with Body Armours requires a combined energetic and psycho-emotional work. In some types of childhood traumas and abuse, Qigong, especially the "Marrow Washing Qigong" is of prime importance. Many modern types of bodywork such as "Structural Integration" also called Rolfing, developed by Ida P. Rolf, or Bioenergetics as mentioned above, or "The emotional Freedom Technique" (EFT), may constitute interesting complements to the acupuncture sinew-release.

4.2 Description of the Segments

4.2.1 Ocular and Crown Segments

Territory
Concerns eyes, sinuses, ears, forehead, the head apex and the occipital regions; the hypophysis (pituitary), hypothalamus (pineal) glands. In the Indian Yoga system, this segment corresponds to the 6th and 7th Chakra centres (▶ Fig. 4.2).

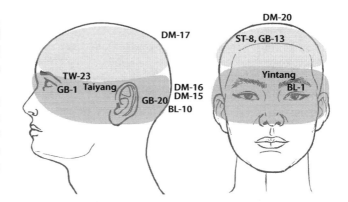

Fig. 4.2:   The Ocular segment (including the apex)

Causes of Armouring of the Ocular Segment

- Light trauma at birth
- Fear of seeing, denial of the right to see
- Rigid belief systems, ignorance
- Spiritual abuse, indoctrination
- Denial of the right to know and to hear the truth

The main cause of the armouring of this segment is the traumatic experience of birth involving the sudden exposure to intense light in the birthing room. Later, the denial of a child's perceptions of the outer world, in particular of what they describe and see, re-enforced by rigid beliefs and indoctrination, progressively produces a state of separation and dichotomy between the infant's own intake and what they should be seeing or hearing. This constant tension may be experienced as a traumatic event by the child and further contribute to the formation of the "ocular" defensive segment.

Pathological manifestations

- Headaches
- Red eyes
- Difficulty to cry
- Anxiety
- Vertigo, tinnitus
- Amnesia
- Psychological traits: rigid belief systems; lack of faith; confusion and hallucinations; nightmares; difficulty in visualising

Treatment

The following points may be used, according to sensitivity, to help release this segment:

- DM-20 *Baihui*, DM-17 *Naohu*, DM-15 *Yamen*
- ST-8 *Touwei*, GB-13 *Benshen*; DM-16 *Fengfu*; GB-20 *Fengchi*
- BL-10 *Tianzhu*, BL-1 *Jingming*
- EP *Yintang;* GB-1 *Tongziliao*; TW-23 *Sizhukong*; EP *Taiyang*

According to constitutional therapy: start with *Chong Mai*; then *Yin* and *Yang Qiao Mai; Du Mai* (▶ Section 2.1)

Exercises for releasing the Ocular segment:

- The Focusing and Expanding the vision exercise (▶ A.4.7)
- Higher self-meditation (▶ A.4.6.3)
- Guided visualisation exercises
- Colour visualisation: white (crown) and violet range (brow) (▶ A.4.5.4)
- Affirmations: I am guided by a higher power/ I am guided by my inner vision/......my higher self/....my inner wisdom; I see clearly; I can manifest my vision
- Processing the belief systems concerning fixed and dogmatic concepts

4.2.2 Oral Segment

Territory

Includes the mouth, tongue, and the jaw (▶ Fig. 4.3)

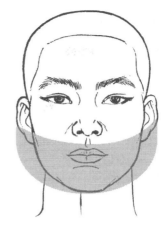

Fig. 4.3:   The Oral segment (see Cervical segment)

Causes of Armouring of the Oral Segment

- Lack of breastfeeding
- Repressed expression
- Addictive family (alcohol, drugs ...)

The oral complex is the basis of many addictive tendencies involving the mouth: smoking, eating or drinking, as well as habits such as nail-biting, or the biting of the lip.

The lack of breastfeeding was previously analysed under the *Ren Mai*, the "Bonding" vessel, and its impact during the first year of an infant's life. This lack of bonding may later manifest with compensation strategies such as eating disorders, dependency and addiction.

Pathological manifestations

- Jaw tension, crooked mouth
- Excess smiling
- Voice problems
- Psychological traits: fear of speaking; excessive talking (logorrhoea); oral complex; addictions

Treatment

The treatment of the oral segment combines the *Ren Mai*: LU-7 *Lieque*; RM-12 *Zhongwan*, RM-24 *Chengjiang*, and the cervical segment points (see below).

4.2.3 Cervical Segment

Territory

Concerns the neck, throat, larynx, thyroid and parathyroid glands and corresponds to the fifth Chakra in the Yoga system (▶ Fig. 4.4).

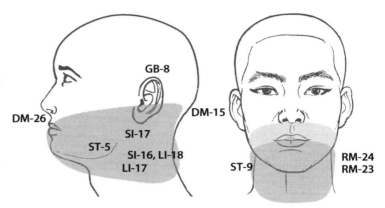

Fig. 4.4:   The Cervical segment

Causes of Armouring of the Neck Segment

- Repressed anger or tears
- Fear of chocking, often due to birth trauma: nucal cord (umbilical cord around the neck)
- Verbal abuse
- Denial of the right to speak (the truth)

Pathological manifestations

- Chronic neck pains or tensions
- Voice problems
- Cough
- Swallowing problems
- Throat problems
- Psychological traits: are the same as for the oral segment

Treatment

The following points may be used, according to sensitivity, to help release this segment:

- DM-15 *Yamen*, DM-26 *Renzhong*
- GB-8 *Shuaigu*; SI-16 *Tianchuang*, SI-17 *Tianrong*, SI-18 *Quanliao*
- LI-17 *Tianding*, LI-18 *Futu*
- ST-9 *Renying*, ST-5 *Daying*
- RM-23 *Lianquan*, RM-24 *Chengjiang*

According to constitutional therapy: start with *Chong Mai*; then *Ren Mai* (▶ see Section 2.1)

Exercises for releasing the Oral and Neck segments:

- Exercises to loosen the neck and shoulders
- Singing and chanting
- Developing communication skills
- Gibberish
- Colour visualisation: blue (▶ A.4.5.4)
- Affirmations: I express myself with authenticity; I have the right to speak the truth
- Processing the belief systems concerning expression and authenticity

4.2.4 Thoracic Segment

Territory

The thoracic segment includes the upper thoracic or shoulder segment and the chest area (▶ Fig. 4.5):

- Territory of the shoulder segment concerns the shoulders, the upper thoracic spine and the arms;

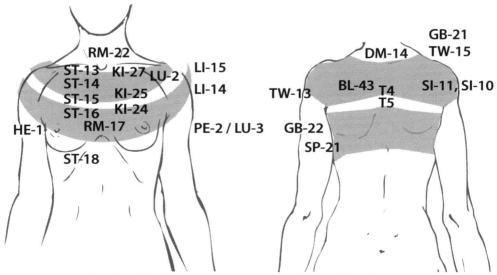

Fig. 4.5:   The Thoracic segment: upper chest and shoulder

- The territory of the chest segment involves the thoracic cage, the breasts, heart and lungs, the mid-thoracic spine, the oesophagus, the thymus gland, and corresponds to the fourth Chakra in the Yoga system.

Causes of Armouring of the Shoulder Segment

- Deceptions
- Injustice
- Expectations: the shoulder area reflects what is expected and demanded of a person symbolically represented by the notions of "fear of the father", "shouldering responsibilities" and the "weight of the world". Quite often a pathological process of the shoulder joint, appearing at a transitional period of a person's life (*Yang Wei or Yang Qiao Mai*) might be in relation with this armouring.

Pathological manifestations

- Shoulder and neck tensions
- Arm tension
- Agoraphobia (fear of crowds)
- Difficulty expressing emotions
- Difficulty assuming responsibility

Treatment
Choose from the following points according to sensitivity:

- DM-14 *Dazhui*; GB-21 *Jianjing*; TW-15 *Tianliao*
- SI-10 *Naoshu*, SI-11 *Tianzong*
- LI-15 *Jianyu*; ST-13 *Qihu*, ST-14 *Kufang*
- RM-22 *Tiantu*; KI-27 *Shufu*
- If the arms are involved add also
- LI-14 *Qimen*; TW-13 Naohui; PE-2 *Tianquan*; LU-2 *Yunmen*, LU-3 *Tianfu*

Causes of Armouring of the Chest Segment Territory

- Unacknowledged grief
- Deceptions; injustice
- Rejection; loveless environment, "broken heart"

Pathological manifestations

- Diseases of the breasts, chest, heart and lungs
- Chronic pain and tension between the shoulder blades
- Psychological traits: Difficulty expressing joy or love; fear of intimacy; lack of self-love; overly sacrificing; co-dependency; anti-social tendency

Treatment

The following points may be used, according to sensitivity, to help release this segment:

- "EP" *Huatuojiaji* of T4–5
- BL-43 *Gaohuang*
- SI-10 *Naoshu*, SI-11 *Tianzong*
- LU-2 *Yunmen*; HE-1 *Jiquan*;
- ST-14 *Kufang*, ST-15 *Wuyi*, ST-16 *Yingchuang*, ST-18 *Rugen*
- KI-24 *Lingxu*, KI-25 *Shencang*
- RM-17 *Shanzhong*
- GB-22 *Yuanye*, SP-21 *Dabao*

According to constitutional therapy: start with *Chong Mai*; then *Yin Wei Mai* and *Yin Qiao Mai* (▶ see section 2.1)

Exercises for releasing the Chest segment:

- Meditation on self-acceptance
- Processing the belief systems concerning relationships
- Colour visualisation: green (▶ A.4.5.4)
- Meditation on forgiveness and self-acceptance
- Affirmations: I am loving to myself and to others

4.2.5 Diaphragmatic Segment

The first armour to form, preventing the breath from descending, it literally cuts a person in half.

Territory

Concerns the solar plexus, hypochondrium, the lower thoracic spine, the stomach, pancreas, liver and Gallbladder, as well as the adrenal glands; it corresponds to the third Chakra in the Yoga system (▶ Fig. 4.6).

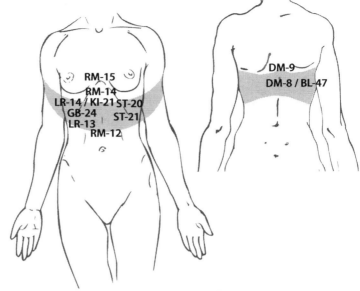

Fig. 4.6:   The Diaphragmatic segment

Causes of Armouring of the Diaphragmatic Segment

- Domination of will
- Intense anger, desire to kill
- Shame
- Early responsibility

Pathological manifestations

- Ulcers, gastritis, nausea
- Eating disorders
- Liver and Gallbladder problems
- Diabetes, hypoglycaemia
- Back pains; scoliosis
- Psychological traits: aggressivity; manipulative; persecuting; victim complex; lack of confidence

Treatment

The following points may be used, according to sensitivity, to help release this segment:

- DM-8 *Jinsuo*, DM-9 *Zhiyang*
- BL-47 *Hunmen*

- GB-24 *Riyue*; LR-14 *Qimen*, LR-13 *Zhangmen*

- ST-20 *Chengman*, ST-21 *Liangmen*; KI-21 *Youmen*

- RM-12 *Zhongwan*, RM-14 *Juque*, RM-15 *Jiuwei*

According to constitutional therapy: start with *Chong Mai*; then *Yin* and *Yang Wei Mai* (▶ see section 2.1)

Exercises for releasing the Diaphragmatic segment:

- Martial arts

- Processing the belief systems concerning power and self-esteem

- Setting goals and finishing projects

- Colour visualisation: yellow (▶ A.4.5.4)

- Meditation on self-confidence

- Affirmations: I honour the power within me; I respect the others

4.2.6 Abdominal Segment

Territory

Concerns the peri-umbilical and lower abdominal regions, lumbar area, intestines and the uterus, corresponds to the second Chakra in the Yoga system (▶ Fig. 4.7).

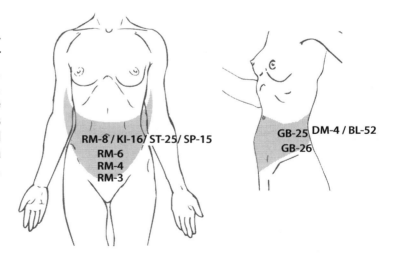

Fig. 4.7:   The Abdominal segment

Causes of Armouring of the Abdominal Segment

- Sexual, physical or emotional abuse

- Fear of being attacked or desire to attack

- Vengeance, hatred
- Neglect

Pathological manifestations

- Fear (often combined with cervical block)
- Abdominal and lumbar diseases
- Sterility and sexual dysfunctions
- Unclear boundaries
- Psychological traits: excessive or lack of clear boundaries; difficulty with socialisation; sexual issues

Treatment

The following points may be used, according to sensitivity, to help release this segment

- DM-4 *Mingmen*
- BL-52 *Zhishi*
- GB-25 *Jingmen*, GB-26 *Daimai*
- SP-15 *Daheng*; ST-25 *Tianshu*; KI-16 *Huangshu*
- RM-8 *Shenque*, RM-6 *Qihai*, RM-4 *Guanyuan*, RM-3 *Zhongji*

According to constitutional therapy: start with *Chong Mai*; then *Dai Mai; Ren* and *Du Mai* (▶ Section 2.1).

Exercises for releasing the Abdominal segment:

- Martial arts
- Belly dancing
- Colour visualisation: orange (▶ A.4.5.4)
- Processing the belief systems concerning spontaneity and pleasure
- Affirmations: I move effortlessly...; I take pleasure in life...; I take pleasure in what I do...

4.2.7 Pelvic Segment

Territory

Concerns the pelvic and sacral regions, the bladder, the genitals and the gonads, the rectum and the perineum; it corresponds to the first Chakra in the Yoga system (▶ Fig. 4.8).

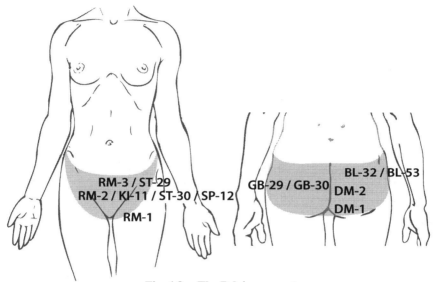

Fig. 4.8:   The Pelvic segment

Causes of Armouring of the Pelvic Segment

- Sexual taboo; early toilet training
- Sexual abuse
- Birth trauma
- Abandonment, malnourishment

Pathological manifestations

- Sexual repression
- Fear of movement
- Obesity or anorexia
- Urinary, genital and rectal dysfunctions
- Intestinal problems, bones, legs and spine disorders
- Psychological traits: Fear and shyness; anxiety; rage; lack of discipline and focus

Treatment

The following points may be used, according to sensitivity, to help release this segment:

- GB-29 *Juliao*, GB-30 *Huantiao*
- BL-53 *Baohuang*, BL-32 *Ciliao* ST-29 *Guilai*, ST-30 *Qichong*; SP-12 *Chongmen*
- KI-11 *Henggu*
- RM-1 *Huiyin*, RM-2 *Qugu*, RM-3 *Zhongji*
- DM-1 *Shangyang*, DM-2 *Erjian*

According to constitutional therapy: start with *Chong Mai*; then *Dai Mai; Ren* and *Du Mai;* possibly the *Yang Qiao* (rooting and empowering); (▶ see Section 2.1).

It is recommended to open this segment last; opening the neck segment helps open the pelvic segment.

Exercises for releasing the Pelvic segment:

- Fitness and exercise
- Dancing
- Colour visualisation: red (▶ A.4.5.4)
- Processing the belief systems concerning the right to exist and be here
- Affirmations: It is safe for me to be here; I feel secure...; I feel grounded...; I am entitled to get what I need...

4.2.8 Body Armours self-test

The following questions help orient the evaluation of the affected body armour:

Segment	Questions	Yes	No
Ocular	• Do I feel lost and need guidance to get back on my spiritual path? • Do I feel like I am on my own, and that I do not get any support from the higher powers? • Do I feel that my life is not in accordance with my destiny? • Do I have a hard time seeing my life any differently than what it is now? • Do I have a hard time changing my point of view? • Do I have a hard time getting in touch with my intuition?		
Oral & Cervical	• Do I have a hard time saying what I think and feel, and doing what I say I would do? • Do I tend to say what I think others want to hear? • Do I feel like other people don't hear me? • Do I have a hard time expressing my ideas clearly? • Do I feel a split between what I want to do and what is required of me to do?		
Thoracic	• Is it hard for me to feel worthy of love? • Is it hard for me to express forgiveness? • Is it hard for me to be gentle and healing towards myself? • Is it hard for me to love and accept myself as I am, and to accept others as they are?		
Diaphrag-matic	• Am I confused about my purpose in life? • Am I lacking self-confidence and need approval? • Am I afraid of "power" because it can be misused? • Do I often tend to delegate my power to others? • Do I often feel powerless to change my circumstances?		
Abdominal	• Do I find it hard to enjoy spending time alone? • Is it difficult for me to be spontaneous and listen to my needs? • Do I feel not respected and utilized by others? • Do I often feel that others are invading my boundaries? • Do I have a hard time taking pleasures in life (food, sex...)? • Do I experience vague feelings of anxiety and fear or unexplained rage?		
Pelvic	• Do I feel like I have a difficult time manifesting what I want? • Do I feel like I do not belong in this world?		

	<ul><li>Do I have difficulties with spending money out of fear of not having enough?</li><li>Do I frequently experience guilt?</li><li>Do I often feel neglected and abandoned?</li><li>Do I experience low libido?</li></ul>		
Please note: The abdominal and pelvic segments have many points in common: both may have resulted from neglect or sexual abuse and may present patterns of frigidity, fear of movement, anxiety and rage.			

4.2.9 Body Armours and Emotional Freedom Techniques (EFT)

EFT was developed by Gary Craig in the late 1990s, most probably drawing from Chinese acupuncture channel theories, Neuro-linguistic programming (NLP) by Bandler and Grinder (1970's), Thought field therapy (TFT) invented by Roger Callahan (1980's) and Tapas Acupressure Techniques (TAT), created by Tapas Fleming (1993). All of these methods, including various types of Energy medicine, have been loosely grouped into alternative and pseudo-medicine, labelled as pseudo-scientific and heavily criticised by the hard-core scientific establishment (▶ see Preface).

The EFT method consists of tapping (stimulating) specific areas and zones while focusing on a particular issue by repeating specific sentences that target the emotional component of the physical or psychological symptom. The tapping areas mainly correspond to the *Jing Jin* ≈ Sinew channels, and their confluent zones.

The EFT has the great advantage that it can be easily self-applied by the patient, on a regular basis, allowing them to subjectively evaluate their progress.

The standard EFT practice is involving all of the Sinew channels indiscriminately. By better adapting the method to the Body Armours, the results may prove even better.

4.2.10 Adapted PAT (Psychology and Acupuncture) exercises for releasing the Body Armours and changing the Beliefs

These exercises have been developed specifically based on the *Jing Jin* ≈ Sinew channel trajectories and confluences, and specially adapted to the various segments of the Body Armours. (Section A.4.2)

The relation between the *Po* ≈ Corporeal soul and the "Body memories", as well as the defensive role of the Sinew channels and the formation of "Body Armours" was discussed above. By helping to liberate these retained body memories via the Sinew channels, involving the *Po*, and by associating a cognitive restructuring, involving the *Hun,* we are calling upon both *Hun* and *Po* subconscious defensive mechanisms.

It has to be understood by the patient, that the goal of this exercise is to free-up the trapped energy. By resisting a painful or uncomfortable situation, one is in fact, giving it more energy, the more the pain, the more effort is needed to contain it. To accept and to stop the resistance will free up all this retained Qi. Two images might serve the purpose of demonstrating this point:

- The image of boiling water; the pressure increases when you put a lid on the pot (image of suppressed feelings)

- The image of two hands struggling one against the other; the more one side is pressing, the more resistance is required by the other side.

4.2.11 Changing the Mind-set

The affirmations, mentioned in section A.4.2 for each segment, are involving the *Shen* (conscious mind) and the *Hun* (subconscious). They allow for consciously replacing the retained subconscious beliefs and memories, with positive and conscious counter beliefs.

The relation between a particular mind-set or belief mechanism and a specific physical or psychological manifestation have been previously covered. Changing a habitual belief mechanism is not always easy. Most belief systems have been incorporated into the personal identity and ego structure. These harmful beliefs, need to be first identified (naming) and then accepted (owning), before they may be changed. In some cases, the individual may resist to let go of some social, cultural or religious beliefs that have been deeply ingrained. The same is also true for beliefs that have once been useful but have now become harmful (▶ see section A.4.3).

4.3   Psychological trauma and the Hun (images, words, sentiments)

The physical sensation of emotions, described as feelings, was explored in Part III.

The outer world is perceived through the sensory functions in the form of vibrations. Each sensory opening is geared to receive a particular frequency:

- The higher light frequencies by the eye,
- The sound frequencies by the inner ear
- Smell and taste need the actual presence of the molecule to be analysed chemically
- The sensory receptors of the skin are programmed to perceive tactile impulses

The emotional responses to outer events are not only physically felt, but also perceived as images, symbols, shapes or colours and frequently relate to the body parts. Many common expressions demonstrate this point:

- Blue with fear; green with shame; burdened with guilt; livid; yellow; black soul; golden ego...
- Blood boiling; getting cold feet; frozen by fear; hair's standing up; head smoking; shivers up the spine...
- Heart-break; heartfelt; gut-wrenching; chocked up; pain in the neck; tight-lipped; tight ass; uptight; spill my guts; antsy feeling...
- Blinded by love; can't see straight; can't stand it; saving face; spineless; gutless; makes me vomit; pisses me off...

The inner representations of feelings and emotions are not universal but quite personal, when some might describe a feeling with an image, others will have shapes and colours to represent a similar sensation. This is even true for other mental functions, such as mathematics or memory and learning, some individuals who excel in these tasks often have a strategy of personal inner imagery.

Images, colours, shapes and impressions are the domain of the *Hun*. Therefore, any emotion will have a particular body sensation together with an inner representation of that feeling. In simple words, an emotion may be associated with a body sensation as well as a sensory perception.

An emotion or a feeling may be mediated and brought on simply by the visualisation of a shape or colour, a particular sound, a smell, even a taste or a spoken word.

Hun registers impressions and verbalised words. Hence there is an association in the mind between a certain word and a particular feeling. This association is strongest for words spoken in the individual's native tongue. Studies have demonstrated that the learning of language in infants is greatly enhanced when associated with touch and in particular a caring touch. (A. Seidl; Purdue University; Indiana).

In fact, during the first developmental months of their life, the infant's brain is unable to clearly distinguish the source of a specific sensory input; vision, hearing, and touch blend into a unitary perceptual experience (D. Levitin; McGill University; Monreal).

4.4   The wrench in the gears (*Gui*)

The *Gui* are the invisible, unconscious parts of all physical or emotional manifestations, hence the term "ghost" or "shadow".

The concept and mechanisms of *Gui* have been previously explored. (▶ Section 1.2.5).

In modern psychology, the *Gui* could be associated with any unexplained behaviour or emotion, concerning a given situation, similar to what Jung refers to as the "shadow".

In the previous comparison between the conscious functioning of the mind and the computer, when the input is properly analysed and stored (*Shen, Yi* and *Zhi*), the information may be retrieved at all times. But at times the file may be corrupted due to a hidden order or defects in the software caused by a computer "virus", inadvertently imported, the so-called "Trojan horse". The program behaves strangely and may even crash.

Every time there is an unexplained mood or emotion, strange thoughts, or when any sensory perception produces an unrelated feeling or even a pain in the body, a *Gui* is present.

4.4.1 Therapeutic indications

The concept of *Gui* may be applied to several clinical situations:

- Unexplained moods or emotional states: oppression, anxiety, panic attacks etc.
- Psychosomatic diseases
- Post-traumatic stress disorders
- Transmitted family trauma
- Faulty belief systems:

- When two unrelated phenomena are associated; this is the basis for many conditioned (Pavlovian) reflexes; but also, may explain several psychosomatic disorders. For example, a certain physical condition such as the common flu in springtime may be associated with the outer manifestations of spring such as the blooming of the plants, making the person recreate the physical flu-like symptoms every springtime; this seasonal occurrence would be then termed as hay fever. This is the case of two linked subconscious programs.

- Or when two contradictory beliefs and opinions co-exist, for example, I like and yet I hate..., I want and yet I am afraid of... etc. This duality makes it impossible for the conscious mind to carry out a chosen task, as the hidden contrary belief will always block the decision.

4.4.2 Therapeutic strategies for clearing the *Gui*

The Chinese acupuncture tradition has described a number of points that contain the term *Gui* in their primary or secondary names, although no mention has been made as how to apply them in clinical practice.

The concept of "being possessed by a ghost" or an evil spirit may be found in all cultures around the world, calling upon sorcerers, shamans or priests for their exorcism. Even in modern times, the concept of evil spirits has been replaced by extra-terrestrials taking possession of a person's psyche.

Therapeutic modalities

The clearing-out of unconscious programs and retained undigested emotional or physical trauma constitutes an important part of treating the roots of disease.

The following approaches may be proposed:

- Working with "Body Armours"
- The Extraordinary Vessels
- Qigong in particular the "Marrow Washing Qigong"
- Cultivation of the mind; working and changing the belief systems; de-programming the *Gui*
- Clearing "Possessions" with protocols proposed by *Sunsimiao*, *Zhangjiebin* and Worsley.

Important note:

There is very little documentation about the use of the following strategies.

It is highly recommended to associate these protocols with an appropriate psychological or psychiatric support, and preferably on stronger patients. It is important to fortify the Blood, in particular Heart and Liver Blood before applying these protocols.

The 13 Gui point protocol by Sunsimiao

Sun Si Miao (7th c.) described a set of thirteen Ghost points to treat "Possessions". He proposed Phlegm as the cause of mental disorders to replace the concept of "Evil spirits". There is no indication of the exact use and the therapeutic protocol for these points.

- LU-11 *Shaoshang* or *Guixin* ≈ Ghost sincerity

- LI-11 *Quchi* or *Guitui* ≈ ghost leg or *Guichen* ≈ Ghost minister

- ST-6 *Jiache* or *Guichuang* ≈ ghost bed or *Guilin* ≈ Ghost forest

- Sp-1 *Yinbai* or *Guiyan* ≈ Ghost eye or *Guilei* ≈ Ghost pile

- BL-62 *Shenma* or *Guilu* ≈ Ghost road

- PE-7 *Daling or Guixin* ≈ Ghost Heart

- PE-8 *Laogong* or *Guiying* ≈ Ghost camp or *Guilu* ≈ Ghost road or *Guiku* ≈ Ghost cave

- RM-1 *Huiyin* or Guicang ≈ Ghost storage

- RM-24 *Chengjiang* or *Guishi* ≈ Ghost market

- DM-16 *Fengfu or Guixue* ≈ Ghost hole or *Guizhen* ≈ Ghost pillow or *Guilin* ≈ Ghost forest

- DM-23 *Shangxing* or *Guitang* ≈ Ghost temple

- DM-26 *Renzhong* or *Guishi* ≈ Ghost market or *Guigong* ≈ Ghost palace or *Keting* ≈ Ghost reception

- *Guifong* (possibly *Taiyang*)

According to Master Yuen and the Daoist oral tradition, these points are to be used in groups of three, with the last set of four points; to be needled bilaterally. The needling order is indicated based on the symptoms and the stage of the mental condition. For example, for a patient describing a feeling of something sitting on their chest, the treatment starts with the second trinity (PE-7, BL-62, DM-16); for the following session the third trinity is needled, then the fourth, ending with group one. Or for dementia, start with group four then in order group one, two and three.

It is further recommended by the tradition to throw the needles on the ground after the session! (probably either to return the *Gui* back to the Earth; or maybe as an indication as not to re-use the needle on another patient?)

Point Combinations	Indications
• DM-26 *Renzhong* • LU-11 *Shaoshang* • SP-1 *Yinbai*	Psychological dysfunction with a change in behaviour; starting to see things; thinking and seeing things differently

• PE-7 *Daling*	Fixity of beliefs and attitudes; indecisiveness; the impression of something sitting on the chest
• BL-62 *Shenmai*	Going places without realising what they are doing; seeking Yin type places (dark and humid); eyes wide open
• DM-16 *Fengfu*	Strange dreams

• ST-6 *Jiache*	Introverted, withdrawing, tendency to hide
• RM-24 *Chengjiang*	Dialogue with imaginary people, schizoid behaviour
• PE-8 *Laogong*	Delusional, paranoid, conspiracy theories

• DM-23 *Shangxing*	Self-mutilating, suicidal, risk-taking
• RM-1 *Huiyin*	Self-mutilating, suicidal, risk-taking
• LI-11 *Quchi*	Paleness, hollow stare, aimless walk; catatonia
• *Gui Fong* or *Yintang*	Hysteria; violent dementia; biting of the tongue; schizophrenia

The Five Ghosts treatment by *Zhangjiebin* (17th c.)

Zhangjiebin describes five types of ghosts and how to treat them:

- If the Liver is weak: there may be an invasion by the "White *Gui*": needle GB-40 *Qiuxu*; followed by BL-18 *Ganshu*

- When the Heart is weak: "Black *Gui*" may invade: treat with TW-4 *Yangchi* (instead of SI-4) and BL-15 *Xinshu*

- When the Spleen is weak: "Green *Gui*" could invade: treat with ST-42 *Chongyang* and BL-20 *Pishu*

- When the Lung is weak: there may be an invasion by "Red *Gui*": treat with LI-4 *Hegu* and BL-13 *Feishu*

- When the Kidney is weak: "Yellow *Gui*" may invade: treat with BL-64 *Jinggu* and BL-23 *Shenshu*

A special three depth needling technic is indicated: insert to the first depth during three breaths, insert to the second depth for one breath, then to the third depth wait for one breath; remove slowly. A special incantation is performed for each *Gui*.

This ancient shamanic treatment could be adapted to modern practice in the following manner:

- The White *Gui*, could be understood as a retained sadness or grief with inability to let go. With the consequence of an exaggerated *Ke* ≈ Control cycle disrupting the Liver. The patient might even describe dreams with predominant white-coloured themes. Treat with GB-40 *Qiuxu* and BL-18 *Ganshu* and the verbalisation of the following affirmations: … I let go of…; I breath-in the present moment (life), and breath-out the past…; …I am forgiving…

- The Black *Gui,* from retained fear affecting the Heart. Treat with TW-4 *Yangchi* and BL-15 *Xinshu;* and the verbalisation of the following affirmations: …I welcome change…; I trust in myself…; …I feel my strength…

- The Green *Gui*, from repressed anger and frustration overacting on the Spleen. Treat with ST-42 *Chongyang* and BL-20 *Pishu*; affirmations: …I go with the flow…; …I am flexible and adapt easily…; …I share of myself…

- The Red *Gui*, from excessive excitement overacting on the Lung. Treat with LI-4 *Hegu* and BL-13 *Feishu*; affirmations: …I radiate joy and love; …I love and accept myself as I am; …I am at peace…

- The Yellow *Gui*, from excessive worry overacting on the Kidney. Treat with BL-64 *Jinggu* and BL-23 *Shenshu*; affirmations: …I trust in existence…; …I appreciate and enjoy life…; …I give and receive…

The 7 Dragons to chase out the internal Demons

This is a protocol proposed by J.R. Worsley (1923-2003). This method is best applied when the patients describe a sense of separation from their actions and behaviours: "something inside makes me do this..." or "I cannot recognise myself..." or "...as though someone else was doing..." or "I cannot help it, it is not in my hands...".

The origin of the protocol remains unknown. There are several variations of the points, but the following seems to be the most accepted consensus.

- RM-15 *Jiuwei* or the Extra point 1/4 *cun* below
- ST-25 *Tianshu*
- ST-36 *Zusanli* or the Extra point *Lan Wei Xue* (2 *cun* below ST-36)
- ST-41 *Jiexi*

It is indicated to Needle in a spiral form, from Right to Left for women, opposite for men; and to remove the needles in the reverse order. For example, for treating a male subject, the needling order should be: RM-15 => ST-25 (left) => ST-25 (right) => ST-36 (right) => ST-36 (left) => ST-41 (left) => ST-41 (right); remove in the reverse order.

The Seven "External Dragons" to expel external Demons

Again, proposed by Worsley, indicated for the impression of something hovering or lurking around or an evil presence:

- DM-20 *Baihui*
- BL-11 *Dazhu*
- BL-23 *Shenshu*
- BL-61 *Pucan*

Remove needles in the reverse order.

4.5 Emotions and Dreams

As elaborated earlier, dreaming is the domain of the *Hun* ≈ Etheric soul, residing in the Liver. The Liver is considered the "record keeper", helping to bring out events from the subconscious into the conscious mind and to keep the "memory of the future" (life curriculum).

The interpretation and significance of dreams was already an integral part of Chinese medicine. *Suwen* chapter 17 and 80 relates specific dreams to organ disharmony patterns:

Dreams of fire	Excess of Yang
Dreams of a large body of water	Excess of Yin
Dreams of mutual destruction	Excess of Yin and Yang
Dreams of flying	Excess above
Dreams of falling	Excess below
Dreams of crowded places	Intestinal short *Gu*-worms
Dreams of fights and arguments	Intestinal long worms
Anger dreams	Liver related disharmony
Crying and sorrow dreams	Lung related disharmony
Dreaming of flowers and fragrance	Liver vacuity
Dreaming of white objects or bloody battles	Lung vacuity
Dreams of raging fires and explosions	Heart vacuity
Starvation dreams or construction, building	Spleen vacuity
Dreams of drowning or swimming	Kidney vacuity

In *Lingshu* chapter 43, dreams are associated with the presence of *Xie Qi* ≈ Pathogenic factors invading the *Zang-Fu* ≈ Viscera and Bowels:

Dreams of anger and irritability	Excess/ repletion in the Liver
Anxiety, fear, crying or flying dreams	Excess in the Lungs
Dreams of laughter, fear or awe	Excess in the Heart

Dreaming of music and singing; or of having a heavy body	Excess in the Spleen
Sexual dreams, or dreaming of the pelvis, or having a loose spine	Excess in the Kidneys
Dreaming of mountains, hills, heights, or fire, and oppressive smoke	Qi Xu ≈ Vacuity with *Xieqi* in the Heart
Dreams of flying, stumbling, or strange metallic or golden objects	Qi Xu with *Xieqi* in the Lung
Dreams of trees, forest, plants, mountains	Qi Xu with *Xieqi* in the Liver
Dreams of ruins, mounds, swamps, fog or rain	Qi Xu with *Xieqi* in the Spleen
Dreaming of a precipice, empty spaces, or drowning	Qi Xu with *Xieqi* in the Kidney
Dreaming of wanderings and travelling	Qi Xu with *Xieqi* in the Bladder
Dreams of large meals (food and drinks)	Qi Xu with *Xieqi* in the Stomach
Dreaming of foreign lands or rice fields	Qi Xu with *Xieqi* in the Large Intestine
Dreams of crowded places, meeting many people; busy roads, or crowded cross roads	Qi Xu with *Xieqi* in the Small Intestine
Dreams of arguments, struggling with choices and decisions; feeling empty, dried out; the idea of self-destruction or suicide	Qi Xu with *Xieqi* PF in the Gall Bladder

Please note: A specific dream may signify a *Zang-Fu* pathology only if accompanied by the relevant physical symptoms, otherwise it should not be considered an invasion of a *Xie* ≈ Pathogenic factor.

Dreams and their significance held a very important place in all cultures and traditions.

The Daoist tradition considered dreams to be means to:

- Express what had been suppressed
- To explore the opposite of an established belief
- To question what is considered reality
- To realise that life itself is like a dream

To quote *Zhuangzi* (4th century BC): when I dream of being a butterfly, is it me dreaming of the butterfly, or is it the butterfly dreaming of being a man?

In the Confucian tradition, dreams were considered as:

- A teaching opportunity and to understand that Qi follows *Li* ≈ Principle directed by the *Zhi* ≈ Will

- Releasing method via the *Hun*; for which it is indicated to treat the Liver and the Kidney. In case of a recurrent dream to treat the related Bladder Back *Shu*, *Ying* ≈ Spring and *Shu* ≈ Stream points. For example, for dreams with a Wood pattern, treat with BL-18 *Ganshu*; BL-19 *Danshu*, LR-2 *Xingjiang* and LR-3 *Taichong*

In the 16th century, *Chen Shi Yuan* (1516-1595) author of *Meng Zhan Yi Zhi* ≈ Analysis and conclusion of dreams, brings more precision to dream interpretation. By the statement:

"Hun knows the future; *Po* conceals the past"

Chen underlines the role of *Hun* in unravelling what is hidden and what is to come (premonitory dreams). He describes the various types of dreams:

- Normal dreams, which are often forgotten: signifying a state of harmony between the five elements and the five emotions; the person wakes up feeling rested.

- Nightmares are unsettling dreams; waking with an uncomfortable feeling; related to the Kidney.

- Dreams concerning thoughts before falling asleep, dreaming that one is awake; related to the Spleen.

- When the dream evolves around words heard before going to sleep, this involves the Heart.

- Happy, celebrating dreams are associated with the Lung

- Fearful dreams involve the Gall Bladder.

4.5.1   Emotions as Internal Pathogenic Factors

All unexpressed, suppressed and denied emotions are retained in the corresponding *Zang* ≈ Organ and will produce an Internal Pathogenic factor (IPF), that will ultimately affect the Heart and produce Heat:

- Anger produces HE-Fire
- Joy and sadness affect HE-Qi
- Worry affects HE-Blood
- Fear and fright disturb the HE-KI communication

All emotions, therefore, will affect the *Shen* and disrupt sleep

The *Hun*, through dreams, helps release these IPF, in the form of disturbing dreams.

When analysing dreams, the following points should be considered:

- The dream scenario;
- The state of the person upon awakening; in particular the dominant emotion which is expressed at the time of waking;
- The factors which influence dreams, "*San Yin*"
  - Environmental
  - Cultural
  - Constitutional

The following dreams should not be interpreted, as recommended by Master Yuen:

- When the subject has gone to sleep in a stressed or emotional state, or with distressing thoughts
- Dreams with a great sense of danger: their interpretation may reinforce the sense of danger
- Interrupted dreams: in which there is no sense of conclusion and no clear emotion
- Partially forgotten dreams

Master Yuen further relates emotions experienced in dreams to specific *Zang-Fu* disharmony patterns and proposes some treatment strategies.

4.5.2 Dreams of Fear, Danger or Threat

- If the fear dream is remembered as a black and white image, it involves the Kidney

- If the dream is distinctly colourful and vivid, it involves Heart (HE-Blood)

- If the dream involves an unknown aggressor, a stranger, a malevolent entity or ghost, it signifies the presence of Phlegm: use *Ren Mai* and *Yin Qiao Mai*

- If the aggressor is a familiar person, it concerns the state of Blood: use *Chong Mai*

- When there are aggressive objects involved: knife, teeth, claws, horns, this signifies the presence of a retained *Xie Qi*: use *Jing* ≈ Well points

- Feeling "Frozen" and inability to move: use the *Jing Bie* (BL-40 *Weizhong*/ KI-10 *Yingu*)

- If there is vague feeling of anxiety or dread, being startled, hateful: use *Gui* ≈ Ghost points: SP-1 *Yinbai*; PE-5 *Jianshi*

General points to be considered in Fear-dreams

- BL-52 *Zhishi* (reduced) with BL-23 *Shenshu* (supplemented) indicated for general fearfulness; retained fear; fear of life; fear of the future, fear of change

- KI-1 *Yongquan*: stabilises *Shen*; indicated for "fright-Wind"; visual dreams; panic attacks, poor memory, loss of will to live

- KI-3 *Taixi*: not finding any resources in the dream; auditory dreams; lacking air and shortness of breath

- KI-6 *Zhaohai*: clears Heat and calms the *Shen*; nightmares before periods and before labour (Blood stasis)

- For insomnia add: KI-21 *Youmen* if tired but cannot sleep, KI-23 *Shenfeng* for a restless mind, KI-25 *Shencang* for insomnia from worry, KI-26 *Yuzhong* for waking in a bad mood, KI-27 *Shufu* for persistent insomnia

TCM patterns in Fear-dreams

- KI-*Jing Xu* from Liver Blood *Xu*; quite common in children: dreams of life-threatening aggression by a person, a monster or an object; confusion, loss of direction, loss of control (HE-Blood)

  Treatment: KI-1 *Yongquan*; KI-3 *Taixi*; KI-6 *Zhaohai*; LR-3 *Taichong*; LR-8 *Ququan*; add LR-1 *Dadun* for anger towards the self

- KI not grasping the Qi; frequent in periods of illness; consider the age of the character in the dream (may represent unfinished traumatic issues at a certain life stage): dreams of injury or death from accident or disease.

  Treatment: add BL-42 *Pohu*; LU-7 *Lieque*; PE-6 *Neiguan*, also choose from *Yin Wei* points: KI-9 *Zhubin*; SP-13 *Fushe*; SP-14; SP-15 *Daheng*; LR-14 *Qimen*

- KI-Qi Xu or Yang Xu with the possibility of sleep-walking; often tired upon waking; fatigue and inability to feel restored: dreams of death from neglect; lack of nourishment and air, suffocation and confinement.

  Treatment: add BL-23 *Shenshu*, BL-52 *Zhishi* and *Dai Mai*

- HE and KI not in harmony: frequent nightmares; dreams of disasters, natural calamities, explosions, wars, chaos; famine

  Treatment: KI-1 *Yongquan*; KI-27 *Shufu*; add according to the type of disaster: tornado (Wind) = KI-24 *Lingshu*; fire, explosion, volcano (Fire) = KI-25 *Shencang*; flood, tsunami (Earth) = KI-23 *Shenfeng*; drought (Metal) = KI-26 *Yuzhong*; cold, blizzard (Water) = KI-22 *Bulang*

4.5.3   Dreams of loss of Home, Property or Territory

In general dreams related to values and possessions concern the Earth;

- The Kidney is also involved if the dreamer tries to save others or to escape
- Loss of valuables through fire (ST-Heat),
- Loss by water (SP-Dampness),
- Damages by cold (SP-Yang Xu);
- Drought (ST-Yin Xu),
- Tornado (ST-Yang rising)

General points to be considered in Property-loss dreams

- BL-49 *Yishe* with BL-20 *Pishu,* for worry and obsessive thinking
- SP-1 *Yinbai*: settles *Shen* and with ST-45 *Lidui* for excess dreaming and nightmares; grief; feeling of something sitting on the chest
- SP-2 *Dadu*: excessive dreaming, obsessive thinking or thinking in circles
- SP-4 *Gongsun*: rectifies Qi; if there is the notion of judgment; guilt, praise, values;
- SP-6 *Sanyinjiao*: regulates Qi, Blood and *Jing*; harmonises SP-LR and KI.

TCM patterns in Property-loss dreams

- SP-Qi Xu: dreams of the inability to secure home, boundary or valuables.

- Treatment: add RM-12 *Zhongwan*; if the dream involves strangers (LR overacting on SP); if it involves known persons (KI insulting SP); which room in the house is being damaged: kitchen= ST; living room or library= SP; bathroom= BL: bedroom= KI; Garden= LR

- SP Qi sinking; occurring often at the onset of sleep; common in elderly or after a trauma; may indicate aggravation of health or finance: dreams of dropping, falling or sinking

- Treatment: if there is a feeling of not being helped or supported add SP-8 *Diji* and KI-2 *Rangu*; falling from a mountain= LU; boat= KI; vehicle= LR; space= HE

- SP-Qi Xu with Dampness: dreams of being submerged, buried; stuck; with a sense of hopelessness; unable to keep up

- Treatment: add SP-9 *Yinlingquan*

4.5.4 Dreams of Control, Direction and Movement

In general, dreams involving mobility relate to Liver: "the free flow of Qi"

- Inability to move to navigate or to stop: LR over-controlling the SP

- Dreams involving malfunction of tools, machines, vehicles or obstacles to reach a destination: LR-Qi stasis

- Dreams of going the wrong way: counter-flow Qi

General points for Control dreams

- BL-47 *Hunmen* and BL-18 *Ganshu*: for frustration and anger

- LR-2 *Xingjian*: regulates Qi, clears Heat, for resentment in taking responsibility

- LR-3 *Taichong*: Regulates Qi, moves Blood, clears Heat, clears Wind and Damp-Heat; for all Liver patterns and Liver body areas

TCM patterns in Control dreams

- LR-Qi stagnation: dreams of frustration from malfunction or inability to move forward

  Treatment: add LR-14 *Qimen*

- LR-Blood stasis; often when the person is physically or emotionally handicapped: dreams of being blocked and not able to overcome the obstacle; loss of control, no sense of direction

  Treatment: add BL-47 *Hunmen*; LR-11 *Yinlian*, LR-5 *Ligou*

- LR-Blood Xu; quite frequent in adolescence and in the pre-menstrual phase: dreams of bad performance, low self-esteem; missing a chance, missing a train etc. Treatment: add LR-8 *Ququan*; BL-43 *Gaohuangshu*

- LR-Yang rising: dreams of over-activity, climbing or flying

  Treatment: add DM-20 *Baihui*

4.5.5   Dreams of Vulnerability and Exposure

- Dreams with themes of lacking protection, concerning the skin, clothing or being caught or exposed, or feelings of imperfection and self-consciousness involve the Metal and Lung.

General points for Vulnerability-dreams

- BL-42 *Pohu* and BL-13 *Feishu*: for sadness, shame and guilt
- LU-3 *Tianfu*: for excessive sadness and grief, talking to oneself
- LU-10 *Yuji*: for Heat in the LU and Blood-Heat

TCM patterns in Vulnerability-dreams

- External Pathogenic Factors: dreams of being vulnerable to nature or aversion to external phenomena
- Treatment: add LI-4 *Hegu* for dreams of flowers and landscapes
- LU Qi Xu or LU-Yin Xu: dreams of nakedness; difficulty connecting with others
- Treatment: BL-13 *Feishu*, LU-1 *Zhongfu*, LU-9 *Taiyuan,* KI-22 *Bulang*, LI-4 *Hegu*
- LU-Heat: insomnia with agitation; dreams of being exposed

Treatment: add LU-5 *Chize*, BL-13 *Feishu*, LU-1 *Zhongfu*, LU-6 *Kongzui*, KI-22 *Bulang*, PE-5 *Jianshi*

4.5.6 Excessive dreaming *Duo Meng* 多梦

Dream-disturbed sleep is a cardinal symptom of Blood-*Xu* ≈ Vacuity particularly Heart or Liver-Blood *Xu*. Excessive dreaming disrupts the quality of sleep hence the subject will wake up feeling tired.

TCM patterns:

- Heart-Blood Xu

- Heart and Spleen-Qi Xu

- Liver-Blood Xu

- Heart- and Kidney-Yin Xu, Empty-Heat (HE and KI not in harmony)

4.5.7 Nightmares *Meng Yan* 梦魇

Nightmares are unpleasant dreams causing the person to wake up with a strong emotional feeling. They are usually related to pathology, stress, post-traumatic conditions or late meals. They occur during REM sleep (dreaming), and are different to night terrors. More common in adolescents, their incidence is less after age 25.

Nightmares are due to the unsettling of the *Hun*: Treat with PE-5 *Jianshi*, SP-1 *Yinbai* + ST-45 *Lidui* and LU-3 *Tianfu*

TCM patterns in Nightmares

- LR-Fire: restless sleep with frequent nightmares

  Treatment: add LR-2 *Xingjian*, LR-3 *Taichong*, GB-44 *Zuqiaoyin*, GB-12 *Wangu*, GB-20 *Fengchi*, BL-18 *Ganshu*, DM-20 *Baihui*, GB-13 *Benshen*, or GB-15 *Toulinqi* together with DM-24 *Shenting*

- HE-Fire: difficulty falling asleep; nightmares; dreams of flying

  Treatment: add HE-7 *Shenmen*, BL-14 *Jueyinshu*, RM-14 *Juque*, KI-23 *Shenfeng*, DM-19 *Houding*, RM-15 *Jiuwei*

- Phlegm-Fire harassing the mind: dreams of feeling responsible for someone's death; guilt; suicidal tendencies

  Treatment: PE-5 *Jianshi*, PE-8 *Laogong*, HE-8 *Shaofu*, ST-40 *Fenglong*, ST-8 *Touwei*, BL-15 *Xinshu*; GB-44 *Zuqiaoyin* and SP-5 *Shangqiu*

- Phlegm misting the mind: dreams of unfinished business; inability to accept someone's death; something hovering around "Floating ghost":

  Treatment: add LU-3 *Tianfu*; also, *Dai Mai* for unresolved issues

- LR and HE Blood-Xu: difficulty falling asleep, frequent waking, anxiety, restlessness, nightmares occurring early in the night; dreams of flying

  Treatment: add SP-6 *Sanyinjiao*, HE-7 *Shenmen*, BL-20 *Pishu*, BL-17 *Geshu*, BL-15 *Xinshu*, BL-18 *Ganshu*, LR-8 *Ququan*, ST-36 *Zusanli*, *Yintang* (extra), *Anmien* (extra)

- LR-Yin-Xu with Yang Rising: restless sleep, vivid dreams, nightmares; early waking; sleep-walking or sleep-talking

  Treatment: BL-18 *Ganshu*, BL-23 *Shenshu*, LR-8 *Ququan* and SP-6 *Sanyinjiao*, GB-20 *Fengchi*, GB-13 *Benshen*, together with DM-24 *Shenting*

- HE- and GB-Qi-Xu: dreams of fear, depression, regret and anxiety; insomnia from insecurity, light sleep

  Treatment: add HE-5 *Tongli*, PE-6 *Neiguan*, RM-17 *Shanzhong*, RM-6 *Qihai,* ST-36 *Zusanli,* GB-40 *Qiuxu* and GB-12 *Wangu*

- ST-Heat: restless sleep; frequent dreams, nightmares, needs to eat or drink to fall asleep, mental restlessness, discontentment, accusing, agitated

  Treatment: BL-21 *Weishu*, RM-7 *Yinjiao*, RM-12 *Zhongwan*, LU-7 *Lieque*, ST-41 *Jiexi*, ST-36 *Zusanli*, ST-21 *Liangmen*, SP-1 *Yinbai*, ST-44 *Neiting*

- Blood stasis: anxiety when lying down, restless sleep, nightmares; sleep-walking or sleep-talking

  Treatment: PE-6 *Neiguan*, HE-7 *Shenmen*, BL-15 *Xinshu*, HE-5 *Tongli*, KI-23 *Shenfeng*, BL-14 *Jueyinshu*, BL-43 *Gaohuangshu*, BL-17 *Geshu*, LI-4 *Hegu*, LR-3 *Taichong*, DM-20 *Baihui* and DM-24 *Sheeting*

4.5.7 Terror dreams, Night-fright (Ghost-fright) *Ye Jing* 夜惊

Technically speaking "Night terrors" are different from nightmares, they do not occur during REM sleep (dreaming) but during SW (slow-wave) sleep. They are common in children between the ages of 2 to 6, and usually appear early in the night (before midnight); there is waking with terror and an inability to regain full consciousness.

Often caused by a feverish pathology, stress, irregular sleep or diet; quite common after Post-traumatic stress. Manifesting as:

- Night Terrors "Ghost fright" and dreams of something sitting on the chest "Ghost oppression"; of dead people; guilt or unfinished matters relate to Phlegm

- Non-acceptance or guilt for someone's death

General points for Terror dreams

- HE-7 *Shenmen*: to quiet and calm *Shen*; agitation, memory loss, sleep-talk

- PE-4 *Ximen*: quiets *Shen*, rectifies Qi; for guilt and shame, fear and fright, sadness; claustrophobia

- PE-6 *Neiguan*: rectifies Qi; eating disorders; for guilt and shame; fright-Wind; poor memory

- PE-7 *Daling*: quiets *Shen*, opens the chest; for fear, grief, anxiety and hysteric laughter

- PE-5 *Jianshi*: quiets *Shen*, clears the Heart's orifices, transforms Phlegm

- To help settle the *Hun*: PE-5 *Jianshi*; GB-4 *Hanyan*; GB-8 *Shuaigu*; GB-23 *Zhejin*; and RM-4 *Guanyuan*

- Sensation of something sitting on the chest: SP-1 *Yinbai* and BL-43 *Gaohuangshu*

TCM patterns in Night-fright

- Phlegm-Fire harassing the mind: see above

- Phlegm misting the mind (Heart orifices): see above

- LR-Fire: see above

- Heart-Fire: see above

4.5.8 Dreams of Flying *Meng Fei* 梦飞

They signify a condition of repletion/excess above and vacuity/deficiency below; quite typical of Heart-Fire and Heart-Blood *Xu*.

TCM patterns:

- Heart-Blood Xu

- Heart-Fire

- Lung-Qi Xu

- Liver-Yin Xu with Liver-Yang rising or Liver-Wind

4.5.9   Dreams of Falling *Meng Zhui* 梦坠

They usually signify a condition of vacuity/deficiency above and repletion below

TCM patterns:

- Kidney and Spleen-Yang Xu
- Kidney-Qi Xu
- Heart-Qi Xu
- Heart and Gallbladder-Qi Xu
- Liver-Qi stagnation (with Blood Xu)

4.5.10   Sexual dreams *Meng Jiao* 梦交

They signify an overactivity of Yang mainly PE-Heat.

When accompanied by spermatorrhoea, it signifies an underlying vacuity.

Standard point combination: BL-10 *Tianzhu*; BL-15 *Xinshu*; BL-23 *Shenshu*

TCM patterns:

- Heart- and Spleen- Qi Xu
- Heart-Qi Xu
- Heart- and Kidney-Yin Xu, Empty-Heat (HE and KI not in harmony)
- Pericardium-Heat
- Liver-Qi stagnation with Liver-Fire

4.5.11   Working with dreams

Dreams constitute a great source of information by providing indications about physical or psychological issues. In general, the same types of messages are received from the body or the psyche during dreams as in wakefulness. While awake, pain and discomfort are the only languages of the body and the psyche; whereas in the dream state, there is an unlimited source of visual and emotional expressions that the *Hun* ≈ Ethereal soul can draw upon, based on personal or collective experiences.

According to the Jungian psychoanalytic school, all emotions, desires and the issues that the subject is dealing with in their daily life can be expressed without censure in a dream.

Energetic and physiological effects of dreams:

During REM sleep (dreaming), the body presents noticeable changes: for example, adrenaline levels rise, blood pressure and heartbeat increase. Actions and feelings in dreams produce electrochemical responses in the body. Most people have experienced waking up and feeling sick from a bad dream or feeling rejuvenated from a good dream. These biochemical changes affect the physical body, and can even help repair it. (Psychosomatic theory of dreams; Shinomiya et al. 1993)

As previously mentioned, Dr Candace Pert demonstrated the chemical interrelation between mind, behaviour, neuroendocrine and the immune systems in the form of neuropeptides. (Pert 1999). In her book "Molecules of emotion", Pert explains the interaction between the human physiology and the emotions. Pert works with dreams and believes that "dreams are direct messages from the body-mind combination, giving the subject valuable information about what is happening physiologically as well as emotionally.

One of the important functions of dreaming appears to be emotional processing, as described in Chinese medicine. Ideally, the best way to initiate change and achieve resolution is by consciously directing one's dream, defined as "lucid dreaming". However, other methods, such as hypnosis, biofeedback, various body-oriented therapies, acupuncture, and guided imagery, appear to trigger the same psychophysiological responses in a patient as during dreaming. In her inspiring article "Dreams: A creative Portal to Healing", Wendy Pannier states: "The limbic system speaks in the language of symbolic imagery: working with dream imagery in the waking state can help change perceptions and resolve conflicts, which are critical keys for mind-body healing." (Pannier 2007)

The place of dreams in modern Psychotherapy:

Fritz Perls (1893-1970), the founder of Gestalt therapy, (Price, 1985), inspired by the theories of Freud and Jung, believed that dreams contained the rejected and disowned parts of the self. Perls rejected the notion of a universal symbolic dream language, rather supporting the idea that each dream is unique to the individual who dreams it. According to Perls, each component of the dream is an aspect of the self. He further established a sort of dialogue in which the dreamer takes on different roles, interacting with the characters or objects of the dream, in order to acknowledge the feelings that had been overlooked or buried.

How to use dreams in therapy:

Since ages, in most traditions, both Eastern and Western, dreams have been considered to be a window into the inner world. In a therapeutic sense, this means that the patient's dreams may provide not only excellent indications as to the origins of their problems but also a means for them to get in touch with hidden aspects of their psyche.

In "Theory of Dreams" published in 1967, psychiatrist Vasily Kasatkin analysed the content of 10,240 dreams from 1,200 subjects over 40 years and made the following conclusions:

- Illness is associated with an increase in dream recall.

- Illness causes dreams to become distressful and nightmarish.

- These dreams generally appear before the first symptoms of the illness.

- Dreams caused by an illness are longer than distress dreams caused by ordinary annoyances and persist throughout the night and the duration of the illness

- The content of the dream can reveal the location and seriousness of the illness.

- (See also Excessive dreaming and Nightmares above).

- Amongst the various categories of dreams three types are particularly important to healing:

- Releasing dreams: during which the subject simply gets rid of the suppressed emotions by experiencing them in a dream scenario;

- Teaching dreams: the subject gets insights into their psycho-emotional patterns;

- Healing dreams: in which the mind regains the power to readjust or heal the body.

Imagery and visualisation

Numerous recent studies on the mind-body connection have demonstrated that imagery and visualisation have definite physiological responses in the body, very similar to the psycho-physiological changes brought about in dreams. (Pannier 2007).

According to Belleruth Naparstek (1995) the main operating principles of visualisation are the following:

- The body does not discriminate between sensory images in the mind and what is considered reality.

- In a relaxed, meditative state, the body is capable of more rapid and intense healing, growth, learning and change.

- Imagery and visualisation work help individuals feel better about themselves, due to a sense of mastery over what is happening to them. Those who are better able to believe that they can cope with problems tend to have better treatment outcomes.

However, visualisation practices have many limitations:

- When the subject is unable to relate to the imagery or to visualise situations;

- If the patient is unable to focus and concentrate;

- When a patient is fixated on the present state of their disease, rather than the desired outcome;

- If the subject is not able to involve all the senses;

- If the person is not able to feel the visualisation in the body;

- When the subject's belief system gives more credibility to the external reality than to the internal healing powers;

- When there is some form of resistance.

For a stronger impact, during a visualisation process, it is important to adapt the visualisation method by using symbols and images that had been previously described by the dreamer. The dream images usually have deep meanings for the subject, to which they can more easily relate to and accept without resistance.

The ideal dream therapy would thus enable the patient to engage in lucid dreaming (see below), during which the consciousness *Shen* would direct the *Hun* as to the content and the unravelling of the dream.

Lucid Dreaming:

Lucid or conscious dreaming is a dream state during which the dreamer is aware that he or she is dreaming, and can therefore, control the dream to a certain extent. In the lucid state, the subject is able to confront threats and, as a result, to become more self-confident and to overcome fears and anxiety. This state of lucidity can be used as a tool to improve skills, to prepare for upcoming challenges, to fulfil fantasies, or to solve problems. There are two types of lucid dreams:

- Dream-initiated lucid dream (DILD) starts as a normal dream during which the dreamer realises that it is a dream.

- Wake-initiated lucid dream (WILD) occurs when the dreamer goes from normal wakefulness directly into a dream state, with no apparent change in consciousness.

Lucid dreaming has been a subject of scientific research (Laberge 1990, Watnabe 2003):

Many aspects of brain activity during the dream state are the same as during waking. What is "learned" or "practised" in a lucid dream state is similar to the type of training and preparation underwent in the waking state.

At least half of all adults have had one lucid dream in their lifetime, and many have reported having lucid dreams without even trying (Snyder & Gackenbach, 1988)

Flying is often associated with lucid dreams. With practice, lucid dreaming can be learned and practised at will. *(La Berge & Levitan 1995)*

As C. Pert's research demonstrated, emotions impact the body's physiology (Pert *1999*). Therefore, transforming nightmarish images into positive, healing images can change the messages sent to the immune system. During dreams, one can bypass conscious resistance and the normal waking logic, to allow the "limbic system logic" to take over and change the image. As the limbic amygdala respond to perceptions, one can change the body's physiology by changing these perceptions.

"Dream Yoga" has been practised by Tibetan Buddhists since the 8th century AD. During Dream Yoga, full waking consciousness is maintained while in the dream state. (Mullin 1997)

Without regular practice, lucid dreaming is sporadic and not easy to enhance at will. From a practical point of view, this means that when a patient is unable to have lucid dreams, the therapist, based on the assessments made on the patient's dream imagery, can propose a combination of active visualisation and guided suggestions. The positive images then reinforce the messages sent to the amygdala, which in turn stimulate the body's healing process. (Colic 2007)

Dream analysis

In analysing dreams, one has to be careful not to rely on dream dictionaries and standardised interpretations. Each dream, like each person, is unique. Although some symbols may be universal, but depending on one's culture and conditioning, they do not always represent the same thing. For example, a dog means something different to someone who dislikes or even hates dogs than it does to someone who loves them. Thus, the personal associations with the subject of the dream, are much more meaningful than any information a dream dictionary might provide.

Otherwise, the presence of a dominant colour may indicate a Five Element disturbance as described by *Zhangjiebin,* as explored earlier (▶ Section 4.4.2).

Acquiring the ability to interpret dreams is a powerful tool for learning about deep secrets and hidden feelings.

When analysing dreams, every detail, even the most trivial symbol, can be significant and must be considered. Each symbol represents a feeling, a mood, a memory, or something from the unconscious. One should look closely at the characters, animals, objects, places, emotions, and even colours and numbers that are depicted in one's dreams. (see above)

Great care and discernment are required when referring to any system in which different body parts or different diseases are related to specific psycho-emotional patterns. The same care should be taken even when approaching Chinese Medicine. For example, a disease located in the lumbar or knee area relates to a Kidney disharmony pattern. As the Kidneys react to fear, it is sometimes assumed that a lumbar pain would signify the fear of change, and that knee pain would mean a fear of death. As every person is unique, every illness or symptom has a different significance. In "You can heal your life" by Louise Hay, a chapter is dedicated to the classification of physical problems, the body parts, the cause of a problem and providing new positive affirmations for healing. (Hay 1999). Such lists may actually prove quite limiting, leading to false beliefs about the cause and cure of a particular disease. They can easily mislead patients and deny them the opportunity to undergo their process of self-discovery.

Searching for the hidden roots of disease is getting involved with the patient's hidden processes, their personal feelings, and interpretations.

Integrating Dream-work into an Acupuncture session:

During the initial consultation, patients are instructed in how to increase their capacity to recall dreams and how to keep a dream journal:

- Self-suggestion in the morning and the afternoon: "I will remember my dreams at night"
- In the evening before going to sleep, the self-suggestion: "Soon dreams will be coming and I will remember them in the morning".
- It is useful to have on the bedside a pen and a writing pad.
- Keep a dated dream journal.
- When possible paint or draw some part of the dream image.

In follow-up sessions, after the acupuncture needles have been removed, the therapist helps patients into a guided fantasy. The theme of this fantasy is inspired by the most relevant dreams and patterns that patients have related.

The therapist aims to guide patients in exploring some of their issues more deeply, especially to replay scenes in a manner in which patients are empowered and can face and deal with the fears and dangers encountered in the dream.

The following points are important when doing this kind of work:

- The therapist should adopt a receptive rather than directive attitude, without making any judgements.

- Keep the integrity of the dream and the dreamer intact. A very useful sentence when making suggestions about the meaning of someone's dreams is: "If this were my dream or my creation...". This acknowledges that anything one says about someone else's dream or creation will be one's own projections.

- Focusing on what the patient is actually experiencing and feeling rather than on objective facts, general considerations, or symbolism. Keep a compassionate attitude without becoming emotionally involved. Not getting fixated on the specific problem allows the therapist to see the context from the patient's point of view.

- Respecting the patient with authenticity and understanding, without prejudice, judgement, solutions, and manipulation. Respecting the dream and the dreamer. The creator of the dream better understands the meaning of their dreams, and to remember that they have all the resources they need to overcome their issues.

- Respecting the limits that a patient might set.

- Facilitating clear and deferent communication. This means that the therapist should help the patient to understand the unconscious messages rather than interpreting them or providing ready-made solutions and advise. Patients know better than anyone what their problems are; the main mistake in trying to help is to believe that we understand what another person is telling us, when in fact we are interpreting or projecting our own ideas on to the situation.

- Heart-to-heart communication is very important in healing. Hence it is very important to maintain a relationship of sharing, respect and equality between patient and therapist.

PART - V
Psychology and acupuncture therapy (PAT)

- **Integrating Acupuncture and Psychology**
    - Searching for the Hidden Causes of Disease
    - Changing the beliefs and the hidden programs
    - Limits of Psychology and Acupuncture Therapy
    - Which medicine to choose from?
    - Practical advice about treatment

- **Psychology and acupuncture therapy (PAT)**
    - Releasing the retained traumatic memories
    - Dealing with emotional release

PART-V

Psychology and acupuncture therapy (PAT)

5.1 Integrating Acupuncture and Psychology

5.1.1 Searching for the Hidden causes of disease

The art of practicing any therapeutic method is to be able to hear, to understand and to search for the true causes of a patient's complaints.

Obviously, this issue is not relevant in acute conditions, *Biao* ≈ Surface diseases, sport injuries and physical traumas.

In TCM, most often a recurrent or chronic complaint is the outer manifestation of an energetic disbalance and hence termed the "Branch" or outer manifestation; the causative factor, the Five Substance and *Zang-Fu* disharmony is the "Knot". The true, often hidden condition which underlies the symptom is referred to as the "Root" (▶ Fig. 5.1). Once a TCM pattern has been diagnosed, a hidden cause, should always be suspected in the following conditions:

- Chronic and recurrent physical complaints: headaches, sleep problems, chronic fatigue, chronic skin pathologies, allergies, etc.

- Recurrent pathologies involving the same area or segment of the body: chest area with heart and respiratory problems; or the pelvic segment urinary tract and genital complaints, etc.

- Pain or other physical manifestations which are not explained by a clear causative factor, often classified as "idiopathic" by allopathic medicine: neck tension, gastritis, lumbar pains, unexplained referred pains, etc.

- And in particular all psycho-emotional issues and harmful lifestyle habits: overwork, lack of exercise, excessive food intake, smoking, drinking, addictions etc.

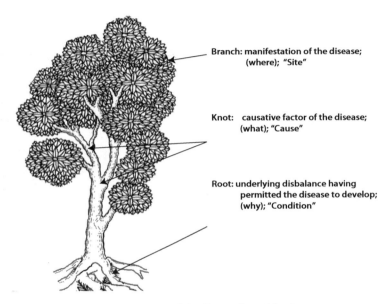

Branch: manifestation of the disease; (where); "Site"

Knot: causative factor of the disease; (what); "Cause"

Root: underlying disbalance having permitted the disease to develop; (why); "Condition"

Fig. 5.1:   Root-Knot-Branch in diagnosis and in therapy

Although at times the hidden cause of a disease might be considerably clear for the therapist, the challenge is to bring the patient to discover the underlying elements of their pathology.

Most often, patients are seeking acupuncture for physical pains or somatic dysfunctions; hence they might be quite reticent in exploring their psycho-emotional issues during the first sessions. It is only through artful and discreet questioning that we may attempt to bring a patient to focus on their psychological issues and repetitive harmful behaviours.

In psychology and acupuncture therapy, two conditions need to be fulfilled before a healing may happen; the patient has to be able to:

- Name their disease: this means shedding light on the dark side, the shadow or the *Gui* ≈ Ghost. In other words, bringing the causative factor from the unconscious into the conscious mind and giving it an identity.

- Own the disease: it is extremely important to recognise that a particular emotion or pain, although caused by an external event, actually is our own response to the outside and that it belongs to us. By owning the disease, the conscious mind is linking with, and accepting the subconscious, rather than rejecting it.

Important note: concerning both patient and therapist.

Owning a disease does not signify that "I am responsible for my pain"..., but rather the recognition that there is a "suffering that belongs to me"..., and not to seek a responsible factor or person on the outside.

At this stage, it is important for the therapist to demonstrate to the patient that their pain or disease is not necessarily bad; that on the contrary it is an indication of something in need of change, and it should be looked at as a stepping stone to healing rather than an obstacle to fight with.

> *Disease is a call for health*
>
> Master Jeffrey Yuen

A common error made by the patients who have understood that they themselves are the creators of their condition, is to assume that they can also undo the disease with their will power. In the *Wu Xing* ≈ Five Phases, the Water phase is about consolidation and concretisation, hence the problem with the *Zhi* ≈ Will, is to further consolidate the ego structure of the person, hence preventing any possible change from taking form.

Part of "owning the disease" is the acceptance that at this stage we need help, be it a higher power, God, a saint, the healer or even allopathic medicine. In fact, the placebo affect is the total trust that a person can allocate to a given healing, the more total the trust, the better the outcome. Hence the importance of seeking out and working on changing the patient's doubts about the healing method that they have chosen to follow.

5.1.2 Changing the beliefs and the hidden programs

The ultimate purpose of any therapy is to relieve the patient of their "dis-ease", in other words what is causing them physical or emotional suffering.

Although many therapeutic modalities may bring momentary symptom relief, it is only by addressing the deeper causes of the problem that a veritable cure may be expected. Aside from congenital defects, accidents and most external causes, the roots of disease are often hidden within the psyche, and constitute the individual's primary belief mechanisms.

The habitual behaviour of a person is a reflection of their belief systems. The "Cognitive Behavioural Therapy" (CBT), clearly describes the relation between emotions, thoughts and behaviour, as being the result of the human core beliefs (▶ Fig. 5.2).

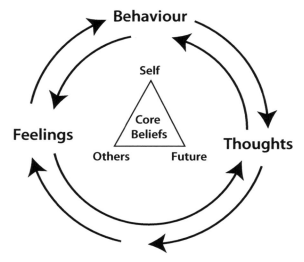

Fig. 5.2:   The Cognitive Behavioural Therapy (CBT) model

As we have explored in the previous chapters, these core beliefs or mental structures are the result of inheritance, conditioning and personal emotional history. Most of these emotional experiences are retained in the body in the form of Qi or Blood stasis, causing further energetic and organic disturbances. Obviously, simply treating the local stasis will not remove the initial causative factor. The mental structure, the belief mechanism, has to be also changed.

The classical psychotherapies or talking therapies, do not always manage to shed the light on the roots of the problem, which may lie buried deeply within the unconscious and not accessible to the conscious mind, in particular ancestral memories or pre-conscious experiences.

Combining acupuncture and energy work with a psychological approach has the potential of providing much faster results.

5.1.3 Limits of the Psychology and Acupuncture therapy

We cannot help everyone!

In the ever-accelerating world of ours, next to fast food and instant coffee, there is also a demand for instant results and instant relief. This explains that world-wide sales of pain-killers and anxiolytics are on top of the list of prescription drugs. Working with psychology and acupuncture therapy is a slow process which involves time and the patient's full collaboration.

Not every person is equipped with the necessary tools to examine the deeper causes of their condition. The naming, owning and changing of the belief systems cannot be applied in the following situations:

- Small children (although quite often changing the parent's perspective has a great impact on the child's behaviour).

- Patients with seriously unsettled or obstructed *Shen.*

- Subjects who cannot or do not wish to make the changes that their suffering is calling for. At times, there is too much fear of the hidden skeletons in the closet preventing the therapist to go any further.

- Individuals who refuse to adopt a new mental framework because their habitual belief system had served them well in the past. This is often the situation when treating patients who have a very strong will power, or have been dedicated to altruistic actions, or have accumulated a lot of information and knowledge about a particular issue, which may be the case when treating another therapist or a medical professional.

Please respect where the patient is at in relation to their life process. It is generally much easier to see what is wrong in another person than see our own shortcomings.

It is counterproductive to have a patient coming into our praxis with a pain and leaving with a burden of guilt, feeling that they are their own cause of suffering!

Our position, as therapists, should be to respond to a patient's complaint (symptoms) and to suggest some lifestyle changes. Only if the right questions are asked, should we attempt to open the door to the hidden roots of their disease, with great circumspection and humility, respecting the patient's limits and life-path.

Respect each individual process; with a piercing Shen concentrate on the patient, the pulses and the points;
part of nourishing life is embracing the good as well as the bad;
To understand this brings longevity...

Sun Si Miao as quoted by J. Yuen, Swiss lectures 2010

5.1.4 Which medicine to choose from?

Today, our patients are often faced with a major dilemma that is, which type of medicine to choose from? In the recent past, allopathic medicine with its great progress in surgery and synthetic pharmacology has been saving lives where older traditional methods were incapable of doing so. However, the price to pay for this rapid evolution is high. Although the general popular belief is still in favour of an all-knowing and omnipotent scientific medicine, the side effects and combined toxicity of chemicals, are taking their toll. It is very unfortunate that in most affluent societies, the "iatrogenic" causes of death are rapidly taking the second position after cardio-vascular factors.

Hence it becomes important to look at the problem differently, not as one approach versus another, but rather, which medicine or method is the most appropriate for a specific person and their condition in a given context. To put it simply, the question should be, who is it we are treating, rather than what are we treating.

For the sake of simplification, we could group all existing therapeutic modalities into three groups (▶ Fig. 5.3):

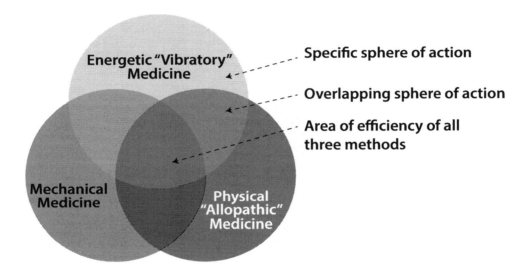

Specific sphere of action

Overlapping sphere of action

Area of efficiency of all three methods

Energetic "Vibratory" Medicine

Mechanical Medicine

Physical "Allopathic" Medicine

Fig. 5.3: Integrative Medicine: Allopathic, Mechanical and Vibrational

- Allopathic medicine, including pharmacology, surgery and radiation therapy.

- Mechanical medicine, including osteopathy, the variety of chiropractic methods, physical therapy, and the more traditional "bone setting" modalities.

- Vibrational medicine, which covers, acupuncture, traditional herbal medicine, homeopathy, Ayurveda, shamanic healing, sound therapy, chromotherapy, and scores of more recent methods.

Each of these groups of medicines has its specific sphere of action, overlapping with the other two. The question then would be: which is the most appropriate approach for the patient at that particular moment? It is obvious that when we break a leg, we seek a surgeon, not an acupuncturist or a bonesetter. But in the presence of a bacterial infection, are antibiotics the only solution? What are the consequences of an infection treated by softer methods that support the immune system of the person, versus the side effects a particular chemical compound that eradicates the infectious agent but decimates the intestinal flora, and further damages the liver and the kidneys? A particular infection might have catastrophic consequences in a small child or an elderly person, and greatly outweigh the side effects of the chemical drug; therefore, the allopathic treatment should be administered. The same infection in a robust and healthy adult could be treated quite differently, supporting the constitution to fight the pathogenic invasion. Understanding the reasons that allowed for the infectious agent to invade the system in the first place and correcting them, would be a more intelligent approach. Ideally in a better health system, patients should have access to all therapeutic modalities, and especially that the practitioners of each of the three medicines should be aware of the other two and may thus better advise the patient as to the best therapeutic modality to choose from. For best results, two or even three approaches may be combined.

The same questions may be asked when confronted with psycho-emotional conditions. What are the limits of psycho-energetic therapy? When should a patient be directed toward a psychiatric institution? Is acupuncture compatible with allopathic, pharmacological treatments?

It should be remembered at all times that a painkiller or an anti-depressant medication does not remove the cause of the disease, but just alleviate the symptoms.

5.1.5 Practical advice about Treatment

Session Frequency

In the West, we are unable to apply the same acupuncture treatment protocols as in China, where patients are often seen on a daily basis. Fortunately, by better adapting the choice of points to the patient rather than to a disease, similar results may be achieved with notably fewer sessions.

When in acute conditions, a daily treatment may be indicated, in chronic conditions, one session per week or even per month would be sufficient.

Number of points/ needles per session

"Less is better"

It is important to keep the number of points to a minimum, multiplying the number of needles not only dilutes the treatment and depletes the Qi of the patient, but also quite frequently puts the patient into unnecessary stress.

In the therapeutic principles, often several points have been indicated; of course, this does not signify that they should all be needled in the same session!

The best and most appropriate points, based on anamnesis and patient typology, has to be chosen, with the option of trying different ones in the follow-up treatments.

By no means should all the indicated points be done in the same session

- Keep the total number of points below 10; even less for children or for the exhausted or the aged patients. When possible, for the elderly, replace the needle with Moxibustion.

- In acute conditions, privilege the distal points, in chronic conditions select from local, proximal and distal.

- Do not treat more than three channels in one session (i.e. HE and KI belong to *Shao Yin* and will be considered as one channel; or SP-4 and PE-6 open the *Chong Mai*, therefore also considered the same channel).

- Do not treat the Extraordinary channels more than once a week.

- **And most importantly, treat the patient and not the symptom or the disease!**

Important notes: It is often quite helpful to give a simplistic indication to the patient as to what a particular acupuncture point or treatment is supposed to do, for example, this point will help you calm down..., or this point will help you sleep deeper..., or this is called the "happy point"..., or this point will help you remember..., etc. Otherwise a simple explanation as to the expected outcome of a treatment, such as: this treatment is aimed at reconnecting you with your body..., or helping to centre you... etc. By doing so, the intention of both therapist and patient are focused on the same issue.

It is also very important for the patient to take stock of their condition, before and after the treatment. A simple method of scoring could be utilised. For example, before and after the treatment, evaluate the intensity of the pain on a scale of 1 to 10. For emotions and mental conditions, the same method could be applied. In case a condition is not present at that moment, for example the stress of passing an exam, the patient may be directed to imagining the stressful situation and scoring it in the same manner.

Treating children

Children respond amazingly fast to treatments. With the exception of inherited conditions, treating children is very easy, providing we respect the delicacy of their constitution.

- Infants and small children have a weak Spleen Qi, therefore very sensitive to dietary factors

- The Kidney Qi is not firm before puberty and has to be protected (avoid points affecting Kidney *Jing* such as DM-4 *Mingmen*)

- The weak Spleen Qi and Kidney Yang is the cause of a weakened *Wei* ≈ Defensive energy and propensity to contracting External Pathogenic Factors (EPF). The usual allopathic treatments (antibiotics), further contribute to the aggravation of Spleen Qi Vacuity.

- Children are quite prone to "Retained Pathogenic Factors", manifesting as recurrent conditions, infections and allergies. The causes could be due to the weakened *Wei Qi* as discussed above, wrong diet, the possibility of in-utero transfer of toxic Heat from the mother, as well as excessive and early immunisation of infants.

Since over thirty years, we have been treating children with a "soft", 40mW Infrared Laser. The results are the same if not even better than with needles, as children are more relaxed and we do not have the habitual stressful relation of Doctor and child.

5.2 Psychology and Acupuncture Therapy (PAT)

In treating mental and emotional disorders, there is no standard protocol. The variety of tools described in the previous chapters should be adapted to each case. In general, the following situation may be encountered in our daily practice:

- Emotional issues:

  - Temporary emotional event due to a specific factor: sadness and grief; frustration, irritability and anger; fear and anxiety; worry… Consider using the *Luo* ≈ Connecting vessels and the "Five *Zhi*" points on the back.

  - Habitual emotions: a tendency to worry, be fearful; irritable… Consider harmonising the "Six Temperaments" and the Extraordinary Vessels

- Traumatic shocks:

  - PTSD: concerning a known traumatic event

  - Suppressed traumatic experiences

  - Hidden trauma: this could involve early childhood, birth or foetal trauma, or ancestral transmitted trauma

- Personality disorders and neurosis: will combine some of the above therapeutic approaches with standard TCM acupuncture therapy

- Psychotic conditions: it is not recommended to take-on psychotic patients in a normal acupuncture setting; these conditions should be treated in a specialised institution.

When a retained emotion or trauma is suspected to have been the cause of a distorted and harmful belief mechanism, the same procedure should be applied as when treating a residual pathogenic factor with acupuncture or herbs, that is:

- First dispel the pathogen

- Then rectify the substances (Qi-Blood...)

Applied to psychological treatments, this signifies:

- Releasing a retained or suppressed traumatic memory

- Helping to re-structure the subject's harmful beliefs and restoring their sovereignty

5.2.1 Releasing the retained traumatic memories

Some traumatic memories are readily accessible to the conscious mind; other memories might have been suppressed or deeply buried.

Some traumatic events may have occurred before the development of the brain's limbic structures and will be embedded in the body in the form of body memories or "Body Armours". In some cases, the trauma might even be epigenetically transferred down several generations, before manifesting itself.

For each of the above cases, a different therapeutic approach is called for.

Important note: Working with Psychology and Acupuncture Therapy (PAT), patient collaboration is fundamental. The patient needs to be committed and to regularly practice the exercises that have been recommended. This point has to be stressed at the onset of therapy. Many patients have become accustomed to bringing their ailments to the therapist, in the same way, that one would take their car to the mechanic to be "fixed". Hence, the therapist has to establish an atmosphere of collaboration, sharing and trust, before attempting to unravel a patient's intimate life-history.

Releasing a traumatic event, especially when the memory has been deeply suppressed, may produce a strong reaction. This reaction may occur during the session or later. See under 5.2.2 how to deal with these situations.

For this reason, it is recommended to always start the therapeutic process by centring and rooting the patient.

- Reconnecting the subject with the "Central Axis" and "Pre- and Post-Heaven" energies: SP-4 *Gongsun* (unilateral); PE-6 *Neiguan*; RM-4 *Guanyuan;* RM-12 *Zhongwan*; RM-17 *Shanzhong; Yintang* and DM-20 *Baihui.*

Explanation: The *Chong Mai* is supporting the Central Axis, which is about rooting the person in their correct position between Heaven and Earth to enhance stability (▶ see further explanation A.4.5.1). The role of *Ren* and *Du Mai* is to help connect the Pre- and Post-Heaven energies, the three Heaters, and the three *Dan Tian* transformational centres. It is recommended to have the subject practice daily the centring exercise before the follow-up session (▶ see section A.4.1).

- The interval between the first and second session depends on the degree of psychological distress. For deep grief and depression, if we suspect that there is a loss of will to live (suicidal tendency), the patient should be treated a few days later with BL-23 *Shenshu* and BL-52 *Zhishi* and BL-44 *Shentang* (supplement all Points); or if there is a loss of passion for life (wanting to die): treat RM-14 *Jiuwei* (supplement) and ST-23 *Taiyi*. It is very important to change the patient's mental frame-work and to find an alternative vision and instigate the life impulse. If after the session, there has been no apparent change in their outlook, it is recommended to direct the patient to a specialist or a specialised institution.

Explanation: The will to live is an attribute of *Zhi*, residing in the Kidney. The passion for life is related to *Shen*; the *Mo* of Heart RM-14, will strengthen this aspect; ST-23 *Taiyi*, helps in re-connecting the Fire-centre with the rest of the body. This point combination, although very simple, is in fact very powerful, and it is not recommended to add any other points.

- In the following session (having eliminated a suicidal tendency), to help release any retained trauma: ST-14 *Kufang* (reduce), stimulate HE-3 *Shaohai* and BL-62 *Shenmai*.

Explanation: *Kufang* as storehouse retains all traumatic events; the Heart's *He* ≈ Sea point helps bring out the memory; the *Yangqiao* helps to see (introspection). It is very important to have the subject write down later any dreams or memories that may surface.

- Consecutive sessions: Repeat *Chong Mai* for all suspected trauma, concerning the gestational period, birth trauma, or early infancy period. SP-4 *Gongsun*; PE-6 *Neiguan*, KI-9 *Zhubin* and DM-20 *Baihui;*

    - For birth trauma: add KI-16 *Huangshu* and RM-6 *Qihai*;

    - For gestational trauma: add RM-1 *Huiyin*, RM-4 *Guanyuan*;

    - For post-natal trauma: add KI-16 *Huangshu*, BL-43 *Gaohuangshu*, BL-51 *Huangmen*;

This treatment may be repeated the following week. During the sessions, a body-oriented guided fantasy may be initiated (▶ A.4.2 / step 4 and A.4.6.3).

Explanation: Pre-heaven trauma (ancestral, constitutional and gestational events) as well as birth trauma and the post-natal period, have a great impact on the psychological construct of the individual. The *Chong Mai* helps to release these retained memories. Quite often one or several Body Armours are also involved, their treatment may be combined with the above points. Specific exercises are given to the patient to perform daily, to help accelerate the releasing process.

- Treat *Dai Mai*: for suppressed traumatic events, particularly involving child abuse and violence: GB-41 *Zulinqi*, TW-5 *Waiguan*, GB-26 *Daimai* or GB-27 *Wushu* or GB-28 *Weidao*.

Explanation: The Belt vessel ≈ *Dai Mai*, is where a person holds traumatic events that could not be dealt with when they initially occurred, hence its name the "Vessel of Latency".

- Treat *Ren* and *Du Mai* for issues with bonding, control and protection during the first years. LU-7 *Lieque*, KI-6 *Zhaohai*, RM-12 *Zhongwan* and RM-1 *Huiyin;* SI-3 *Houxi*, BL-62 *Shenmai*, and DM-20 *Baihui*

Explanation: As described earlier, both the lack or an exaggerated bonding, care and protection, are experienced by the infant as stressful, with deep psychological and compensation issues later in life. Regulating and re-harmonising the *Ren* and *Du* constitute an important phase in constitutional therapy. Combining the "Infinity" protocol, starting with SI-3 on the left for men, followed by BL-62 on the opposite side, then KI-6 (left), followed by LU-7 (right). For women start with LU-7 on the right, KI-6 on the opposite side, BL-62 (right) and SI-3 (left), add RM-12 and DM-20 (pre- and post-Heaven Qi).

- Consider *Yin* and *Yang Wei Mai* and *Yin* and *Yang Qiao Mai* for traumatic events during transitional periods of life: PE-6 *Neiguan*, SP-4 *Gongsun,* KI-9 *Zhubin*; TW-5 *Waiguan,* GB-41 *Zulinqi,* and BL-63 *Jinmen.*

Explanation: The *Wei* and the *Qiao* regulate the physical and mental development of the individual according to specific cycles, symbolically referred to as the cycles of 7 and 8. Certain recurrent physical ailments or difficulties with life transitions may reflect on the disturbances of these vessels (the Seven Gates page…). Aside from the presence of characteristic psycho-emotional patterns, the palpation of the four *Xi* ≈ Cleft points (KI-9 *Zhubin*; KI-8 *Jiaoxin*; BL-59 *Fuyang*; GB-35 *Yangjiao*), is of great diagnostic support.

- The identification and the release of body memories constitutes an important stage in "releasing therapy". The affected Body Armour may be identified by the supplied questionnaire and the presence of physical symptoms (▶ see section 4.1). The treatment will combine acupuncture with visualisation work and specific personal exercises. (▶ see section A.4.1). For a stronger impact, releasing the Body Armours is often combined with the Extraordinary Vessels.

Explanation: Almost all early or repeated traumatic events will be retained by the *Jing Jin* ≈ Sinew channels and will get organised into a local protective armouring. Although the *Chong Mai* deals with these early issues in general, most Body Armours may benefit from the regulation of the other Extraordinary vessels, which are chosen either based on anatomical or symptomatic consideration. For example, *Dai* for the pelvic issues or for a fearful and indecisive personality; *Du* for spinal problems and a weak character; *Yin Qiao* for throat problems and expression etc. (▶ see section 2.1)

- For certain neurotic conditions the releasing of *Gui* may be indicated (see under pathologies): choose from the following protocols:

  - *Sunsimiao* 13 Ghost points: for psychotic behaviours

  - Worsley 7 Internal Dragons: for feelings of having two wills, something inside making one do things…

  - Worsley External Dragons: a feeling of something lurking around…

Explanation: There is very little information in the classical texts concerning the release of *Gui*, although the concept is very relevant to modern psychotherapy. When the indication is appropriate, I have found both protocols extremely efficient, although the 7 Dragons is easier to apply, the 13 Ghost points has the greater advantage of having very specific mental and psychological indications.

- Working with dreams is an important stage of therapy; dream-work not only helps identify the psychological issues but also it is an excellent monitor for the therapeutic progress. (▶ Section 4.5 and Appendix-IV)

Explanation: As discussed earlier, *Hun* ≈ Etheric soul attempts to release the hidden and suppressed traumas and emotions through dreams. The interpretation and significance of dreams for the patient are of great importance, allowing them to get in touch with the suppressed parts of their psyche and to acknowledge and to name them. With some training, the patients can start remembering their dreams. The acupuncture treatments may further be geared to the dream scenario. (▶ see Section 4.5)

- Emotional release with the *Luo* points (▶ see Section 2.3)

Explanation: *Luo* ≈ Connecting vessels are not only indicated for releasing retained emotions, but they are also extremely important in the management of temperaments and behaviours. (see page…)

- Emotional release with the Five *Zhi* points (▶ see Section 1.1)

Explanation: This is an important diagnostic as well as the therapeutic stage of the releasing phase. The palpation of the outer branch of the *Zutaiyang*-Bladder channel will reveal tension areas or even lumps or nodules, which are felt subjectively as painful by the patient. Aside from the five "Will" or "Spirit" points (*Shen, Po, Hun, Yi* and *Zhi*), BL-43 *Gaohuangshu*; BL-45 *Yixi*; BL-51 *Huangmen* and BL-53 *Baohuang*; also have important diagnostic significances. (see chapter…) The painful and reactive points should be needled with a reducing (dispersing) technique. This reduction should be repeated until the point is no more manifesting a state of repletion.

- Additional points for helping remember and speak about a trauma:
    - PE-6 *Neiguan*: memory enhancing
    - HE-5 *Tongli*: helps to speak about traumatic events
    - LU-7 *Lieque*: helps to let go
    - PE-4 *Ximen*: helps to remember
    - KI-21 *Youmen*: helps to bring out memories from the sub-conscious
    - RM-17 *Shanzhong*: helps to express
    - DM-10 *Lingtai*: difficulty with introspection
    - BL-62 *Shenmai*: introspection
    - SP-2 *Dadu*: lack of concentration and synthesis

5.2.2 Dealing with emotional release

Traumatic memories that have been retained in the body or the subconscious, often manifest in the physical body as localised tension or even muscular knots and pain. These muscular knots are present either in an area corresponding to the Body Armour, or a specific point in relation to a particular emotion (back *Zhi* or *Luo* points, etc.) or again on the trajectory of the *Luo* channel. The palpation of these areas is frequently painful and helps in orienting the diagnosis and especially in consciously connecting the patient with that particular body-part. It is recommended to massage the point before needling it. Most traditions needle these muscle knots directly, although Dr Wang Ju-Yi advises to needle next to the nodule.

An emotional release may occur during the session or later.

Emotional release during an acupuncture treatment:

For most acupuncture treatments, after the needles have been inserted, the patient is usually left alone for the necessary duration of time. But for treating psycho-emotional issues, it is very important to remain with the patient and help and accompany them during their process.

Frequently emotional release may occur during a session manifesting with:

- Tears: establish a dialogue with the patient; it is important that they identify and "name" what is coming up. Reassuring the patient that what is happening is very positive and not to suppress the feelings.

- Fear or anxiety: having the patient breath into their lower abdomen, or counting their breath, helps to settle these emotions.

- Very rarely a stronger cathartic reaction, such as anger or a panic attack, may occur. Holding or pressing KI-1 *Yongquan* while having the patient breath slowly down to the lower belly helps to settle the mind.

Emotional release after an acupuncture treatment

It is very important to explain to the patient that any feelings, emotions or dreams that might come up, are extremely crucial and should be noted down, so that they may be explored during the next session. Reminding them, not to transfer their negative feelings onto their family members, but rather share it with them, for example: …please don't take it personally, but this treatment has brought up a lot of rage in me which has nothing to do with you…., please be patient with me for the next few days…, just help me and forgive me…

When a condition of Liver-Heat or Liver-Qi stagnation has been diagnosed, the releasing treatments may bring up a lot of frustration and anger that may prove to be socially inappropriate. Patients need to be instructed as how to release this energy by channelling it into regular exercise, sports or dancing;

although later this energy could also be transferred into creativity and art, but not at this early stage.

To fully involve the patient in their therapeutic process, it is important to have them keep a diary, and especially to write down any memories and souvenirs that come up, in full detail.

5.2.3 Restructuring the Psyche

Constitution and Temperament are the basis for the belief mechanisms. Traumatic events do not necessarily produce the same psychological issues and personality disorders in every subject. The traumatic impact mainly depends on the temperament of the individual. Based on their constitution, some subjects manage to handle stressful situations better than others. Individuals that can better adapt their behaviour to a given situation will experience less the stress of a traumatic event.

When the behaviour is repetitive and not flexible, it will automatically lead to psychological and emotional distress due to a lack of adaptability to outer changes.

In restructuring the psyche, it is important to give the person the full access to their psycho-emotional potential:

- Supplementing and re-connecting the temperament with its complementary level. An evaluation of the person's temperament during one of the initial sessions (see questionnaire), helps in orienting the follow-up treatments and especially the best choice of the acupuncture points (see chapter…). After the initial releasing steps, reconnecting the temperament helps to change the behaviour and give the person more options and flexibility.

- Changing the beliefs by positive affirmations through a mind and body integration process: This helps in seeing oneself liberated from a physical or psychological burden. The purpose of the self-treatments and exercises described in sections A.4.1 through A.4.6 is to integrate certain body sensations and specific acupuncture point stimulations, with mental affirmations to help replace a limiting belief with a new self-empowering counter-belief. The stimulation of specific points and certain body segments assists in disconnecting retained disruptive body memories (*Po*) and subconscious beliefs, words or concepts (*Hun*), and supplanting these mindsets with positive affirmations, similar to an antidote.

- Guided fantasy; changing the story (the memory): ideally, this process is conducted during each acupuncture session. Certain points can help this process:

  - GB-20 *Fengchi*, DM-16 *Fengfu*: for changing of beliefs.

- BL-1 *Jingming*; GB-14 *Yangbai*, and *Yintang*: for changing the vision.

- GB-13 *Benshen*, DM-24 *Shenting*: help to let go of fixed ideas and assumptions

- GB-18 *Chengling* and DM-20 *Baihui*: for assuming one's spirituality

- At all times the *Yin* and *Yang Qiao* are important to consider concerning how the subject sees or relates to themselves or the outer world.

- TW-18 *Qimai*: fear of change

- BL-52 *Zhishi*: fear of the future, fear of life

• To further consolidate the character of the person the "Will" or "Spirit" points (*Shen, Po, Hun, Yi* and *Zhi*), would now be supplemented. In general BL-23 *Shenshu* and BL-52 *Zhishi*, are added to the treatment. For example, a patient manifesting a weak *Hun* (shyness, indecisiveness, lack of direction in life....), the treatment will include BL-18 *Ganshu*; BL-47 *Hunmen*; as well as BL-23 *Shenshu* and BL-52 *Zhishe*.

• During a traumatic event, when the *Shen* was disconnected (no memory of the trauma), there is a loss of communication between the fore-brain and the limbic structures. The restructuring of the psyche should also include establishing the communication between the pre-frontal cortex and the limbic areas as well as the left (logical) brain with the right (emotional) brain:

- DM-24 *Shenting and* GB-13 *Benshen* with DM-17 *Naohu*, GB-18 *Chengling* and DM-20 *Baihui*: for connecting the fore-brain and the mid-brain

- SP-21 *Dabao* and *Yin* and *Yang Qiao* (infinity method: KI-6 *Zhaohai* => LU-7 *Lieque* => SI-3 *Houshi* => BL-62 *Shenmai*) with DM-20 *Baihui*: for connecting the right and left hemispheres. Some exercises that the patient may perform daily are extremely beneficial (► see A.4.5.5).

PART - VI
Common Psychological issues

- **Depression**
    - TCM patterns
    - Treatment strategies for Depression

- **Sadness and Grief**
    - TCM patterns
    - Treatment strategies for Grief

- **Stress and Anxiety**
    - TCM patterns in Stress and Anxiety
    - Treatment strategies for Stress and Anxiety
    - Management of Panic attacks
    - Post-traumatic Stress Disorder (PTSD)
    - Burn-out syndrome

- **Insomnia**
    - Sleep in Chinese medicine
    - Diagnosis of Insomnia
    - Treatment strategies for Insomnia
    - Other sleep disturbances

- **Addictions and Compensation issues**
    - Co-dependence
    - Addictions
    - Eating disorders: Anorexia; Bulimia; Orthorexia

- **Bipolar disorders**

- **Memory and Attention**
    - Amnesia
    - Attention Deficit Hyperactivity Disorder (ADHD)

- **Autism/ Autism spectrum disorder (Asperger syndrome)**

- **Tourette's syndrome**

- **Personality disorders**
    - Split personality or Dissociative Identity disorder (DID)
    - Avoidant Personality disorder
    - Obsessive-compulsive disorder (OCD)
    - Paranoid Personality disorder (PPD)
    - Histrionic Personality disorder (HPD)
    - Narcissistic Personality disorder (NPD)
    - Passive-aggressive Personality disorder
    - Schizophreniform disorder

Part-VI

Common Psychological issues

6.1 Depression

Depression is medically defined as a mental condition characterised by a state of low mood, of hopelessness and inadequacy accompanied by an aversion to activity, a loss of motivation and interest in life, which may consequently lead to suicidal thoughts. Depressive states affect a person's thinking ability, with difficulty in concentration and of creative thought, as well as changing their outlook on life, and consequently their behaviour. The depressive state may also include sadness, an increased desire for sleeping, and reduced or increased desire for food. It is by far the most frequent psychological complaint worldwide, affecting by predilection women, young people and the elderly.

In Chinese medicine, all of the above mental and physical manifestations are found under the heading of "Qi vacuity/ deficiency". Therefor the depressive state may accompany each organic Qi vacuity, to a higher or lesser degree.

In TCM, the depressive condition is referred to as *Yu Zheng* 郁证, although certain depressive aspects may also be found in the following psychological conditions: Lilium syndrome *Baihe Bing* 百合病, Plum-stone syndrome (globus hystericus) *Mei He Qi* 梅核气, or in the depressive phase of a bipolar condition: *Dian* 癫; or in some more agitated conditions: *Zang Zao* 脏燥.

Causes of Depression:

- Sadness and grief, usually due to loss, qualified as "true depression" (see further)
- Qi-vacuity due to life-style (over activity; lack of rest, chronic insomnia; diet...), sickness or ageing
- Qi-stagnation, "false depression" due to repressed feelings and frustrations

Differential diagnosis:

- In Qi deficient patterns of depression, the subject feels worse after effort, better with rest. The pulses are Weak or Empty.

- In Qi stagnation, the patient feels much better after effort or exercise; the pulses are Wiry.

- It is very important to clearly establish the causative emotion: sadness through loss, sadness through fear of death, loss of self-esteem, feelings of guilt and shame, or suppressed anger. Obviously, the treatment strategy is not the same.

6.1.1 TCM patterns in Depression

Heart and Lung-Qi Xu: True Sadness affecting the HE and LU

Symptoms:

- Sadness and tears; depression
- Superficial sleep, insomnia from anxiety
- Asthenia, easily tired and the need to rest
- No desire to move or to speak
- Palpitations; shortness of breath
- Spontaneous sweating

Heart and Spleen-Qi Xu

Symptoms are the same as above, with:

- Extreme lassitude; feeling of heavy limbs
- Loss of appetite
- Bloating and soft stools

Heart-Blood Xu

Symptoms:

- Sadness, sudden tears, over sensitivity; dysphoria (general dissatisfaction with life); shyness
- Absent-minded, poor memory; trembling with emotion
- Palpitations, dizziness, blurred vision; fatigue

Heart-Yin Xu

Symptoms:

- Anxiety and fear; sadness and melancholia; weak character, shyness; misanthropic tendency
- Agitation, insomnia; restless sleep
- Five-Heart Heat; thirst

Heart and Kidney Yang Xu

Symptoms:

- Depression; anxiety and fear, easily startled; sadness and melancholia; weak and introverted character, shyness and indecisiveness; misanthropic tendency; cold with emotions
- Superficial sleep, insomnia from anxiety

Phlegm misting the Heart

Symptoms:

- Mental confusion, lack of concentration, disorientation; emotional numbness; apathy
- If more severe: psychosis, mania dementia or coma
- Reduced sensory functions

Liver Qi stagnation

Symptoms:

- Feeling stressed, frustrated, moody, depressed (false depression)
- Chest oppression and flank pains; premenstrual pain and tension; neck and shoulder tension; plum pit feeling in the throat
- Irregular periods and bowel movements

Liver-Fire

Symptoms:

- Irritability and anger, envy, jealousy; hysteria; false depression
- Restless sleep, nightmares, insomnia between 1-3 am, waking early
- Headaches, red eyes

6.1.2 Treatment strategies for Depression

Please adapt the following treatment strategies to the TCM pattern and the causative factor (▶ see A.1.1 and A.4)

Yin temperaments are more prone to depressive patterns: *Taiyin; Jueyin* and *Shaoyin*.

Do not use more than ten points (needles) per session.

Start with two sessions weekly, then once a week. Usually, results may be expected after 6-8 sessions, otherwise examine and work with the belief mechanisms (▶ see A.4)

If a suicidal tendency is suspected, always start with RM-14 *Juque* with ST-23 *Taiyi*; the follow-up acupuncture treatments should preferably be done in collaboration with appropriate psychiatric support.

- Supplement Shen: He-7 Shenmen, BL-44 *Shentang*, KI-25 *Shencang*, RM-17 *Shanzhong*, RM-15 *Jiuwei*, BL-15 *Xinshu*, DM-11 *Shendao*, also HE-3 *Shaohai*, ST-36 *Zusanli* and DM-20 *Baihui*

- Release the retained emotion
  - Sadness: BL-42 *Pohu*, LU-7 *Lieque*, LI-6 *Pianli*, KI-24 *Lingxu*, KI-21 *Youmen*,
  - Deception, rejection, loss of self-esteem: BL-43 *Gaohuangshu*
  - Fear, fear of death, fear of change: BL-52 *Zhishi*, KI-8 *Jiaoxin*
  - Severe depression: add BL-23 *Shenshu*, BL-52 *Zhishi*, BL-47 *Hunmen*
  - Loss of desire to live: RM-14 *Juque* with ST-23 *Taiyi*
  - Loss of will to live, death thoughts: BL-23 *Shenshu*, BL-52 *Zhishi*, BL-44 *Shentang*

- Supplement Qi: RM-6 *Qihai,* ST-36 *Zusanli*

- Raise the Qi: SP-4 *Gongsun,* DM-20 *Baihui*; also, the *Jingbie* of ST and SP to raise the clear Yang: ST-30 *Qichong*, SP-12 *Chongmen*, RM-12 *Zhongwan*, ST-9 *Renying* and DM-20 *Baihui*

- Supplement HE-Qi, LU-Qi, SP-Qi, KI-Qi ... (according to the pattern; (▶ see A.1.1)

- Clear Phlegm: PE-5 *Jianshi*, ST-40 *Fenglong*; DM-20 *Baihui*; ST-8 *Diji,* DM-18 *Qiangjiang*; also, the *Jingbie* of ST and SP (see above)

- Move Qi: LR-3 *Taichong,* LI-4 *Hegu*, LR-14 *Qimen*, PE-6 *Neiguan*

- Open the chest: (see below)

6.2 Sadness and Grief

Deep sadness, grief and mourning are the main causes of depression. In the management of depressive states, it becomes imperative to clear out this emotion.

In Chinese many terms designate the states of sadness:

- "*Bei*" 悲: Sadness, sorrow, grief, mourning, misery
- "*Ai Si*" 哀思: Grief, deep sorrow, mourning
- "*Sang*" 喪: funeral, mourning
- "*Tong Ku*" 痛苦: anguish
- "*You*" 憂: oppression
- "Hui" 悔: regret

The causes of sadness and grief are quite varied and would necessitate a different therapeutic approach:

- Loss, mainly through death
- Loss of a relationship; separation
- Loss of a job or social position (redundancy, retirement)
- Ageing; menopause
- Personal health issues (cancer…)
- Loss of any particular attachment (pet, object, or a particular situation)
- Regrets (also shame)

Consequences: prolonged sadness and grief are mainly harmful to the Lung:

- Blocking the Qi in the chest affecting the circulation of *Ying* ≈ Nourishing and *Wei* ≈ Defensive Qi: shortness of breath; oppression; weak voice, tiredness;
- Reduced *Wei Qi*: loss of instinct of preservation
- Affecting the Heart Qi (deficiency and stagnation); loss of joy; lack of communication
- Depression
- Heat in the chest due to Qi stasis: drying the fluids but also destroying Yang-Qi

- Qi stagnation in the chest may lead to tumours or breast lumps in women
- In women grief may cause Liver Blood-Xu
- Sadness and Grief may affect the Liver and the *Hun*:
  - Confusion
  - Aimlessness and loss of direction in life
  - Inability to make choices
- Unexpressed sadness (loss of joy) may affect the Kidneys
  - Loss of will to live: suicidal tendencies
  - Disturbed Water metabolism
- Produces a Short or Weak pulse in both *cun* positions

6.2.1 TCM patterns in grief

- Heart and Lung Qi *Xu* (see above)
- Heart Yin or Blood Xu (see above)
- Liver-Fire (see above)

6.2.2 Treatment strategies for grief

Please consider the same therapeutic indications as described for depression (▶6.1.2).

- Release Sadness: BL-42 *Pohu,* LU-7 *Lieque,* LI-6 *Pianli,* RM-17 *Shanzhong,* KI-24 *Lingxu,* KI-21 *Youmen,* LU-3 *Tianfu*
- Open the chest: RM-17 *Shanzhong,* RM-15 *Jiuwei,* RM-22 *Tiantu,* KI-25 *Shencang,* BL-43 *Gaohuangshu,* BL-17 *Geshu,* BL-46 *Geguan,* PE-6 *Neiguan*
- Treat depression: see above + supplement LU-Qi
- Severe grief, suicidal tendencies: RM-14 *Juque* with ST-23 *Taiyi*; BL-44 *Shentang* with BL-23 *Shenshu,* BL-52 *Zhishi*; or BL-13 *Feishu,* BL-42 *Pohu* and DM-12 *Shenzhu*
- Loss of job or separation: add BL-43 *Gaohuangshu*; BL-47 *Hunmen*; KI-26 *Yuzhong*
- Regrets: KI-24 *Lingxu*; LU-7 *Lieque*
- Importance of the "Cultivation of the mind": acceptance and letting go = forgiveness (self and others); see exercise on forgiveness in Annex page…

- To help let go of a shameful or guilty feeling: LU-7 *Lie Que;* KI-24 *Ling Xu;* HE-4 *Ling Dao*

- To help let go of retained emotions, sorrow and regret: PE-6 *Neiguan;* KI-9 *Zhubin;* RM-17 *Shanzhong*

Importance of observing cultural customs and ceremonies; tears; expressing the pain.

6.2.3 Dealing with Death and Dying

Fear of death is probably the first emotion experienced by the human being at birth. Rooted in the instinct of survival and genetically transferred, it involves the *Po* and the "Survival instinct", *Shen* and the "Passion for life" and *Zhi* the "Will to live".

Fearing death is as inevitable as dying itself, although its intensity and impact greatly depend on cultural and particularly on religious and spiritual beliefs.

Believing in reincarnation and life after death greatly attenuates this fear. In the Buddhist tradition, dying is like going to sleep, with the difference that upon waking up, one assumes a whole new identity.

Obviously, in cultures that believe this life to be finite, death is considered a great tragedy.

In our Western Judeo-Christian societies, the topic of death is taboo. We give our children a great amount of knowledge to prepare them for active life, but nothing about death. So, when the time is up for them or their loved ones, naturally they have no preparation for this final voyage.

The fear of death is in fact the fear of the unknown, and it probably constitutes the biggest obstacle that prevents many humans from living their lives fully.

As therapists, we come up against the fear of death and disease in our patients on a daily basis. It is important to understand and to be able to help them at the various stages of their emotional evolution. When faced with a terminal disease for oneself or a family member, there are a number of common emotional reactions. For example, taking the Kübler-Ross model:

- Denial: no, it is not true, they made a mistake; this is simply not possible...

- Anger: at oneself for causing the condition or at society or at god; guilt or blame...

- Bargaining: usually with the higher powers, I will do this... if you save me...

- Depression: it is hopeless; what is the point of going on?; I am doomed...

- Acceptance: dissolution of fear, the welcoming of the disease and of death; "thy will be done"...

In practice, patients do not experience the above phases in the same order, for example, the first reaction upon being diagnosed with a fatal disease could be depression, then bargaining, leading to anger when the dealing with superior powers did not bring the expected results etc...

The acceptance phase may take many forms. Some patients might never manage to attain this acceptance and simply sink deeper into despair, or revolt by stopping all treatment, or outright rage, expressing this anger to their family and the medical staff. Some even decide to shorten the suffering by choosing suicide.

Our role as therapists, is to help the patient go through the above stages as smoothly as possible. Obviously, the patient seeks and even demands to be cured of their condition, which is not always possible, but at least accepting this fact, brings a state of peace to the terminally ill patient.

Preparing for Death

Aside from the imminence of death in terminally ill patients or in extreme life-threatening situations of natural catastrophes or war, we all need to face our mortality at some stage of our lives and to come to terms with it.

In the same manner that the Eight Extraordinary Vessels organise the various physical transformational stages of life, they also coordinate the mental and spiritual evolutions of the individual.

These changes are reflected in the natural ageing process. At the start, the totality of the human energy is directed towards the growth and the construction of the body according to a pre-established plan. At puberty, the Kidney-Fire via the Fire-minister ≈ *Xin Bao*, directs the energy towards the outer world, primarily reproduction, followed by worldly pursuits and passions. By the middle ages, the Kidney-*Jing* starts waning, the outer-world should normally lose its impact and the *Shen* ≈ Emperor should start moving from its "Earthly" palace to its "Heavenly" residence. This signifies that by following the natural rhythms and life seasons, the human beings should direct their energies toward spiritual matters.

In most Western cultures, the ageing process, the diminishing of physical capacities and the waning interest for the outer world are considered pathological. This point is evidenced by the great solicitation for surgical and pharmacological alternatives to postpone the inevitable outer signs of ageing.

The loss of passion and interest for the outer world is often experienced as a depressive state, and again chemically treated.

The Daoist belief about the human existence, offers an alternative way of understanding the ageing process. The human being comes into this world with a *Ming* ≈ Life Curriculum that needs to be realised. The *Ming* is brought by the *Shen* after conception and deposited together with *Yuan, Jing,* and *Zong* in the lower *Dantian* in the form of *Dong Qi* ≈ "Moving Qi" between the Kidneys. The Extraordinary Vessels, all rooted in the *Dong Qi*, disseminate this information and coordinate the individual's life cycles accordingly. The *Hun* ≈ Ethereal Soul, is the record keeper and the link between the *Ming* and the *Shen*. Throughout life, the *Hun* directs the choices and events to comply with this curriculum, and through dreams, it reveals facets of the *Ming* to the consciousness ≈ *Shen*. As life draws closer to its natural end, there is an urgency for the individual to take stock of their life achievements and to finalise this curriculum. Dreams become more persistent and intense, in an attempt of the *Hun* to focus the mind's attention on unresolved issues and unfinished programs.

From a Daoistic point of view, the much-rejected signs of ageing could be seen differently. The reduced physical activity, is forcing one to do less and to retire into the inner sanctum. The diming of vision is an opportunity to lessen the outer distractions and an invitation to look within. The loss of the mental capacities and memory is like the pruning of the tree before winter, to get rid of all the unnecessary baggage and accumulated information, even to forget painful events and to help focus and concentrate on the essentials and the "here and now". The identifications that one has made with the ego, the worldly accomplishments, and the idea of separation from the whole, all slowly start dissolving as the snowflake reaches the ocean… As time starts running out, a great anxiety sets in, the mind and the will lose their control over the outer world. In the absence of a spiritual belief and support, the fear of dissolution and disappearance is a source of confusion and anguish.

> *Death is when we have no more questions…*
>
> Daoist saying

The hidden roots of most pathologies can be said to be the non-acceptance of these laws of life and the faulty beliefs that stem from it. Helping our ageing patients to understand and to come to terms with these life facts is the most important stage of therapy.

Example of some disruptive common beliefs:

- We are separate from existence and need an Ego to survive…
- The Ego needs to be defended…
- Having and accumulating equals happiness…
- We have to "fight" against death and disease…

- Life and death, health and illness are opposite enemies…

- Our spirit and soul need a physical body to exist…

- Security is possible (a place where no change may occur)…

Many such beliefs need to be identified and changed (▶A.4.1.1 and A.4.1.3).

Working with dreams and assisting the person to unravel the dream messages, and to attend to unresolved matters, will automatically reduce the desperation and urgency that is experienced by patients as they sense the approach of the end (▶Section 4.5.11).

Most importantly, to awaken the spiritual dimension of the person and to remind them of their eternal *Shen* and their oneness with the whole. To re-establish their connection with their higher self, their guardian spirit or their God.

Some of the exercises in the Annex-IV are indicated for this: (▶A.4.6.1 and A.4.6.2).

Dealing with cancer

After cardiovascular incidents, cancer is the second cause of fatality worldwide, representing roughly 20% of deaths. With the progress that medicine has made, both in the area of detection and treatment, the death rate by cancer has been slowly diminishing. Today half of the diagnosed patients may hope to recover completely from their disease.

Two similar persons having been diagnosed with the same type of cancer, and having received identical treatments, do not have the same chances of recovery. Obviously, this remains an open question; can it be genetics, lifestyle or the psyche of the patient?

Understanding the significance of cancer:

Billions of cells are being daily reproduced in the body, and some could be faulty or abnormal.

These abnormal cells are eliminated by the immune system, in particular the circulating white blood cells, that can recognise a foreign body or an abnormal cell and eliminate it by a phagocytic process.

Therefore, for a cancer cell to survive, to grow, and to invade, implies a breakdown of the immune functions.

Medical science considers that it takes years for an abnormal cell to become an invasive tumour. So, what are the reasons that allow for this anomaly to continue unchecked for such a long time? Aside from an ageing body, with its natural process of general physiological decline, or with the exception of genetically transmitted cancers, what are the reasons for younger patients to develop a faulty protective system?

Any chronic disease process is an expression of something gone wrong. The various psycho-physical dysfunctions are expressed by minor signals, maybe pain or discomfort, that have been ignored or misinterpreted, sometimes for years.

In Chinese medicine, cancer is a disease of stagnation involving long standing stagnation of Qi, Phlegm, Blood or *Jing*. Any type of stagnation manifests with specific symptoms, pain in particular. In part 1.2.7, "pain" as the body's language has been explored. When a painful signal is not caused by an external irritant it is often an expression of the hidden shadows of the unconscious mind.

When a minor signal is ignored long enough, the local stagnation of Blood and Qi slowly transforms into a more condensed, organic form, expressed by the context of "Invisible Phlegm". This invisible Phlegm may take the form of calcification in the joints, or stones in the kidney or gallbladder, atheroma in the arteries, or various types of lumps and tumours.

The process of "accepting a disease", is to hear and to come to terms with what the unconscious has been trying to signal over the years.

To understand, to name and to own one's disease nemesis, is true acceptance. At times it is even possible to respond to the call of the subconscious and to rectify the pathological process, in which case physical healing may occur. Otherwise, at least the patient might find a sense of conclusion and inner peace.

Therapeutic strategies

- Always start with supporting the life principle: RM-14 *Juque* with ST-23 *Taiyi*

- Or the will to live, presence of death thoughts: BL-23 *Shenshu,* BL-52 *Zhishe*, BL-44 *Shentang*

- Release the predominant emotions: fear (Bl-52 *Zhishe* and BL-58 *Feiyang*); sadness (BL-42 *Pohu* and LI-6 *Pianli*); anger (BL-47 *Hunmen* and GB-37 *Guanming*); worry (BL-49 *Yishe* and ST-40 *Fenglong*)

- Changing the belief system about cancer being a terminal disease (▶ see A.4.1.3 and A.4.2)

- Changing the beliefs about cancer treatments being toxic (▶ see A.4.2)

- Changing the beliefs about death: accepting help and enhancing trust in higher powers (▶ see A.4.2)

- For cancer patients, it is extremely important to have an atmosphere of positive support at home. If the family is not validating the patient's choice of therapy, or if the surrounding people (family, friends and doctors), are convinced that there is no hope for the patient, the chances for healing are greatly reduced.

- Supporting acupuncture treatments during a standard allopathic protocol is very important. Most treatments such as chemotherapy or radiation, deplete the Qi, Blood, Yin and the *Jing*. It is very important to supplement the body's substances by regular, even daily supportive treatments, by implicating the patient or the family. For example, daily Moxa on RM-12 *Zhongwan,* RM-6 *Qihai* and ST-36 *Zusanli*; or teaching a family member to do 2-3 times per week Moxa on BL-17 *Geshu*, BL-19 *Danshu,* BL-20 *Pishu* and BL-23 *Shenshu*; or the "four flowers": BL-17 *Geshu*, BL-19 *Danshu,* BL-43 *Gaohuangshu* and *Huanmen* (Extra: 0.5 *cun* above BL-15 *Xinshu*). Patients who have regular Moxa therapy during their cancer treatments, show fewer side-affects, and the fact of getting self-help or family support, is psychologically empowering. (▶ A.4.2)

- A great mistake that most cancer patients make is to trivialise their disease and expect to go back exactly to their previous habits and life-style, disregarding the important message that their sickness was trying to convey. It is fundamental to establish a dialogue with the patient on this issue. This point is also valid for any other life-threatening condition.

- In case of cancer metastasis or relapse, the information is frequently experienced as a shock and should then be treated accordingly (see below).

- When a fatal outcome is inevitable, helping the patient to let go with LU-7 *Lieque* (also helpful for close companions), BL-60 *Kunlun*, TW-5 *Waiguan* (with BL-63 *Jinmen*), PE-7 *Daling* and KI-24 *Ling Shu* (▶ see also A.4.6.4 and A.4.6.5)

6.3   Stress and Anxiety

- **Stress** is the feeling of pressure or strain resulting from the body's response to an outer event, perceived as a threat or a challenge. Physiologically it involves the sympathetic nervous system when the stressful event is acute, with the release of adrenalin (fight or flight hormone) in the first stage, or the hypothalamo-pituitary regulatory axis resulting in the release of cortisol in the second stage.

Short-term stress is considered positive, helping to improve adaptation, performance and even motivation and is termed "eustress". Otherwise chronic stress, called negative or "distress" is the result of experiencing an external event as being above one's resources to cope with.

The causes of stress may be roughly grouped into:

- Natural disasters or wars; combat stress; violent personal assault; violent accidents: often at the origin of Post-traumatic-stress disorders

- Major life events, relationship issues, loss of a job, major life changes, disease and death

- Daily life and job pressures: increased demands in the workplace, mobbing; school pressure on children to perform better, bullying; daily decisions; public performance; personal conflicts; examination stress; and travel pressure...

- Environmental factors: noise, light, pollution, radiation, traffic and crowds.

Chronic stress has become the leading cause of disease in the modern world. The higher levels of sympathetic nervous activation have numerous detrimental effects on the body:

- Higher risk of cardiovascular disease; hypertension

- Sleep disruption: further contributing to the exhaustion of resources

- Compromised immunity: susceptibility to physical illness and reduced healing capacities

- Depression and anxiety; reduced cognitive performance and memory impairment

- Change of behaviour: smoking, eating, drinking; compensations

- Ulcers

- Cancer

- Burn-out syndrome

- **Anxiety** is the emotion that is experienced when a future outer event is subjectively perceived as menacing. Anxiety differs from fear, which is the natural response to a real and immediate threat. The anxiety condition greatly depends on personal beliefs, constitution and conditioning. The main causative factor for anxiety is stress, in particular the anticipation of a stressful event. Anxiety disorders may manifest in various forms:

- General anxiety
- Phobia (in relation to a particular object or animal)
- Panic attacks without an external causative factor
- Obsessive-Compulsive behaviour

Chronic anxiety may cause numerous physiological and psychiatric symptoms:

- Restlessness and tension; jumpiness, irritability, anticipating the worst; stress; panic attacks; depression; obsessive worry; suicidal tendencies
- Sleep disruption; nightmares
- Neurological symptoms: headaches, vertigo, tinnitus, fainting, paraesthesia
- Heart: palpitations; chest pain
- Digestive: nausea, diarrhoea, indigestion; irritable bowels
- Lung: shortness of breath; sighing
- Skin: excessive sweating; pruritus
- Urogenital: urinary frequency, urgency; impotence

In Chinese medicine, stress involves Liver energetics. Liver, as the "general of the army", is in charge of dealing with a threatening situation: fight or flight. *Hun* ≈ Ethereal soul is responsible for modulating the psycho-emotional responses to the outer world. An overactive *Hun*, will cause a person to over-react to external stimuli and may even be responsible for maintaining a constant state of vigilance.

In chronic stress, the *Zhi* is also involved, manifesting as a permanent state of fearfulness and anxiety.

Anxiety may also relate to future worry, the *Po*, or obsessional worry, the *Yi*.

In the diagnostic evaluation, it is important to palpate the six points on the outer Bladder channel: BL-42 *Pohu*, BL-43 *Gaohuangshu*, BL-44 *Shentang*, BL-47 *Hunmen*, BL-49 *Yishe*, and BL-52 *Zhishi*

The long-term effects of stress and anxiety on the Kidney will overtax the Yang (Adrenaline), deplete the reserves, Kidney Yin, and ultimately damage the Kidney-*Jing*.

6.3.1 TCM patterns in Stress

Although Chinese medicine has not specifically identified stress, the condition may be found under several TCM patterns:

- Liver Qi stagnation
- Liver-Blood *Xu*
- Liver-Yang rising
- Heart and Kidney-Yin *Xu* (Heart and Kidney not in harmony)
- Kidney-Qi Xu

6.3.2 TCM patterns in Anxiety

Anxiety may be found in a number of Chinese disease headings: anxiety, worry ≈ *You Si* 优思; fear ≈ *Jing* 惊; agitation ≈ *Zao* 躁; panic attack (running piglet) ≈ *Ben Tun* 奔豚; fearful throbbing (palpitations) ≈ *Zheng Chong* 怔忡

- Liver-Qi stagnation with Liver-Yang rising
- Heart and Kidney-Yin *Xu* (Heart and Kidney not in harmony)
- Heart and Kidney-Yang *Xu*
- Heart and Spleen-Qi *Xu*
- Heart-Qi *Xu* (often associated with GB-Qi *Xu*)
- Heart-Blood *Xu*
- Lung-Qi *Xu* or Lung-Heat
- *Chong Mai* counter-flow Qi

6.3.3 Treatment strategies for Stress and Anxiety

- Calm or quiet Shen: HE-7 *Shenmen*, PE-6 *Neiguan*, PE-7 *Daling*, DM-20 *Baihui*, DM-19 *Houding*
- Move Liver-Qi: LR-3 *Taichong*, LR-14 *Qimen*, LI-4 *Hegu*
- Harmonise Heart and Kidney-Yin: HE-7 *Shenmen*, HE-6 *Yinxi*, KI-3 *Taixi*, KI-7 *Fuliu*, RM-14 *Juque*, RM-4 *Guanyuan*
- Open the chest: RM-17 *Shanzhong*, RM-15 *JiuWei*, BL-43 *Gaohuangshu*, PE-6 *Neiguan*
- For Heart-Yang Xu: add BL-15 *Xinshu*, DM-14 *Dazhui*
- For Heart-Blood Xu: add SP-6 *Sanyinjiao*, BL-17 *Geshu*

- For GB-Qi Xu: add GB-40 *Qiushu*, HE-5 *Tongli*, KI-8 *Jiaoxin*

- For Lung-Qi Xu: add LU-9 *Taiyuan*, LU-7 *Lieque*, BL-13 *Feishu*, DM-12 *Shenzhu*

- For *Chong Mai* counter-flow Qi: SP-4 *Gongsun,* PE-6 *Neiguan,* LR-3 *Taichong,* PE-7 *Daling,* RM-18 *Yutang* and DM-20 *Baihui*

- Clear the emotion; select from: BL-47 *Hunmen,* BL-44 *Shentang,* BL-52 *Zhishi,* (also BL-49 *Yishe,* and BL-42 *Pohu*)

- Many Luo points that are indicated for personality disorders, specifically deal with stress and anxiety:

  - PE-6 *Neiguan*: stress and anxiety with palpitations, fear and fright
  - LI-6 *Pianli*: anxiety
  - HE-5 *Tongli*: emotional over-reactivity; hysteria
  - SI-7 *Zhizheng*: anxiety and terror; hysteria
  - KI-4 *Dazhong*: settles emotions; fear of people; hysteria, panic attack
  - LR-5 *Ligou*: excessive worry and fear; hysteria; panic attacks
  - RM-15 *Jiuwei*: anxiety, mania, hysteria

6.3.4 Management of Panic attacks

Panic attacks are described in the Chinese classics as the "Running piglet syndrome" ≈ *Ben Tun* 奔豚. These are sudden feelings of intense fear, frequently starting in the lower abdomen and rushing upward toward the chest and the head, accompanied by palpitations, difficulty breathing or hyperventilation, sweating, cold or numb extremities, heat in the head and the conviction of imminent tragedy and loss of control.

The symptom description is consistent with the counter-flow Qi in the *Chong Mai*. The condition may occur in many psychological disorders or with drugs.

The incidence of panic attacks increases with the stress level of a given society (3% in Europe, 11% in the US), and more frequently in women.

Treatment:

- For *Chong Mai* counter-flow Qi: SP-4 *Gongsun,* PE-6 *Neiguan,* LR-3 *Taichong,* PE-7 *Daling,* RM-18 *Yutang* and DM-20 *Baihui*

- KI-4 *Dazhong:* settles emotions; fear of people

- LR-5 *Ligou*: excessive worry and fear; hysteria; panic attacks

- Breathing exercises are quite useful in the management of the condition

- Treatment of the cause: anxiety, depression, PTSD, drug abuse, ...

6.3.4 Post-Traumatic stress disorder (PTSD)

PTSD is a mental disorder that develops after a major traumatic event, in particular involving personal aggression, rape or child abuse, it may also develop after natural catastrophes, warfare, accidents, unexpected death of a loved one, disease-related or pregnancy-related trauma.

The incidence of PTSD varies between 1 and 3.5%, more frequent in women and higher in combat and conflict regions.

Symptoms:

- Recurrent feelings, thoughts or dreams related to the traumatic event

- Physical or psychological distress triggered by trauma-related memories

- Anxiety and increased reactiveness

- Depression

- Risk of self-harm and suicide

From a classical Chinese medical perspective, PTSD could be related to a non-processed (undigested) traumatic event during which the Conscious mind ≈ *Shen* was totally or partially disconnected, hence the *Yi* ≈ Intellect could not properly analyse and digest the sensory input. *Hun* ≈ Ethereal soul and *Po* ≈ Corporeal soul had to take over the defensive mechanisms, storing the totality of the physical and psychological experience together in one location, thus creating a *Gui* ≈ Ghost or unnamed entity. Each time any part of the traumatic event is stimulated, such as a touch, a word, a feeling or a smell etc., the whole experience is re-lived in totality, with the corresponding physiological defensive responses (adrenaline and cortisol). The body is in a permanent state of alert. The *Hun* attempts to release these subconscious and unprocessed memories through dreams, which often take the form of nightmares.

Important traumatic events provoke a great release of *Wei* ≈ Defensive Qi, which will drain the Kidney-*Jing* and the *Yuan* Qi. The *Jing Bie* ≈ Divergent channels are in charge of supplementing the surface *Wei Qi* from the deeper reserves of *Yuan Qi*.

Traumatic events involving sudden fear and shock (fright) or gradual fear, disrupt the flow of Qi and Blood resulting in *Shen* disturbances, ranging from confusion to mania. The harmonisation of Blood is recommended in the treatment strategy.

The impact of a given trauma on two individuals is not the same and greatly depends on their constitution. Traumatic shocks involving interpersonal and sexual aggression are more likely to cause PTSD than natural catastrophes.

6.3.6 Treatment strategies for PTSD

There is no standard treatment protocol; the following strategies should be adapted to each case. Please see guidelines under "Psychology and Acupuncture Therapy PART-V".

Shocks involving great danger to the self and physical or sexual aggression may deplete the *Jing*, making the treatment much more difficult. In these cases, the practice of "Marrow washing *Qigong*" is recommended. All shocks will have an impact on Qi and Blood that need to be harmonised. The stasis of Qi often causes an accumulation of Phlegm, further obstructing the *Shen* producing neurosis.

It is difficult to propose a standard protocol, but some general concepts may be adapted to most:

- Releasing the body memories: PAT exercises for releasing the *Jingjin* ≈ Sinew channels. Releasing the *Gui* (see below);

- Harmonising the substances: *Jing; Shen; Xue* ≈ Blood; clearing Phlegm;

- Bringing the traumatic event into the conscious mind: working with dreams.

- Transformation of the emotions: acupuncture and PAT exercises

The following are some therapeutic guidelines:

- First root the *Shen* (Life principle): RM-14 *Juque* with ST-23 *Taiyi*

- Help release any traumatic event: ST-14 *Kufang,* HE-3 *Shaohai,* BL-62 *Shenmai*

- For sexual aggression treat *Dai Mai*: GB-41 *Zulinqi,* TW-5 *Waiguan,* GB-26 *Daimai* or GB-27 *Wushu* or GB-28 *Weidao.* Master Yuen recommends the SI and BL *Luo* for parental abuse, LR and KI *Luo* for rape.

- Release fear and fortify the Kidneys: BL-52 *Zhishi,* BL-23 *Xinshu,* DM-4 *Mingmen* and RM-4 *Guanyuan*

- Traumatic events at life transitions: *Yin* and *Yang Wei Mai*

- Helping to express emotions: HE-5 *Tongli,* LU-7 *Lieque,* PE-6 *Neiguan*; RM-17 *Shanzhong*

- For connecting the fore-brain and the mid-brain (loss of memory of the traumatic event): DM-24 *Shenting* and GB-13 *Benshen* with DM-17 *Naohu,* GB-18 *Chengling,* and DM-20 *Baihui*

- Clearing the habitual mood or emotion with the *Luo*: (▶ Section 2.3); in particular the *Luo* of *Taiyang*: SI-7 *Zhizheng* and BL-58 *Feiyang.* The *Taiyang* is the outer-most defensive layer, and in PTSD, it is permanently in a reactive state.

- Indication of *Jing Bie* ≈ Divergent channels, Master Yuen recommends:

    - For trauma depleting the *Jing*: war, surgery, severe accident: use BL-KI *Jing Bie*: BL-40 *Weizhong,* KI-10 *Yingu,* BL-10 *Tianzhu* and DM-20 *Baihui*

    - For birth trauma (child) or post-partum (mother), head trauma or after a stroke: use TW-PE *Jing Bie*: DM-20 *Baihui,* PE-1 *Tianchi,* TW-16 *Tianyou* and TW-17 *Yifeng*

    - For situations with severe blood-loss: add GB-LR *Jing Bie*: GB-30 *Huantiao,* LR-8 *Ququan,* SI-17 *Tianrong* and DM-20 *Baihui*

    - For severe dehydration: ST-SP *Jing Bie*: ST-30 *Qichong,* SP-12 *Chongmen,* RM-12 *Zhongwan,* ST-9 *Renying* and DM-20 *Baihui*

- Harmonise Blood: move Blood with HE-6 *Yinxi;* invigorate Blood with LR-8 *Ququan*; dissipate Blood with PE-4 *Ximen*

- Help to "digest" bad news: ST-44 *Neiting*

- Help to let go and to forgive: LU-7 *Lieque,* LI-18 *Futu,* KI-24 *Lingxu*; BL-47 *Hunmen*

- Body Armours for releasing the somatic *Gui* (▶ Section 4.2)

- Standard protocols for releasing *Gui:* Sunsimiao; Worsley (▶ Section 4.4)

- Dream-work for identifying and releasing the psychological issues (▶ Section 4.5)

- Changing the "Belief system" and cultivation of the mind: (▶ Appendix-IV)

6.3.7 Burn-out syndrome

One of the consequences of chronic stress is the Burnout syndrome. Most often the stress is work-related, hence the term "occupational burnout". But burnout can affect any individual having difficulties with daily life management, in setting priorities and adapting their resources to the tasks at hand. Usually, persons with higher ambitions, perfectionists, having greater demands on themselves, or individuals having difficulties in setting limits or saying "no", are more prone to burnout.

Burnout symptoms manifest when the resources are exhausted, "burned-out" manifesting with:

- Exhaustion
- Sleep disorders
- Concentration and memory problems; difficulties in deciding, setting priorities or taking initiatives...
- Physical complaints: tension, oppression, easy sweating, palpitations, headaches, dizziness, tinnitus, back pain; digestive, respiratory and urogenital disorders, etc.
- Depression, indifference, sadness, lack of desire to communicate, loss of self-esteem, anxiety, bitterness...
- Tongue: often red and peeled or with a red tip, possibly a Heart-crack
- Pulse: Thin and Rapid, or Weak and Empty or Floating

6.3.8 Treatment strategies for Burnout

Although the chief complaints are fatigue and exhaustion, it would be a great mistake to start by supplementing Qi. In fact, in the burnout syndrome, the main concern is the exhaustion of Yin through having spent too much Qi (Yang), and not enough recovery through rest and sleep.

- Calm *Shen*: HE-7 *Shenmen,* DM-20 *Baihui*
- Harmonise sleep (see below)
- Supplement Yin (Heart and Kidney Yin): HE-7 *Shenmen,* KI-3 *Taixi,* HE-6 *Yinxi,* KI-7 *Fuliu,* RM-4 *Guanyuan,* and SP-6 *Sanyinjiao*
- Fortify the Kidney and relax the Will: BL-23 *Xinshu,* BL-52 *Zhishi*
- Help set priorities: LU-3 *Tianfu*
- Supplement Qi (only after the Yin has been restored): RM-6 *Qihai,* RM-12 *Zhongwan,* ST-36 *Zusanli*
- Clear the emotion; select from: BL-47 *Hunmen,* BL-44 *Shentang,* BL-52 *Zhishi,* BL-49 *Yishe,* and BL-42 *Pohu*; and the related *Luo* points
- Changing the "Belief system" and cultivation of the mind (▶ App.-IV)

6.4 Insomnia

In humans and a substantial majority of animals, regular sleep is as essential for survival as is air, food and water.

Sleep takes up about one-third of our lives of which 1/4th is spent in dreaming. Science has demonstrated that regular sleep is essential for survival, although the purpose and mechanisms of sleep are only partially understood.

Normal sleep is defined by a condition of rest for the body and the mind. In TCM terms this would mean a somatic stillness of the *Jin* ≈ Sinews and mental quietness of the *Shen* ≈ Mind.

Various studies on sleep deprivation have shown two stages of sleep to be most important for physical and mental regeneration: deep sleep classified as N3 or slow-wave sleep, during which the body recovers from fatigue, and REM (Rapid eye movement) or paradoxical sleep, which represents the dreaming stage, important for the recuperation and regeneration of the mind.

During the dreaming stage, the body is in total inertia, but certain parts of the brain are very active, in particular the visual cortex, the limbic areas, as well as great portions of the hind-brain. This explains the fact that while dreaming, the person is visually and emotionally experiencing the dream scenario, and that the autonomic nervous system is reacting to the emotional experiences, while the physical body remains in complete inertia.

In normal conditions, sleep is perfectly balanced with activity. When the activity has been more intense, sleep is adapted in consequence; not necessarily by increasing the length of sleep, but rather by increasing its quality. Neuroscience defines this as sleep efficacy, measured by the brain's "delta activity" in relation to the total sleeping time. In fact, after a period of sleep deprivation, the system recovers by increasing the deep-sleep (N3) and the REM sleep (dreaming) time without increasing the overall sleep duration.

Sleep disturbances, in particular insomnia, have been steadily increasing in numbers, affecting almost 40% of the population and disturbingly a large proportion of children.

In psycho-emotional pathologies, disturbed sleep is amongst the first manifestation of the condition.

Sleep disorders are roughly grouped into:

- Dyssomnia: including insomnia, narcolepsy (excessive sleepiness), sleep apnoea, restless legs syndrome, chrono-biological sleep disorders (altered sleeping rhythms) as observed in delayed sleep phase syndrome, but also in jet lag or shift-work.

- Parasomnia: sleep disorders involving abnormal occurrences during sleep causing partial arousal and disrupting the sleeping process, these include night terrors, sleep-walking, sleep-talking, sleep-sex, bruxism, nycturia, tinnitus, pruritus, and painful conditions...
- Secondary to psychiatric conditions

6.4.1 Sleep in Chinese medicine

Daytime and activity are considered Yang, and adapted to night time and sleep, the Yin.

In a state of health, there is equilibrium between the two, in which the sleep time and especially the sleep quality is adjusted in response to an increased need for Yang.

Sleep is the most representative of the body's circadian rhythms, hence an excellent indicator of the inner equilibrium of Yin, Yang and the Five substances. The Eight Extraordinary vessels, acting as inner regulators, maintain the inner balance and the adaptation to external changes. Hence, a detailed assessment of sleep patterns and dreams can supply an accurate evaluation of a person's overall psycho-energetic state.

When analysing sleep, it is not the length, but the quality of sleep that is the most important factor and defines the efficiency of sleep.

In chronic sleep problems, often several TCM patterns are present, making the treatment that much more complex.

In TCM, sleep could be analysed in three ways:

- In relation to the Five Substances, mainly *Xue* ≈ Blood and *Shen* ≈ Spirit/mind;
- In relation to the movements of *Wei Qi* ≈ defensive energy;
- In relation to the internal synchronisers: Extraordinary vessels.

Xue ≈ Blood

During sleep, *Shen* ≈ Mind and the *Hun* ≈ Ethereal soul retire into the Blood. The state of Blood plays a central role in the physiology of sleep.

Blood vacuity will affect the *Shen* and *Hun* and may cause sleep disturbances with difficulty falling asleep, classified as:

- Calm insomnia ≈ *Zao* 躁: with mental agitation or irritability, involving Heart-Blood.

- Restlessness ≈ *Fan* 烦: vexation with muscular restlessness involving Liver-blood.

When blood is deficient and cannot contain *Shen* and *Hun*, there will also be easy and frequent waking and dream disturbed sleep. The person will also manifest emotional vulnerability, be easily startled and overly sensitive, needing to fidget and presenting memory loss, usually of the most recent events.

Other conditions which disturb the Blood, would also disrupt sleep:

- Blood-Heat: causes an agitated sleep with a tendency to depression, irrationality and impulsiveness.

- Blood stagnation: produces an agitated sleep, quite common among those with severe psychological conditions, manifesting as extreme worry, anxiety or depression coupled with eating disorders or addictive behaviours as seen in alcoholism, drugs or sexual-addictions. Blood stasis often leads to forgetfulness, dementia and even *Kuang* ≈ mania.

Wei Qi ≈ Defensive energy

Ling Shu ≈ spiritual axis (chapter 8), describes the cyclic movements of *Weiqi*:

> *Weiqi circulates on the surface 25 times during the day (predominantly in the sinew channels), penetrating at the ankle in the evening, to circulate in the Zangfu 25 cycles during the night, following the Ke- control cycle of the Five movements, and emerging at the corner of the eye, (probably at Jingming BL-1), allowing for the eyes to open.*

This passage relates to the sleep and wake cycle and to the movements of *Weiqi,* strongly evoking the role of *Yin Qiao Mai* Motility Vessel and its synchronisation with *Yang Qiao Mai* ≈ Yang Motility Vessel to manage the nyctemeral (day-night) sleep cycles.

Weiqi, during the day, is maintaining muscle tone and mobility, hence its internalisation, which allows for the muscles to relax, is considered the first stage of sleep.

Weiqi is also responsible for the surface body temperature.

Interestingly, science has demonstrated that the internal synchronisation of sleep follows a 25-hour cycle and not the expected 24 day-night rhythms. The deepest sleep time, corresponds to the highest levels of melatonin secretion from the pineal gland, coinciding with the lowest body temperature. Falling asleep and deep sleep occur during the lowest temperature dip, whereas waking occurs during the ascending phase of the curve. In fact, drowsiness and sleep onset are enhanced by the progressive increase in melatonin secretion in response to the stimulation by the suprachiasmatic nucleus, which is receptive to the waning of ambient light (▶ Fig. 6.1 and 6.2). Exposure to bright light sources at night, disrupts this natural rhythm, and is amongst the main environmental causes for insomnia.

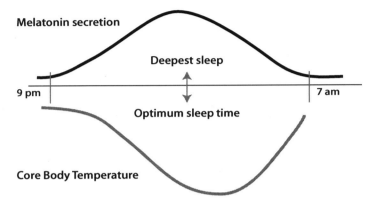

Fig. 6.1:   **Melatonin secretion, body temperature and sleep**

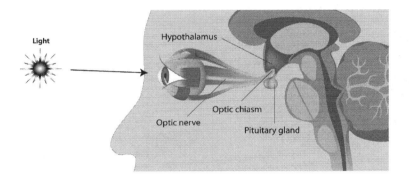

Fig. 6.2:   **Melatonin secretion by the Pineal (Hypothalamus) gland, when the light starts waning**

In the normal sleeping process, as *Weiqi* starts moving inward, the mind becomes drowsy and:

- The portals start closing down: eyes, nose and ears: as the eyes start closing, breathing gets deeper, and the hearing is reduced. When the portals cannot relax, there may be intense visual perceptions, snoring or tinnitus during the sleep onset.

- Then *Weiqi* passes through the chest before moving to the *Fu* before moving to the *Zang*

Shen ≈ Mind

Sleep is a condition of rest for the body and the mind. The body-rest reflects on the relaxation of the sinews and the movements of *Weiqi*. As the *Weiqi* moves inwards, the sinews relax and the mental activity slows down. This process involves the functions of the Liver and Heart. Hence the statement that at night *Shen* and *Hun* retire into the Blood.

Periodically *Hun* is released and is said to "wander". This is the dreaming phase, during which either pathogenic factors and accumulated and un-resolved emotions are released, or through which the challenges of one's *Ming* ≈ Life Curriculum are being examined. If there is a brief waking after a dream, portions of the dream are remembered. When the *Shen* accompanies the *Hun*, the entire dream may be recalled. Lucid dreaming occurs when the *Shen* directs the *Hun* during the dream.

When strong emotions are expressed during this processing, the dream is experienced as a nightmare.

Shen also represents the sum total of our emotions and is responsible for their manifestation. Therefore, all emotions, whether they are excessive, repressed or in-adapted, will affect the Heart and disrupt the *Shen* ≈ Mind and, cause sleep disturbances.

Calming the mind constitutes a major stage in the treatment of insomnia. The main challenge is to identify the offending emotion, through the analysis of the dreams and their symbolism, and to treat the emotion by addressing the underlying cause (▶ Section 4.5.11).

Eight Extraordinary vessels ≈ *Qi Jing Ba Mai*

All Yin and Yang phenomena reflect on the "Eight Extraordinary vessels", acting as reservoirs, organising the Yin and the Yang, maintaining the internal balance and harmony as well as adapting the inner milieu, the microcosm, to the outer variations, the macrocosm.

Four of these channels participate mainly in modulating (regulating) the Yin-Yang, day-night and life cycles (called the cycles of 7 or 8).

- *Yin* and *Yang Wei Mai* ≈ Binding vessels regulate variations in Yin and Yang spaces

- *Yin* and *Yang Qiao Mai* ≈ Stepping or heel vessels regulate variations in Yin and Yang rhythms (times). The *Yin* and *Yang Qiao Mai* have traditionally been indicated for sleep pathologies, more specifically for symptoms associated with day and night.

Yin Qiao and *Yin Wei* collaborate in sleep organisation in maintaining sleep length and depth. They are naturally in equilibrium with *Yang Qiao* and *Yang Wei* in charge of the activity.

Hence, in the assessment of sleep disorders, the complementary Yang vessels should also be considered.

6.4.2 Diagnosis of Insomnia

The following points should be clarified before an adapted treatment could be proposed:

- Total length of sleep-time: the time between going to bed and getting up

- General condition upon waking: rested or tired; the presence of a particular emotion

- The disturbed part of sleep-time: initial phase, middle or terminal phase

- To determine if the sleep is disturbed in its timing or quality: consider the mental and physical state during the awake time:

  - Clear mind: calm insomnia usually reflects a disturbance of the *Yin Qiao Mai*

  - Agitated with restlessness or other physical manifestations that disrupt the quality of sleep: restless leg syndrome, pruritus, hunger, night sweating, disturbing dreams, sleep apnea, sleep walking or sleep talking, etc... may be due to a disharmony of *Yin Wei Mai.*

  - When both synchronisers are affected, the person may present two types of insomnia, for example, difficulty falling asleep with a clear mind (*Yin Qiao),* as well as waking early with hot flashes, night sweats and restlessness (*Yin Wei*).

- Palpation of the four *Xi* ≈ Cleft points to confirm the Extraordinary vessel dysfunction:

  - KI-8 *Jiaoxin* for the *Yin Qiao*

  - KI-9 *Zhubin* for the *Yin Wei*

  - BL-59 *Fuyang* for the *Yang Qiao*

  - GB-35 *Yangjiao* for the *Yang Wei*

- The state of Blood: confirmed by the tongue and pulse

- The movement of *Weiqi* inward.

  - When the portals cannot relax, there may be intense visual perceptions, snoring or tinnitus during the sleep onset.

  - When the chest cannot relax: waking with a feeling of heat, sweating and oppression; also snoring

- If the passage in the *Fu* is hampered, there may be some somatic symptoms:

  - ST: difficulty falling asleep, night-time food craving, irritability
  - LI: teeth-grinding, neck and shoulder tension
  - BL: difficulty falling asleep, restlessness, muscle cramps, night sweating
  - SI: dry mouth, night thirst, enuresis
  - GB: head pruritus, neck tension, bitter taste
  - TW: drooling; crusting around the eyes

- Dream analysis: in particular the presence of a specific emotion (see...)

- Zang-Fu disharmony patterns: please note that the disturbed timing may help to orient the identification of the Zang-Fu dysfunction implicated in the insomnia process

- When "timing" Yin Qiao is involved (confirmed by the clear state of mind and reactivity of KI-8):

  - The initial phase (difficulty falling asleep) corresponds to Shao Yin: Heart and Kidney disharmony patterns
  - The middle phase (waking in the middle of the night with a clear mind) corresponds to Tai Yin: Lung and Spleen patterns
  - The terminal phase (early waking) reflects on Jue Yin: Liver and Pericardium patterns

- If the sleep quality is affected, with restlessness, confirmed by KI-9 reactivity:

  - The initial phase corresponds to *Taiyin*: Lung and Spleen patterns
  - The middle phase corresponds to *Jue Yin*: Liver and Pericardium patterns
  - The terminal phase corresponds to *Shao Yin*: Heart and Kidney disharmony patterns

Please note: the analysis of sleep disharmony patterns based on the Extraordinary Vessels is quite unusual and not well known in the habitual TCM *Zang-Fu* approach. This method has the great advantage of supplying very rapidly valuable information about the overall condition of a patient and especially indicates the most appropriate choice of points and the best therapeutic strategies adapted specifically to the subject.

6.4.3 Treatment strategies for Insomnia

The difficulty in treating chronic insomnia lies in the fact that quite often several patterns may be present which all need to be corrected. Furthermore, patients with chronic insomnia have been frequently taking medication for years, which makes the treatment that much more complicated.

Ideally, based on the typology of the patient and of insomnia, a tailored treatment has the best chances of bearing results:

- Calming *Shen*:
  - *An Shen* ≈ Calm the mind: HE-7 *Shenmen;* indicated for in all cases with Blood *Xu*
  - *Qing Shen* ≈ Quiet the mind; only when Blood is sufficient: PE-4 *Ximen*, PE-5 *Jianshi*, PE-6 *Neiguan*, PE-7 *Daling*
  - *Ding Shen* ≈ Settle the mind; to root the *Shen,* when the mind is very agitated (presence of nightmares): KI-1 *Yongquan*, SP-1 *Yinbai*, ST-45 *Lidui*, LR-1 *Dadun*, LU-5 *Chize*

- Supplement Blood: SP-6 *Sanyinjiao*, BL-17 *Geshu*, BL-20 *Pishu*, ST-30 *Qichong*
  - For Heart-Blood: add HE-5 *Tongli*, BL-15 *Xinshu*
  - For Liver-Blood: add LR-8 *Ququan*, BL-18 *Ganshu*

- Harmonise the Liver: LR-3 *Taichong*, LR-14 *Qimen*, LI-4 *Hegu*

- Harmonise the movement of *Weiqi*:
  - To relax the portals: BL-1 *Jingming*, BL-62 *Shenmai*
  - To relax the chest: BL-17 *Geshu* and TW-7 *Huizong*
  - For *Fu* somatic disturbances: *Sishencong* or DM-20 *Baihui*; ST-12 *Quepen*; add the appropriate lower *He* ≈ Sea points (ST-36 for the Stomach; ST-37 for the Large Intestine; ST-39 for the Small Intestine; BL-40 for the Bladder; BL-39 for the Triple Warmer or GB-34 for the Gallbladder) and the related *Jing* ≈ Well point.

- Reset the synchroniser:
  - *Yinqiao:* KI-6 *Zhaohai*, LU-7 *Lieque*, KI-8 *Jiaoxin*, BL-1 *Jingming*
  - *Yangqiao:* BL-62 *Shenmai*, SI-3 *Houxi*, BL-59 *Fuyang*, BL-1 *Jingming*
  - *Yinwei:* PE-6 *Neiguan*, SP-4 *Gongsun*, KI-9 *Zhubin*, appropriate confluent point
  - *Yangwei:* TW-5 *Waiguan*, GB-41 *Zulinqi*, GB-35 *Yangjiao*

- Reset the inner clock:

    - Re-harmonising pre and post Heaven Qi: RM-12 *Zhongwan;* LU-1 *Zhongfu*; LR-14 *Qimen*; DM-20 *Baihui* (needled in a specific order, see (▶ Fig. 6.3)

    - Resetting the *Yin* and *Yang Qiao Mai*: KI-6 *Zhaohai*; BL-62 *Shenmai*; and BL-1 *Jingming* (or *Yintang*)

    - Jet-lag or shift work: TW-5 *Waiguan*; LI-4 *Hegu*

- Treat the *Zang-Fu* pattern, selecting the appropriate points based on the pattern (▶ Appendix-I)

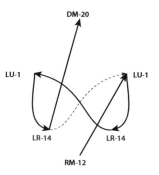

Fig. 6.3: **Re-setting the clock**

- *Shaoyin* patterns (HE and KI): difficulty falling asleep or early waking

    - HE-7 *Shenmen*: for all insomnia, frequent waking and dreams, sleep talking

    - HE-8 *Shaofu:* insomnia with mental restlessness

    - KI-1 *Yongquan:* anxiety, hysteria

    - KI-3 *Taixi*: insomnia with fear, helps to stabilise the emotions

    - KI-6 *Zhaohai*: insomnia with agitation, irregular cycles

    - KI-21 *Youmen*: tired but cannot sleep, (infants needing carrying)

    - KI-22 *Bulang*: feelings of injustice

    - KI-23 *Shenfeng*: restless mind, anxiety when lying down

    - KI-24 *Lingxu*: psychic stress, anxiety; suspicious

    - KI-25 Shencang: insomnia from worry, restless mind; negativity

    - KI-26 *Yuzhong*: insomnia, waking in a bad mood; feeling unloved; touchiness

    - KI-27 *Shufu*: persistent insomnia, agitation; apprehension, expecting a misfortune

- *Jueyin* patterns (PE-LR):

    - PE-1 Tianchi: restlessness

    - PE-5 Jianshi: insomnia, night terrors; with PE-7 *Daling* in menopause

    - PE-6 *Neiguan*: insomnia, anxiety, stress

    - PE-7 *Daling*: insomnia, anxiety, panic; with PE-5 *Jianshi* in menopause

- PE-8 *Laogong*: mental restlessness, anxiety, cannot sleep at all
- PE-9 *Zhongchong*: night crying in children, fear of the dark, anxiety
- LR-3 *Taichong*: insomnia, nervousness
- LR-8 *Ququan*: restless leg syndrome
- LR-10 *Zuwuli*: insomnia

- *Taiyin* patterns
  - LU-1 *Zhongfu*: insomnia, waking at 3 am (solar time)
  - LU-2 *Yunmen*: insomnia, waking at 3 am (solar time)
  - LU-3 *Tianfu*: restless sleep, ghost talk (sleep-talking)
  - LU-9 *Taiyuan*: insomnia from over excitement
  - LU-10 *Yuji*: insomnia, grief
  - LU-11 *Shaoshang*: insomnia in children, sleeping with half-open eyes
  - SP-1 *Yinbai*: restless sleep, nightmares, ghost oppression
  - SP-2 Dadu: insomnia, worry, dreams of narrow passes or ruins
  - SP-3 *Taibai*: laziness upon waking
  - SP-4 *Gongsun*: insomnia, restlessness
  - SP-5 *Shangqiu*: nightmares, children who need to be carried
  - SP-6 *Sanyinjiao*: insomnia from fatigue

- Other points affecting sleep:
  - LI-2 *Erjian*: the tendency to fall asleep
  - LI-3 *Sanjian*: likes to lie down
  - LI-4 *Hegu*: insomnia from weakness, influences sleep quality
  - LI-13 *Shouwuli*: likes to lie down
  - ST-9 *Quepen*: insomnia from nervousness
  - ST-21 *Liangmen*: insomnia after midnight, needs to eat to fall asleep
  - ST-27 *Daju*: insomnia from worry
  - St-36 *Zusanli*: insomnia
  - ST-44 *Neiting*: nightmares, restless extremities at night
  - ST-45 *Lidui*: dream disturbed sleep, nightmares, sleepiness
  - SI-3 *Houxi*: dream disturbed sleep, dreams of narrow passages

- BL-1 *Jingming*: insomnia or sleepiness
- BL-2 *Zanzhu*: nightmares
- BL-10 *Tianzhu*: insomnia from overwork, nightmares
- BL-15 *Xinshu*: insomnia, dream disturbed sleep, dreams of the dead
- BL-20 *Pishu*: light sleep
- BL-43 *Gaohuangshu*: insomnia
- BL-44 *Shentang*:   insomnia
- BL-45 *Yixi*: insomnia from fatigue
- BL-47 *Hunmen*: a vague feeling of fear at night
- BL-60 *Kunlun*: emotional insomnia, infantile insomnia (dentition)
- BL-62 *Shenmai*:   insomnia or sleepiness
- BL-15 *Xinshu;* BL-18 *Ganshu;* BL-20 *Pishu*: insomnia from Blood-xu, superficial sleep
- DM-10 *Lingtai;* DM-18 *Qiangjian;* DM-20 *Baihui;* DM-22 *Xinhui*: insomnia
- DM-13 *Taodao*: insomnia from fatigue
- DM-17 *Naohu*: insomnia before midnight
- DM-19 *Houding*: insomnia, severe anxiety
- RM-4 *Guanyuan*:   insomnia, night fears
- RM-6 Qihai: insomnia
- RM-15 *Jiuwei*: insomnia, anxiety

- Extra Points for insomnia:
  - *Yintang*: insomnia
  - *Yiming / Anmien*: insomnia, agitation and restlessness; waking easily from sound or light
  - *Anmien* I and II: insomnia, sleepwalking
  - *Sishencong*: insomnia

- Auricular points for insomnia:
  - *Shenmen*
  - Relaxation (Tranquiliser) point
  - Insomnia 1; Insomnia 2 (Nogier points)
  - Omega (Master Cerebral) point
  - also: Temple, Endocrine, Sympathetic...

6.4.4 Other sleep disturbances

✦ **Nightmares *Meng Yan* 梦魇** (▶ see Section 4.5.6)

✦ **Excessive dreaming *Duo Meng* 多梦**: often accompanies light sleep, increasing toward the middle and end of the night, having a detrimental impact on sleep quality, hence the *Yin Wei Mai* (check the reactivity of KI-9 *Zhubin*). As a result, the subject wakes up feeling tired or even distressed.

Most common patterns are:

- Heart-Blood *Xu*
- Liver-Blood *Xu*
- Liver-Yin *Xu*
- Heart and Gallbladder-Qi *Xu*
- Heart and Kidney-Yin *Xu* (Heart and Kidney out of Harmony)
- Liver-Fire
- Phlegm-Fire Harassing the mind

The most common points for excessive dreaming:

- HE-7 *Shenmen*: frequent waking, excessive dreaming, agitation, sleep-talking
- SP-1 *Yinbai*: restless sleep, excessive dreaming, agitation, nightmares
- ST-45 *Lidui*: dream-disturbed sleep, nightmares
- SI-3 *Houxi*: dream-disturbed sleep, dreaming of narrow passages
- BL-15 *Xinshu*: dream-disturbed sleep, dreaming of the dead
- GB-13 *Benshen* (with DM-24 *Shenting*): excessive dreaming, nightmares
- GB-44 *Zuqiaoyin*: excessive dreaming, nightmares

✦ **Night-Fright (Night Terror or Ghost fright) *Ye Jing* 夜惊**: (▶ see Section 4.5.7).

✦ Sleep-walking (somnambulism) *Meng You* 梦游:

Is classified as a parasomnia occurring mostly during the N2 stage of sleep, and not during the REM sleep. It is considered to be a sort of acting out of the last portion of a previous dream, often dreams of confinement or threat. Sleep-walking disturbs sleep quality, involving primarily the *Yinwei Mai* but also *Yangwei*.

Most common patterns are:

- Heart-Blood *Xu*
- Liver-Blood *Xu* with Liver-Qi stagnation
- Liver-Fire
- Phlegm-Fire Harassing the mind
- Heart-Blood stasis
- Heart and Kidney-Yang *Xu*

The most common points for somnambulism: *Anmian* I and *Anmian* II

✦ Sleep-talking / Ghost-talk (somniloquy) *Meng Yi* 梦呓:

Similar to sleep-walking, it occurs during the transitional phase following REM sleep, it may at times manifest during REM sleep when there has been a breakdown of the normal motor atonia as seen in "REM behaviour disorder".

Most common patterns are:

- Heart-Fire
- Heart-Blood stasis
- Food stagnation

The most common points for sleep-talking: HE-7 *Shenmen*, HE-5 *Tongli*, LU-3 *Tianfu*

✦ Sleep apnoea *Shui Mian Hu Xi Zhan Ting Zong He Zheng* 睡眠呼吸暫停綜合征

Characterised by repeated pauses of breath during sleep producing partial arousal as well as reduced blood oxygen saturation. This condition has only been recently identified by polysomnography and classified as either a central sleep apnoea or an obstructive apnoea in which there is a physical blocking of the airflow. The latter is often the result of an accumulation of Phlegm, frequently accompanied by other related manifestations: snoring, obesity, daytime sleepiness and tiredness. Sleep apnoea affects sleep quality and daytime activity (Yin and Yang *Qiao Mai*).

Most common patterns are:

- Phlegm misting the mind

- Spleen-Qi *Xu*

- Kidney and Spleen-Yang *Xu*

- Blood stasis in the upper parts

The most common points for obstructive sleep apnoea (OSA):

- PE-5 *Jianshi*: clears portals blocked by Phlegm

- To help move *Weiqi* down and clear local obstruction from the nose: BL-1 *Jingming* (or *Yintang*), LI-20 *Yingxiang,* BL-62 *Shenmai* or KI-6 *Zhaohai*

- To help loosen the chest: BL-17 *Geshu,* TW-7 *Zonghui,* RM-17 *Shanzhong,* BL-43 *Gaohuangshu,* RM-22 *Tiantu*

- For central sleep apnoea: add DM-16 *Fengfu,* DM-17 *Naohu,* DM-20 *Baihui,* GB-20 *Fengchi,* and RM-9 *Renying*

✦ **Hypersomnia (narcolepsy)** *Shi Shui* 嗜 睡:

Excessive sleeping or somnolence, ranges from an increased need for sleep to a condition known as narcolepsy in which the subject is constantly falling asleep. This condition may be associated with poor quality of sleep at night, but not necessarily.

Generally, somnolence is due to an accumulation of Yin above (Dampness, Phlegm or Blood) preventing the rising of the clear Yang to the head. Reflecting on the repletion of *Yin Qiao Mai* and the vacuity of *Yang Qiao Mai* (check KI-9 *Zhubin* and BL-59 *Feiyang*)

Most common patterns are:

- Phlegm misting the mind

- Blood stasis in the upper parts

- Spleen-Qi *Xu*

- Heart and Spleen-Qi *Xu*

- Kidney Yang *Xu*

The most common points for hypersomnia:

- To help open the portals: LI-2 Erjian, LI-3 *Sanjian,* TW-8 *Sanyangluo,* TW-10 *Tianjing*;

- To clear Dampness and Phlegm: PE-5 *Jianshi,* LU-5 *Chize,* SP-5 *Shangqiu* and KI-4 *Dachong*;

- Regulate Yin and Yang *Qiao Mai*: KI-6 *Zhaohai* (reduce), BL-62 *Shenmai* (supplement), and BL-1 *Jingming*

- To help carry clear Qi to the head *Jingbie* of ST and SP (ST-30, SP-12, RM-12, ST-9, DM-20)

- LI-13 *Shouwuli*: desire to lie down

- ST-45 *Lidui:* sleepiness, excessive dreaming

- GB-24 *Riyue*: sleepiness

6.5 Addictions and Compensation issues

Both conditions reflect strongly on *Ren Mai*, considered the bonding vessel and the vessel of compensations, dealing with unresolved and unfulfilled issues by a holding pattern, often in the form of Phlegm. Many of the *Ren Mai* points deal with Yin and Phlegm accumulation.

In Chinese medicine, the concept of "Hungry Ghosts" also referred to as the "Three Worms", relates to these issues:

- Hungry Ghost: concerns unresolved material desires

- Sexual Ghost: resulting from unfulfilled or over indulged sexuality

- Wandering Ghost: relates to frustrated emotional needs

When there is an inability to properly assimilate and to feel fulfilled, the unconscious seeks compensations, which can never replace the initial lack of bonding, therefore they are never appropriate or enough. (▶ see Section 2.1.11).

6.5.1 Co-dependence

During the first year of life, over bonding or lack of bonding with the mother, may later manifest with compensation issues in an attempt to either replace the maternal matrix or because nothing seems to be sufficient.

The psychological profiles for *Du* and *Ren Mai* are complementary, a weakness of *Du Mai* (lack of identity) is accompanied by and repletion of *Ren Mai* (over-dependence), and vice versa.

Co-dependency most often is the result of excessive bonding by the mother during the first year or a lack of a paternal presence in the second year. This makes the person overly dependent on the mother or the partner, seeking relationships of total dependence, delegating their power to the partner, therapist or leader (guru) even taking on victim roles.

Co-dependence is the basis for addictions

Therapeutic orientations:

- *Ren Mai*: LU-7 *Lieque,* KI-6 *Zhaohai,* RM-12 *Zhongwan*
- *Chong Mai* (▶ see Section 2.1.10): SP-4 *Gongsun,* PE-6 *Neiguan*
- *Gao Huang* points concerning a lack of nourishment and compensation issues
  - KI-16 *Huangshu*: the early severance of the umbilical cord; may be the cause of a permanent state of anxiety and worry.
  - BL-51 *Huangmen*: lack of sufficient breastfeeding; at the origin of all addictions or compensations related to the "oral complex": smoking, drinking or eating disorders.
  - BL-43 *Gaohuangshu*: lack of chest-to-chest bonding with the mother, early weaning, rejections and deceptions; could be at the origin of lack of self-love and self-respect driving the person to seek situations and relationships that will reproduce or repeat this pattern.
  - BL-53 *Baohuang*: possibly from early toilet training, or sexual taboo, or even child-abuse; may cause issues with sexuality and sexual nourishment. Sexual addiction is quite often an attempt to artificially nourish this aspect.
  - RM-6 *Qi Hai* (but also *Huangzhiyuan*); similar causes as with BL-53, but may also combine an overall lack of maternal nourishment, provoking a lack of incentive, weak will power, no desire to live and eating disorders.

- Feeling of vulnerability: ST-15 *Wuyi*
- Vulnerability from guilt or shame: LU-9 *Taiyuan*
- Lack of self-trust: KI-8 *Jiaoxin*
- Lack of roots and direction: BL-47 *Hunmen*
- "Body Armours": Oral; Thoracic; Abdominal or Pelvic segments

6.5.2 Addictions

The relation between co-dependence, addictive personality types and *Ren Mai* was explored above.

Acupuncture combined with the appropriate psychological support has yielded great results in various types of addictions. But it is also important to analyse and to correct the energetic impact of each addictive substance concerning each individual. In other words, a person may be unconsciously seeking to harmonise a certain un-balance through the use of an addictive substance; for example:

- Tobacco addiction:
  - Nicotine has a stimulating action, the bitter taste of tobacco, stimulates the Heart-Qi: supplement Heart-Qi with HE-7 *Shenmen* or HE-9 *Shaochong*; nicotine also increases the brain dopamine levels (the motivational hormone) in this case add: DM-4 *Mingmen*, BL-52 *Zhishi* and DM-20 *Baihui*
  - The hot smoke puts the Lung in a state of momentary repletion, helping to control a condition of Liver repletion or stagnation: harmonise Liver-Qi with LR-3 *Taichong* and LI-4 *Hegu* or LR-14 *Qimen*
  - Nicotine has also a calming action: calm *Shen* with HE-7 *Shenmen*, or with PE-7 *Daling* or PE-6 *Neiguan* and DM-20 *Baihui*
  - For all oral addictions (tobacco, alcohol, food...): GB-8 *Shuaigu* with GB-9 *Tianchong*
  - Otherwise, numerous protocols have been proposed for tobacco addiction, just to name a few:
    - Extra point (possibly *Xiawenliu)*; lateral and proximal to LU-7 *Lieque*, on the lateral border of the radius, using an intradermal needle.
    - St-9 *Renying* and BL-10 *Tianzhu*

- LU-7 *Lieque*; LI-4 *Hegu*; LI-20 *Yingxiang*, *Yintang* and Ear *Shenmen*

- GB-1 *Tongzi*; GB-8 *Shuaigu*; GB-6 *Xuanli*; *Yintang*; *Bitong* and ear "Zero" point; all points to be reduced three times at 10-minute intervals. The treatment needs to be repeated every 3-4 days until the patient describes the appearance of a metallic (coppery) taste in the mouth during the session. When successful, this protocol produces a strong tobacco dislike in 80% of cases. Unfortunately, the patient's will power is still required to maintain the tobacco withdrawal.

- After the withdrawal: for bulimia add ST-45 *Lidui*; for nervousness add He-7 *Shenmen*; move LR-Qi with LR-3 *Taichong* and LI-4 *Hegu*...

- Alcohol addiction: alcohol helps to release Liver-Qi stagnation and hence alleviate stress and help to relax; always harmonise the Liver: LR-3 *Taichong* with PE-7 *Daling* and LI-4 *Hegu*

- Cannabis: also has a calming action, by increasing the parasympathetic activity, relaxing the muscles and the mind and bringing down the blood pressure: calm *Shen* and harmonise the Liver and supplement Spleen-Qi: BL-20 *Pishu* and BL-49 *Yishe*

- Cocaine and methamphetamine: both increase the brain dopamine; add DM-4 *Mingmen*, BL-52 *Zhishi* and DM-20 *Baihui*, DM-17 *Naohu*

- Heroine and other opiates: increase the endorphin release by the pituitary; this is the antalgic and joy-inducing hormone; add HE-7 *Shenmen*; HE-3 *Shaohai*; RM-17 *Shanzhong*; DM-20 *Baihui*; *Yintang* and SP-21 *Dabao*

- Ecstasy: its amphetamine base also increases the dopamine levels, helping, in particular, the feeling of openness, sharing and expression; add RM-17 *Shanzhong*; PE-6 *Neiguan* and HE-5 *Tongli*

- Gambling and computer games addiction: both involve dopamine (expectation and reward mechanism) and endorphin (feeling of happiness); add DM-4 *Mingmen*, BL-52 *Zhishi* and DM-20 *Baihui*, DM-17 *Naohu* and *Yintang*

- Sexual addiction: involves endorphin and oxytocin stimulation; add DM-4 *Mingmen*, DM-20 *Baihui*, DM-17 *Naohu*; *Yintang* and BL-10 *Tianzhu*; LR-4 *Zhongfeng*

Therapeutic orientation:

In all addictions, the root treatment is the *Ren Mai*: LU-7 *Lieque;* KI-6 *Zhaohai*; and RM-12 *Zhongwan*. The following points have been traditionally indicated:

- LI-6 *Pianli* (repletion): addictive personality; manic-depression; talkativeness

- ST-40 *Fenglong* (vacuity): addictive tendencies

- BL-58 *Feiyang* (vacuity): addictive tendency; inability to set limits

- GB-8 *Shuaigu* with GB-9 *Tianchong*: for all dependencies; the "oral complex"

- To help strengthen the will power: BL-23 *Shenshu;* BL-52 *Zhishi;* KI-8 *Jiaoxin*; GB-6 *Xuanli;* GB-8 *Shuaigu*; GB-9 *Tianchong* and RM-6 *Qihai*

Acupuncture should be combined with an appropriate therapy to help change the mindset and belief mechanisms. An excellent method that has proven its efficacy is the 12 Step program, which was originally presented by Alcoholics Anonymous (AA) and later modified for various types of addictions:

1. Admitting powerlessness over the addiction

2. Believing that a higher power (in whatever form) can help

3. Deciding to turn control over to the higher power

4. Taking a personal inventory

5. Admitting to the higher power, oneself, and another person the wrongs done

6. Being ready to have the higher power correct any shortcomings in one's character

7. Asking the higher power to remove those shortcomings

8. Making a list of wrongs done to others and being willing to make amends for those wrongs

9. Contacting those who have been hurt, unless doing so would harm the person

10. Continuing to take personal inventory and admitting when one is wrong

11. Seeking enlightenment and connection with the higher power via prayer and meditation

12. Carrying the message of the 12 Steps to others in need

The classical 12-steps could be modified and adapted to Chinese medicine:

1.   Naming the problem: admitting that there is a dependence (addiction) and the harm that it is doing us and the surrounding

2.   Owning the problem: the dependence is a compensation for a deeper issue; recognising that this problem is beyond our control (will) and that, we "need help"...

3.   Healing stages:

   • Accepting to surrender and accepting to, be honest and sincere

   • Taking the necessary steps (it takes time to heal)

   • Balancing *Ren* and *Du Mai*: LU-7 *Lieque* / KI-6 *Zhaohai*; SI-3 *Houxi* / BL-62 *Shenmai*; DM-9 *Zhiyang* (reduce); supplement: RM-4 *Guanyuan*; RM-12 *Zhongwan*; and RM-23 *Lianquan* (or RM-22 *Tiantu*)

   • Rectifying the harms done to self and to others: *Dai Mai* (GB-41 *Zulinqi*; TW-5 *Waiguan;* GB-26 *Daimai*); to let-go and to forgive (LU-7 *Lie Que;* KI-24 *Ling Xu;* HE-4 *Ling* Dao); for retained emotions, sorrow and regret (PE-6 *Neiguan*; KI-9 *Zhubin*; RM-17 *Shanzhong*)

   • Importance of belonging to a group (*Ren Mai*)

   • Recognising the connection to the whole (*Chong Mai*)

Practical exercises: see Appendix: Central Axis (▶ see A.4.5.1); Changing the Beliefs (▶ see A.4.2 and A.4.3); Forgiveness (▶ see A.4.6.1 and A.4.6.2).

6.5.3 Eating disorders

Eating disorders may be roughly grouped into three categories:

   • Excessive food intake: over-eating, obesity and bulimia nervosa

   • Selective food intake: sugar addiction; salt, fats...

   • Insufficient nourishment: anorexia nervosa; orthorexia nervosa; food intolerance

✦ Over-Eating:

Characterised by excessive hunger, frequent eating and night binging:

   • Stomach-Heat or Stomach-Fire

- Blood stasis and Heat in the Stomach (stomach ulcers and cancer)
- Liver-Qi stagnation

Treatment orientation:

- Clear ST-Heat, quell ST-Fire: ST-44 *Neiting,* ST-45 *Lidui*; RM-12 *Zhongwan*; ST-21 *Liangmen*

- Blood stasis add: RM-15 *Jiuwei*; KI-21 *Yaomen*; KI-18 *Shiguan*; ST-34 *Liangqiu*

- LR-Qi stagnation: add LR-14 *Qimen*; KI-21 *Yaomen*

- Waking at night to eat: DM-20 *Baihui*; ST-21 *Liangmen*; ST-36 *Zusanli*; ST-45 *Lidui*

- Excessive eating: ST-19 *Burong;* SP-17 *Shidou*

- Bulimia: ST-45 *Lidui*

- Thinking about food: BL-57 *Chengshan*

- For food obsession: BL-20 *Pishu* (supplement), BL-49 *Yishe* (reduce)

- Over-eating to suppress sadness: SP-17 *Shidou*

✦ **Bulimia Nervosa *Shan Shi Yi Ji* 善食易饥**

Bulimia manifests as eating without hunger, binge eating (large amounts in a short time) and purging through forced vomiting or excessive use of laxatives and diuretics, which further causes an important loss of minerals and other nutrients. Bulimic behaviour seems more prevalent in social groups concerned with physical appearance or sports.

Psychologically, bulimia may be considered a compensation pathology involving the *Ren Mai* and the lack of bonding.

Treatment orientation:

- *Ren Mai*: LU-7 *Lieque;* KI-6 *Zhaohai* (self-image) and RM-12 *Zhongwan*

- Compensation issues, *Gao Huang* points: KI-16 *Huangshu*; BL-51 *Huangmen*; BL-43 *Gaohuangshu*; BL-53 *Baohuang*; RM-6 *Qi Hai* (see explanation above)

- LR-5 *Ligou*: hungry Ghost (treats 3 worms: hungry, lusty, wandering)

- Bulimia: ST-45 *Lidui*

- Feeling of vulnerability: ST-15 *Wuyi*

- Vulnerability from guilt or shame: LU-9 *Taiyuan*

- Lack of self-trust: KI-8 *Jiaoxin*

- Lack of roots and direction: BL-47 *Hunmen*

- Oral complex: GB-8 *Shuaigu*

- Excessive appetite: ST-19 *Burong*

- Over-eating: ST-19 *Burong*; SP-17 *Shidou*

- Hunger but unable to digest: LI-10 *Shousanli*; ST-36 *Zusanli* and RM-12 *Zhongwan*

✦ Selective food intake

Manifesting as an exaggerated intake of specific foods or tastes, often reflecting the body's attempt at supplementing an organic dysfunction:

- Excessive intake of sweets: to supplement a SP-Qi vacuity or for calming

- Excessive intake of salty foods: for KI-Qi vacuity or for raising the blood pressure

- Excessive intake of spicy foods: for LU-Qi vacuity or for moving Liver-Qi stasis

- Excessive intake of sour foods: for LR-Qi vacuity or for astringing

- Excessive intake of bitter foods: for a HE-Qi vacuity or for purging

- Excessive intake of starch or fat: Dampness as a means in helping to suppress unresolved issues; consider *Daimai* (GB-41 *Zulinqi*, TW-5 *Waiguan* and GB-26 *Daimai*)

Treatment orientation:

- Supplement the appropriate *Zang*: use Back *Shu*; *Ying* ≈ Spring and *Shu* ≈ Stream points

- For obsessive and fixed habits: BL-20 *Pishu* (supplement) and BL-49 *Yishe* (reduce)

- Self exercises changing the Beliefs and habits: (▶ Appendix-IV)

✦ Obesity:

Obesity is considered today as one of the most serious health problems worldwide, representing the leading preventable cause of death. It concerns over 10 % of the population, and its progression in the past decades has reached epidemic proportions, particularly in children. Although the causes may be due to genetic transmission, hormonal dysfunctions (thyroid, pancreas, adrenal) or fluid retention, the condition mainly reflects the increased sedentary life-style and excessive food, in particular sugar intake. It also seems that the loss of intestinal flora through antibiotic treatment in early childhood might be a contributing factor in the increase of obesity in children.

These social and medical factors often combine with the psychological causes as discussed in the above conditions of over-eating, bulimia or an excessive intake of sugar or starchy foods, necessitating psycho-therapeutic support in the management of obesity.

Treatment management: see above

✦ Anorexia nervosa *Bu Yu Shi* 不欲食 or *Shi Yu Bu Zhen* 食欲不振

Anorexia is manifesting with low weight, at times to the point of starvation; reduced food intake from fear of weight gain; and an unrelenting self-image of being overweight. There is quite often binge eating and purging as with bulimia and a denial of their condition. The incidence worldwide varies between 1-4% and is 10 times higher in women. Anorexia is the cause of numerous medical complications, higher mortality rate and risk of suicide.

Psychologically, anorexia may be considered a control issue involving the *Ren Mai*; refusal to self-nourish is a loss of the vital impulse *Shen* (RM-14 *Juque*), which may stem from a feeling of not being wanted or loved (BL-43 *Gaohuangshu*). Or a loss of the will to live (BL-52 *Zhishi*). A similar condition is also observed in patterns often wrongly diagnosed as pyloric stenosis, in which the infant vomits the mother's milk, symbolically refusing to live. When in pyloric stenosis there is, in fact, a mechanical problem necessitating surgery, the child's refusal of the mother's milk may be a subconscious manifestation of feeling unwanted.

Some TCM patterns may accompany the psychological disorder:

- ST-Yin vacuity
- Retained Heat in the *Ying* level or Damp-Heat in the middle TW
- LR-Qi stagnation
- SP-Qi vacuity
- SP and KI-Yang vacuity

Treatment orientation:

- Help return the vital impulse: RM-14 *Juque* with ST-23 *Taiyi;* ST-41 *Jiexi*

- Control issues involve the *Ren Mai*: LU-7 *Lieque;* KI-6 *Zhaohai* (self-image) and RM-12 *Zhongwan*

- Help change the self-image: *Yin Qiao Mai* and RM-12 *Zhongwan* with ST-23 *Taiyi*

- Rectify the *Zang-Fu* disharmony (when applicable)

- No desire to eat: ST-41 *Jiexi*; BL-21 *Weishu*; KI-21 *Yaomen*

- Loss of appetite: ST-19 *Burong;* ST-21 *Liangmen*; ST-22 *Guanmen*; SP-3 *Taibai*; LR-13 *Zhangmen*; RM-11 *Jianli*

- Self-exercises (▶ Appendix-IV)

✦ **Orthorexia Nervosa**

Although this condition is not officially recognised as an eating disorder, yet the increasing preoccupation with food quality to the point of obsessiveness on the choice and restriction of foods, has been an increasing source of health issues, even malnutrition, as well as social segregation.

Quite often food intolerance might have been at the origin of orthorexia. Food hypersensitivity is not a true food allergy and may be due to a lack or diminished digestive enzymes or a reduced ability to absorb a particular food substance. Quite often, the food intolerance is further re-enforced by the subject's belief that they have a food allergy.

Therapeutic orientation:

- Harmonise the centre (*Li Dong Yuen's* protocol): RM-12 *Zhongwan* with ST-36 *Zusanli*; RM-13 *Shangwan* with PE-6 *Neiguan*; RM-10 *Xiawan* with ST-25 *Tianshu* and RM-6 *Qihai*

- Obsessive thinking: BL-20 *Pishu*; BL-49 *Yishe*; SP-2 *Dadu*

- Hunger but unable to digest: LI-10 *Shousanli*; ST-36 *Zusanli* and RM-12 *Zhongwan*

- Thinking about food: BL-57 *Chengshan*

- PAT exercises (▶ Appendix-IV)

6.6   Bi-Polar disorders/ Manic-depression *Dian Kuang* 癲狂

Manic-depression is a mental disorder characterised by phases of depression (Yin-type psychosis) and manic behaviour (Yang-type psychosis). In less severe forms, the psychotic element might be absent and the subject will manifest periods of hyperactivity, irrational optimism and reduced sleep, alternating with depressive phases, sadness and negative thoughts. Bipolar disorders concern 3% of the world population and represent a common cause of disability, with equal incidence in women and men.

In Chinese medicine, the bipolar condition, mainly reflects on the instability of *Hun* ≈ Ethereal soul: the manic phase manifests as an excessive movement of *Hun*, un-bridled by *Shen*; when the depressive state corresponds to a weakness of *Hun*, with a total absence of direction, inspiration and incentive. The main causative factor is "Phlegm obstructing the Heart orifices".

TCM patterns:

- Liver-Qi stagnation producing Phlegm
- Heart and Spleen-Qi vacuity with an accumulation of Phlegm
- *Yangming*-Fire (manic phase): from retained external pathogenic factors or from Liver-Fire over-controlling the Earth
- Phlegm-Fire harassing the mind (manic phase)

Therapeutic orientation:

- Resolve Phlegm: PE-5 *Jianshi*, ST-40 *Fenglong*, DM-20 *Baihui,* DM-18 *Qiangjian*; GB-13 *Benshen*
- *Yangming*-Fire: ST-40 *Fenglong*; ST-8 *Touwei*; ST-36 *Zusanli*; ST-42 *Chongyang*; ST-45 *Lidui*
- Phlegm-Fire: PE-5 *Jianshi*, PE-8 *Laogong*, HE-8 *Shaofu*, BL-14 *Jueyinshu*, RM-12 *Zhongwan*, RM-9 *Shuifen*, ST-40 *Fenglong*
- LI-6 *Pianli*: Manic-depression, talkativeness
- Obsessive thoughts: GB-17 *Zhengying*; GB-18 *Chengling*
- SP-4 *Gongsun*: Manic-depression
- The treatment strategy depends also on the stage during which a patient is seen:
  - Manic phase: treat Phlegm-Fire; add DM-20 *Baihui*; DM-14 *Dazhui*; or *Sunsimiao's* 13-Ghost protocol (see page...)

- Mania: LI-5 *Yangxi*; LI-7 *Wenliu*; SI-16 *Tianchuang*; BL-10 *Tianzhu*; DM-19 *Houding*; DM-26 *Renzhong*
- Depressive stage: see under depression

6.7   Memory and Attention

The memory process is the conscious function of the mind to store, to retrieve and to process information.

Memory is subdivided into:

- Explicit or Declarative memory (conscious storage of data), which involves sensory perception, analysis and storage. In Chinese medicine. this would imply the coordination between *Shen* ≈ Mind/ Spirit, *Yi* ≈ Intellect/ Thought and *Zhi* ≈ Will.

- Implicit or non-declarative memory is the unconscious storage and recollection of information, this includes "Procedural" memory (unconscious performance of tasks) and "Priming" (subliminal programming). The implicit memory would involve the *Hun* ≈ Ethereal soul and *Po* ≈ Corporeal soul.

The five aspects of memory were discussed in section 1.2.8.

In general, the memory banks are related to Kidney-*Jing*. The Liver (time keeper) is in charge of retrieving this memory to bring it into the consciousness (relation between Kidney-*Jing* and Liver-Blood).

The components of normal working memory are:

- Explicit or Declarative memory: defined as the conscious, intentional recollection of information and previous experiences. It is further sub-divided into "Episodic memory" (personal experiences) and "Semantic memory" (accumulated knowledge). The concept of *Shen* represents this aspect of memory.

- Working memory: which involves reasoning, decision-making and behaviour. *Yi* manages the working memory by analysing and classifying the new information. Some consider this to be the short-term memory.

- *Zhi* represents the memory bank or "Long-term" memory. This includes Episodic and Semantic memories, as well as implicit memories, and the inherited and transmitted information. Although the latter are not readily available to the conscious mind, they do influence the sub-conscious and consequently the behaviour.

✦ Weak memory:

To enhance the memory and to help focus:

- General points to strengthen the memory: BL-20 *Pishu*; BL-49 *Yishe*; SP-2 *Dadu* and SP-3 *Taibai*; *Sishencong*; DM-20 Baihui; BL-10 *Tianzhu* KI-26 *Yuzhong*

- Poor memory and concentration: BL-23 *Shenshu;* HE-7 *Shenmen*

- Forgetfulness: HE-3 *Shaohai*; KI-1 *Yongquan*; KI-24 *Lingxu*

- Reduced memory in the elderly: BL-23 *Shenshu;* BL-52 *Zhishi*; BL-43 *Gaohuangshu*; DM-17 *Naohu*

- Forgetting words: PE-6 *Neiguan*; HE-5 *Tongli*

6.7.1 Amnesia *Jian Wang* 健忘

Amnesia is a memory dysfunction concerning the partial or total loss of memory. It is further sub-divided into retrograde (involving the past) or anterograde amnesia (inability to form new memory). Amnesia is often associated with brain damage, secondary to head trauma, cerebrovascular incidence and infections, tumours and other types of brain lesions.

TCM patterns:
- Heart and Spleen-Qi vacuity
- Heart-Blood vacuity
- Kidney-*Jing* vacuity
- Heart and Kidney Yin vacuity (HE and KI not in harmony)
- Phlegm misting the Heart portals
- Blood stasis

Therapeutic orientation:

Adapt treatment to the pattern.

Please note that all the *Du Mai* points from DM-14 to DM-26; as well the GB channel points from GB-13 to GB-20 have a strong impact on the brain and help to open the mind's portals.

- Supplement HE-Qi and Blood: HE-7 *Shenmen;* BL-15 *Xinshu;* BL-20 *Pishu;* DM-20 *Baihui;* ST-36 *Zusanli;* SP-6 *Sanyinjiao; Sishencong*

- Supplement KI-*Jing:* add BL-23 *Shenshu;* BL-52 *Zhishi;* KI-3 *Taixi*

- Supplement the "Sea of Marrow": DM-16 *Fengfu;* DM-17 *Naohu;* DM-20 *Baihui;* and *Dumai* (SI-3 *Houxi;* BL-62 *Shenmai*); also DM-15 *Yamen*

- HE- and KI Yin vacuity: add HE-6 *Yinxi;* KI-6 *Zhaohai*

- Phlegm misting the portals: PE-5 *Jianshi,* ST-40 *Fenglong,* DM-20 *Baihui,* DM-18 *Qiangjian;* GB-13 *Benshen*

- Blood stasis: add BL-43 *Gaohuangshu;* SP-10 *Xuehai;* GB-20 *Fengchi;* DM-22 *Xinhui;* also DM-26 *Renzhong*

- Bring "Clear Yang" to the head: *Jing Bie* of ST and SP: ST-30 *Qichong;* SP-12 *Chongmen;* RM-12 *Zhongwan;* ST-9 *Renying;* DM-20 *Baihui*

6.7.2 Attention Deficit and Hyperactivity (ADHD)

ADHD is a mental disorder typically combining a lack of attention with excessive activity, impulsiveness and difficulty in regulating the emotional responses. It is frequently diagnosed in early childhood. The exact causes remain unknown, although certain food additives and sugar are being suspected.

From a Chinese medical perspective, the condition reflects an overactivity of *Hun* ≈ Ethereal soul, which explains the hyperactivity and impulsiveness; and weakness of *Yi* ≈ Intellect, responsible for difficulties in focusing and maintaining attention. An over-stimulation of *Du Mai* during the second developmental year may be the causative factor. (▶ see section 2.1.12)

Hyperactivity frequently concerns blocked *Shaoyang* temperaments having lost the connection with their complementary Yin level, the *Jueyin.* To re-establish this connection: combine the *Luo* of *Shaoyang* with the *Yuan* of *Jueyin:* add RM-18 *Yutang* (knot point) and supplement *Jueyin.*

TCM patterns:

- Liver-Yin or Liver Blood vacuity with Liver-Yang rising or Liver-Fire

- Heart and Spleen-Qi vacuity

- Heart and Kidney Yin vacuity with Heart-Fire

- Phlegm or Phlegm-Fire

Therapeutic orientation:

Please note that all the *Du Mai* points on the head from DM-14 to DM-26; as well the GB channel points from GB-13 to GB-20 have a strong impact on the brain and help to open the mind's portals.

- Settle *Hun*, calm *Shen*: BL-47 *Hunmen* with BL-18 *Ganshu*; HE-7 *Shenmen*

- Stimulate *Yi*: add BL-20 *Pishu*; BL-49 *Yishe*

- Clear LR- and HE-Fire: add LR-2 *Xinglian*; LR-3 *Taichong*; RM-15 *Jiuwei*; HE-8 *Shaofu*; DM-24 *Shenting*

- Supplement HE-Blood: add SP-6 *Sanyinjiao*; BL-20 *Pishu*; BL-15 *Xinshu*; BL-17 *Geshu*; BL-43 *Gaohuangshu*

- Supplement LR-Yin or LR-Blood: add LR-8 *Ququan*; LR-3 *Taichong*; GB-13 *Benshen*; DM-24 *Shenting*

- Supplement KI and HE-Yin: add HE-6 *Yinxi*; KI-3 *Taixi*; RM-4 *Guanyuan*; SP-6 *Sanyinjiao*; RM-15 *Jiuwei*

- Clear Phelgm-Fire: PE-5 *Jianshi*, PE-8 *Laogong*, HE-8 *Shaofu*, BL-14 *Jueyinshu*, RM-12 *Zhongwan*, RM-9 *Shuifen*, ST-40 *Fenglong*

- Impulsiveness: add DM-5 *Xuanshu*

- Emotional over-reaction: HE-5 *Tongli*; KI-26 *Yuzhong*

- Restlessness: LI-4 *Hegu*; SP-6 *Sanyinjiao*; KI-9 *Zhubin*; KI-23 *Shenfeng*; KI-25 *Shencang*; *Yiming* (Extra)

- Self-exercise: re-connecting the brain (▶ Appendix-IV)

6.8 Autism/ Autism spectrum disorder (ASD)

ASD involves 1% of the world population (2% in the US), and is four times more frequent in men.

Autism spectrum disorders include a wide variety of characteristics in various degrees:

- Slow development of social and communication skills: difficulties creating connections with other people; lack of empathy; aggravated by a state of anxiety and depression;

- Slow learning of language and problems keeping a consistent speech rhythm;

- Abnormal responses to sensations including sights, sounds, touch, and smell.

The social dysfunctions may vary from the total impairment, being completely disconnected from the outer world to the high functioning individual, even with superior mental capacities (in restricted areas: splinter skills), but with odd social behaviour, and often a pedantic speech. The social deficit manifests as a lack of attention and response to the outer world, or on the contrary, restricted interest and exaggerated reactions to touch or sound etc. The repetitive behaviours may also greatly vary: body movements; compulsive or ritualistic behaviours; resistance to changing routines and patterns; unusual eating; and behaviours that may cause self-injury.

To date, there has been no concrete evidence of any particular causative factor, several theories have been proposed:

- Genetic transmission

- Pre-birth or birth trauma

- Parental age and mother's health and nutrition

- Alteration of the intestinal flora

From a neurological perspective, there seems to be un-equal development of the brain, over-developed in some areas and under-developed in other zones.

The classical Chinese texts have not defined this condition, although, from the symptom description, autisms may be related to two patterns of behaviour corresponding to:

- Blocked *Taiyin* temperament: (▶ Section 2.6)

- Blocked *Shaoyin* temperament (▶ Section-2.2)

Both patterns may explain the social disconnection and lack of empathy; the obsessive and compulsive repetitive movements and eating habits and the over-reaction to touch (*Po*) are more resonant with the blocked *Taiyin*; the speech difficulties and lack or abnormal responses to stimuli are more evocative of *Shaoyin* (*Shen*).

6.8.1 Asperger's syndrome

This is a milder form of the Autism spectrum, characterised by social difficulties and restricted interests and repetitive behaviours.

Therapeutic orientation:

- Start with *Chong Mai*: Deals with inherited factors and birth and pre-birth trauma; helps the centring of the personality:

    - SP-4 *Gongsun* and PE-6 *Neiguan*

    - Due to birth trauma: add KI-16 *Huangshu* and RM-6 *Qihai*

    - Due to gestational trauma: add RM-1 *Huiyin*, RM-4 *Guanyuan* and DM-20 *Baihui*

    - Due to post-natal trauma: add KI-16 *Huangshu*, BL-43 *Gaohuangshu*, BL-51 *Huangmen*;

- Mobilise and open *Taiyin*:

    - RM-12 (Knot point) with LU-2 *Yunmen* and SP-12 *Chongmen* to help open the *Taiyin* level outward.

    - *Luo/Yuan*: LU-7 *Lieque* with LI-4 *Hegu*; SP-4 *Gongsun* with ST-42 *Chongyang*

    - To help express feelings RM-17 *Shanzhong*, PE-7 *Daling*

    - For obsessions and worry: BL-49 *Yishe*

- Mobilise and open *Shaoyin*:

    - HE-8 *Shaofu*; HE-6 *Yinxi*; KI-2 *Rangu* and KI-5 *Shuiquan*; add RM-23 *Lianquan* (Knot point), KI-15 *Zhongzhu*; KI-26 *Yuzhong* and move Yin with RM-4 *Guanyuan* or LR-13 *Zhangmen*

    - Luo/Yuan: HE-5 Tongli with SI-4 Wangu; KI-4 Dazhong with BL-64 Jinggu

- Other points:

    - HE-5 *Tongli* (repletion): difficulty interacting with others; issues with empathy and compassion

    - PE-6 *Neiguan* (vacuity): inability to feel

    - LI-6 *Pianli* (repletion): repetitive behaviour; talkativeness

- PAT exercises: (▶ Appendix-IV: A.4.5.5: re-connecting the brain)

6.10 Tourette's Syndrome

Tourette's is part of a spectrum of tic disorders, which includes transitory or chronic tics; it involves multiple motor tics (blinking, coughing, throat clearing, sniffing, body or facial movements), and at least one vocal tic. In some rare cases, it is accompanied by "coprolalia", which is the utterance of inappropriate or insulting words.

It appears in early childhood and may often disappear by adolescence; concerning 1% of the world population and four times more frequent in men.

In Chinese medicine, tics, in general represent internal Wind.

TCM patterns:

- Liver-Yang rising from Liver-Heat or Liver-Qi stagnation
- Liver-Yin or Liver Blood vacuity with Liver-Yang rising or Liver-Fire
- Kidney Yin vacuity with Liver-Heat
- Heart and Kidney-Yin vacuity with Heart-Fire
- Phlegm or Phlegm-Fire

Therapeutic orientation:

- Treat the TCM pattern
- Settle Wind: LR-2 *Xingjian*; LR-3 *Taichong*; GB-20 *Fengchi* etc.
- Talking to oneself: LU-3 *Tianfu*; HE-5 *Tongli*; ST-32 *Futu*; ST-41 *Jiexi*
- Needing to swear: KI-24 *Lingshu*; LR-13 *Zhangmen*
- Incoherent speech: SI-7 *Zhizheng*; LR-5 *Ligou*; DM-26 *Renzhong*
- Raving: TW-2 *Yemen*

6.11 Personality disorders

In general, personality disorders involve the "Temperaments" and concern the blockage or lack of communication of the Six Levels (▶ Section 2.2).

6.11.1 Split personality or "Dissociative identity disorder" (DID)

A mental condition characterised by the presence of multiple personalities accompanied by significant memory gaps. In the majority of cases, there is a history of abuse in childhood. DID is quite frequently accompanied by other psychological and mental conditions such as:

- Borderline personality disorder (BPD): the tendency to unstable or reckless behaviour, and difficulty controlling emotions and thoughts

- Post-traumatic stress disorder (PTSD): see above

- Depression; anxiety; addictions or self-harm: see above

DID, seems to concern 1.5% of the world population, six times more frequent in women.

In Chinese medicine, the split personality may correspond to a disturbance of the social development reflecting on the *Luo* of Liver and more frequent in the *Jueyin* blocked personality. Otherwise, it may be the result of an acquired *Gui* ≈ Ghost during a traumatic event with the total or partial disconnection of *Shen* ≈ *Conscious mind* and *Yi* ≈ *Intellect* (▶ see Section 4.4).

Therapeutic orientation:

- Release the Gui: Sunsimiao's 13 Ghost points: start with the third triad (see page...)

- Mobilise *Jueyin* and re-connect it with *Shaoyang*.

  - Mobilise *Jueyin*: PE-8 *Laogong;* PE-4 *Ximen*; LR-2 *Xingjiang*; LR-3 *Taichong*; LR-6 *Zhongdu*; also, PE-5 *Jianshi*; LR-14 *Qimen*; and RM-18 *Yutang* (Knot point).

  - *Luo/Yuan*: PE-6 *Neiguan* with TW-4 *Yangchi*; LR-5 *Ligou* with GB-40 *Qiuxu*

  - To help reconnect the above and below: GB-41 *Zulinqi* with TW-5 *Waiguan*

  - To harmonise social relations: BL-47 *Hunmen*; BL-23 *Shenshu*; BL-52 *Zhishi*

- LR-5 *Ligou*: Talking to oneself, schizophrenia; daydreaming; multiple personality disorders (palpate the point, reduce/bleed if the point is in repletion, or supplement if there is a condition of vacuity)*.

*According to Master Yuen, when the LR-*Luo* is in repletion the subject is unaware of their split personality; but when the *Luo* is in vacuity, the subject remains aware of their split behaviour.

Important note: The patient's mental condition has to be evaluated by the therapist in order to decide for the most appropriate self-exercises described in Appendix-IV

6.9.2   Avoidant personality disorder

Characterised by severe social anxiety and inhibition, extreme shyness, with extreme sensitivity to negative feelings; extreme lack of self-confidence and feelings of being inadequate and an inferiority complex. They desire intimacy, but fear being rejected or humiliated and rather choose isolation. Their fear of abandonment may lead to excessive co-dependence and drug abuse, or self-hate and even suicide. This condition is frequently described in patients with anxiety disorders; it concerns about 2% of the population, with equal frequency in men and women.

In Chinese medicine, the avoidant personality may correspond to a disturbance in the social development stage corresponding to the *Luo* of Kidney and Heart and more frequent in the *Shaoyin* blocked personality; but also, the *Luo* of GB.

Therapeutic orientation:

- Mobilise and open *Shaoyin*:
  - HE-8 *Shaofu*; HE-6 *Yinxi;* KI-2 *Rangu* and KI-5 *Shuiquan*; add RM-23 *Lianquan* (Knot point), KI-15 *Zhongzhu*; KI-26 *Yuzhong* and move Yin with RM-4 *Guanyuan* or LR-13 *Zhangmen*
  - Luo/Yuan: HE-5 Tongli with SI-4 Wangu; KI-4 Dazhong with BL-64 Jinggu

- KI-4 *Dazhong*: inferiority complex; fear of people

- HE-5 *Tongli* (repletion): Heart pain: betrayal, broken Heart, disappointment; difficulty in interaction and contact with the others

- GB-37 *Guangming* (vacuity): Loneliness, hopelessness; suicidal tendency

- Recommended self-exercises: Central Axis (▶see A.4.5.1); Changing the beliefs (▶see A.4.2 and A.4.3)

6.9.3   Obsessive-compulsive disorder (OCD)

Manifesting with obsessive and uncontrollable thoughts and the deliberate repetition of certain routine actions (washing of hands, counting objects, switching the light on and off, checking if the door is locked...). OCD is frequently associated with tics and anxiety disorders; it may also include compulsive hoarding, as observed in the Diogenes syndrome (without the element of self-neglect and squalor).

OCD involves about 2.3% of the population with equal frequency in men and women.

In Chinese medicine, obsessions and compulsions correspond to a disturbance of *Yi* ≈ Thought/ intellect and in the social developmental stage, it relates to the *Luo* of LI and is more frequent in the *Taiyin* blocked personality. It may also reflect on the *Luo* of Kidney, the repetitive (familiar) compulsive behaviour being a strategy to control fear.

Therapeutic orientation:

- Mobilise and open *Taiyin*:

  - RM-12 (Knot point) with LU-2 *Yunmen* and SP-12 *Chongmen* to help open the *Taiyin* level outward.

  - *Luo/Yuan*: LU-7 *Lieque* with LI-4 *Hegu*; SP-4 *Gongsun* with ST-42 *Chongyang*

  - For obsessions add: BL-49 *Yishe*

- LI-6 *Pianli* (repletion): need to be repetitive; addictive aspects

- Mobilise and open *Shaoyin*:

  - HE-8 *Shaofu*; HE-6 *Yinxi;* KI-2 *Rangu* and KI-5 *Shuiquan*; add RM-23 *Lianquan* (Knot point), KI-15 *Zhongzhu*; KI-26 *Yuzhong* and move Yin with RM-4 *Guanyuan* or LR-13 *Zhangmen*

  - *Luo/Yuan*: HE-5 *Tongli* with SI-4 *Wangu*; KI-4 *Dazhong* with BL-64 *Jinggu*

- KI-4 *Dazhong* (repletion): obsessive-compulsive behaviour

- SP-5 *Shangqiu* and RM-12 *Zhongwan*: obsessive-compulsive behaviour

- Recommended self-exercises: Central Axis (▶see A.4.5.1); General releasing (▶see A.4.1.1) and Changing the beliefs (▶see A.4.2 and A.4.3).

6.9.4 Paranoid personality disorder (PPD)

Characterised by deep paranoia, delusions, mistrusting others, and a general suspicion and guardedness towards the world. Often oversensitive, misinterpreting other people's intentions, holding conspiratorial theories, and a tendency to holding on to grudges.

PPD affects about 2% of the population, predominantly men.

Chinese medicine relates fearfulness to a weakness of *Zhi* ≈ Will and in the social developmental stage it relates to the *Luo* of Kidney.

Therapeutic orientation:

- Fortify the *Zhi*: BL-23 *Shenshu*; BL-52 *Zhishe;* DM-4 *Mingmen*
- Supplement *Du Mai* and the character: SI-3 *Houshi*; BL-62 *Shenmai*; DM-1 *Changqiang*; DM-20 *Baihui*
- Mobilise and open *Shaoyin*:
  - HE-8 *Shaofu*; HE-6 *Yinxi;* KI-2 *Rangu* and KI-5 *Shuiquan*; add RM-23 *Lianquan* (Knot point), KI-15 *Zhongzhu*; KI-26 *Yuzhong* and move Yin with RM-4 *Guanyuan* or LR-13 *Zhangmen*
  - *Luo/Yuan*: HE-5 *Tongli* with SI-4 *Wangu*; KI-4 *Dazhong* with BL-64 *Jinggu*
- KI-4 *Dazhong*: inferiority complex; fear of people
- HE-5 *Tongli* (repletion): Heart pain: betrayal, broken Heart, disappointment; difficulty in interaction and contact with the others
- GB-37 *Guangming* (vacuity): Loneliness, hopelessness; suicidal tendency
- Kidney *Luo* vacuity: supplement KI-4 *Dazhong*
- Feeling of being mistreated: BL-11 *Dazhu*
- Feeling of doom: RM-15 *Jiuwei*
- Feeling of injustice: KI-22 *Bulang*
- Recommended self-exercises: Central Axis (►see A.4.5.1); General releasing (►see A.4.1.1) and Changing the beliefs (►see A.4.2 and A.4.3).

6.9.10   Histrionic personality disorder (HPD)

The Histrionic personality presents with excessive emotions that seek attention, such as seduction, excessive vivacity and dramatic, exhibiting strong and provocative behaviour, egocentrism and self-indulgence; they tend to be extremely manipulative.

HPD Affects 2-3% of the general population, four times more frequently in women.

From a Chinese medical perspective, the histrionic personality corresponds to the overactivity of *Hun* ≈ Ethereal soul; a blocked *Jueyin* level and particularly a disturbance of the *Luo* of Pericardium.

Therapeutic orientation:

- Harmonise the *Hun*: BL-18 *Ganshu*; BL-47 *Hunmen*

- Mobilise Jueyin and re-connect it with Shaoyang.

  - Mobilise *Jueyin*: PE-8 *Laogong;* PE-4 *Ximen*; LR-2 *Xingjiang*; LR-3 *Taichong*; LR-6 *Zhongdu*; also PE-5 *Jianshi*; LR-14 *Qimen*; and RM-18 *Yutang* (Knot point).

  - *Luo/Yuan*: PE-6 *Neiguan* with TW-4 *Yangchi*; LR-5 *Ligou* with GB-40 *Qiuxu*

  - To harmonize social relations: BL-47 *Hunmen*; BL-23 *Shenshu*; BL-52 *Zhishi*

- PE-6 *Neiguan* (repletion): inability to control emotions (sociopathic)

- Recommended self-exercises: Central Axis (▶see A.4.5.1); General releasing (▶see A.4.1.1) and Changing the beliefs (▶see A.4.2 and A.4.3 and A.4.3).

6.9.11   Narcissistic personality disorder (NPD)

This condition presents with, an exaggerated sense of self-importance, of self-admiration and a need to be admired. Thinking about achieving fame, power and success, a typical social climber, with a lack of empathy toward other people and a tendency to take advantage of them. They tend to be controlling and generally intolerant of criticism and easily pass the blame. NPD seems to concern about 1% of the population and predominantly men.

In Chinese medicine, this personality profile corresponds to a blocked *Taiyang* having lost the connection with the complementary Yin level. In some aspects: the need to be admired, absorbed with self-image, manipulativeness and envy also reflect on a blocked *Jueyin* level. Fixation on past physical appearance or social positions implies a disturbance of *Yin* or *Yang Wei Mai*. The causative factors seem to do with parental excessive and unjustified adoration of the child; or on the opposite, an inappropriate criticism causing a feeling of not being wanted or valued; hence the construction of an inflated self-image as a compensation.

Therapeutic orientation:

- Re-connecting *Taiyang* with *Shaoyin*: Luo/Yuan: SI-7 *Zhizheng* with HE-7 *Shenmen*; BL-58 *Feiyang* with KI-3 *Taixi*

- Mobilise *Jueyin* and re-connect it with *Shaoyang*.

    - Mobilize *Jueyin*: PE-8 *Laogong;* PE-4 *Ximen*; LR-2 *Xingjiang*; LR-3 *Taichong*; LR-6 *Zhongdu*; also, PE-5 *Jianshi*; LR-14 *Qimen*; and RM-18 *Yutang* (Knot point).

    - *Luo/Yuan*: PE-6 *Neiguan* with TW-4 *Yangchi*; LR-5 *Ligou* with GB-40 *Qiuxu*

    - To harmonise social relations: BL-47 *Hunmen*; BL-23 *Shenshu*; BL-52 *Zhishi*

- Excessive self-love: KI-10 *Yingu*

- Recommended self-exercises: Central Axis (▶see A.4.5.1); General releasing (▶see A.4.1.1) and Changing the beliefs (▶see A.4.2 and A.4.3).

6.9.12   Passive-aggressive personality disorder

Combines the tendency to procrastinate, obstruct others, of passive resistance, of negativity and being extremely stubborn. Although the passive-aggressive character may present great self-assertion to the others, internally they feel quite ambivalent, lacking self-confidence and having difficulty in making choices and taking decisions.

According to the Chinese temperaments, the blocked *Taiyin* Earth-type corresponds to the procrastinating and passive resistance and pretending to comply attitude and hide their emotions of the passive-aggressive. The sly, backhanded attitudes and playing the victim and blaming others is more representative of a blocked *Shaoyin*.

Therapeutic orientation:

- Mobilise and open *Taiyin*:

- RM-12 (Knot point) with LU-2 *Yunmen* and SP-12 *Chongmen* to help open the *Taiyin* level outward.

- *Luo/Yuan*: LU-7 *Lieque* with LI-4 *Hegu*; SP-4 *Gongsun* with ST-42 *Chongyang*

- Mobilise and open *Shaoyin*:

  - HE-8 *Shaofu*; HE-6 *Yinxi;* KI-2 *Rangu* and KI-5 *Shuiquan*; add RM-23 *Lianquan* (Knot point), KI-15 *Zhongzhu*; KI-26 *Yuzhong* and move Yin with RM-4 *Guanyuan* or LR-13 *Zhangmen*

  - *Luo/Yuan*: HE-5 *Tongli* with SI-4 *Wangu*; KI-4 *Dazhong* with BL-64 *Jinggu*

- Recommended self-exercises: Central Axis (▶see A.4.5.1); General releasing (▶see A.4.1.1) and Changing the beliefs (▶see A.4.2 and A.4.3).

6.9.13   Schizophreniform disorder

Presenting with symptoms of delusion, hallucination and paranoia, but the signs of disruption don't present the frequency and thinking difficulty consistent with a diagnosis of schizophrenia.

Therapeutic orientation:

- ST-40 *Fenglong*: hallucinations; phobia; *Yangming* type mania

- HE-5 *Tongli*: talking to oneself

PART - VII
Microcosm-Macrocosm
The Human and the World

- **Impact of modern life-style on human psychology**

- **Collective Belief Systems and Ecology**

Part-VII

Microcosm-Macrocosm: The Human and the World

Mental disorders are rapidly increasing worldwide.

The "Diagnostic and Statistical Manual of Mental Disorders" (DSM), was first published in the fifties with a compilation of over 100 mental and mood disorders. The latest version the DSM-V (2013) contains over 400 mental disorders with their diagnostic and statistical criteria.
Psychiatric disorders or mental illnesses are defined as behaviours or thoughts that cause significant distress and disrupt the individual's functioning. Worldwide, one out of three people qualify for at least one mental disorder at some point of their lives; this percentage seems even higher in the US (46%). The incidence seems to correspond to the degrees of social and economic changes brought on by the shift from an agrarian to an industrial society, hence the modification of the environment and of lifestyle. The root cause of the problem seems to be the physical and psychological alienation of humans from their natural world (Les Convivialistes, 2013). This disconnection from nature has been linked to a growing load of stress and mental health challenges in modern societies (Rosa; Theory of Acceleration 2014).

7.1 Impact of modern life-style on human psychology

Our modern industrial society seems to have been detrimental to humans and their environment through the changes that it has brought on:

- Urbanisation: the displacement from smaller village life to populated settlements and towns and the inevitable over-crowding and proximity issues. This expansion of human habitation is at the detriment of the natural surroundings, the flora and the fauna as well as a great loss of quality of life for the human being.

- Changes in family structures: from older family structures extending several generations to nuclear families, consisting only of the parents and their children. Older people find themselves quite often isolated and relegated to specialised institutions, rather than being naturally surrounded by their family, with the inevitable consequence of dreading old age and its psychological issues, prevalent in urban societies.

- Industrialisation, which at this time is mainly dependent on fossil energy with its indisputable disastrous ecological impact. In fact, urbanisation and industrialisation have been responsible for the extinction of numerous species of animals and plants through the destruction of their natural habitat and through the climatic changes, partly imputed to the human technological progress. According to scientific data, the rate of biological extinction has reached alarming levels (Pimm et al. 2014). Furthermore, the industrialisation of agriculture has had a catastrophic effect on biodiversity, disrupting the nature's symbiotic equilibrium.

- Loss of contact with nature and the natural rhythms: In fact, the human has been striving to dominate nature; the notion of day and night has been abolished by artificial light; the cold of winter or the heat of summer are mastered by technology. But even as the outer natural rhythms and changes may be artificially altered to fit the social needs, the inner cycles cannot be harnessed in the same manner. The human being will still get old and die and no scientific technology can modify the inner seasons.

The split between the human psyche and nature is linked to both, the current ecological crisis (Jordan, 2009) and the mental health of humanity (Chalquist, 2009).

7.2 Collective Belief Systems and Ecology

In the first chapter of *Nei Jing Su Wen*, the Yellow Emperor ≈ *Huang Ti* is asking the question of why are people living shorter life spans and becoming decrepit? *Qi Bo* answers:

> **In ancient times, those who understood the Dao,**
>
> **lived in harmony with the natural rhythms...**

Following the Chinese concept of the human (microcosm) being a reflection of its environment (macrocosm), it becomes quite clear as to why mental disorders are affecting an ever-increasing number of individuals on the planet.

But the reverse is also true; the outer world is a reflection of the inner human state; in other words, we create the world that we live in. Explicitly, the collective mental framework or belief systems are at the origin of our present-day reality.

Industrialisation stems from beliefs such as:

- More is better...
- Success in life is to have...
- Happiness is to own....
- Money is power...
- A progressive society is one that produces more...
- If I am rich enough nothing can happen to me...
- If I am rich enough, I can do whatever I want...

Which naturally leads to beliefs about superiority and inferiority, competition and power struggles, rich and poor etc.; and unfortunately leads to the justification of abnormal and dehumanising acts of domination, war, invasion, genocide and terrorism.

The collective belief, predominant in the world today, is that happiness is money and that money is power and vice versa. As the economic growth in the world seems to correspond to the industrialisation and productivity, it leads to the belief that only through industrial growth a society may reach happiness and well-being.

It seems that real poverty is encountered more in affluent areas of the world and in larger agglomerations. In the so-called poor rural areas, there is a natural support for the needy, by their community.

This explains the fact that in a clinical setting, the most central of our patient's complaints is the issue of insecurity and fear, stemming from financial or affective concerns.

Historically, the invention of currency as a medium of exchange was to facilitate trade. Various objects and mediums where used to be later replaced by coins. Paper money appeared first in China around the 7th century to become popularised by the 13th century. The concept of currency refers to a current, something fluid and in motion. When a river's fluidity is blocked, there is an accumulation (excess) on the up-stream and a deficiency down-stream. This also happens with wealth and resources that are accumulated in one place rather being distributed evenly worldwide. The result of this discrepancy can be clearly seen in the geo-political situation of today's world.

It is not difficult to see the disturbing parallels between the human physical and mental disorders and the conditions of the world, namely nature, ecology and the human society.

Health Issues in TCM	Changes in Nature and in Society
Hot and Yang-type diseases: bacterial and viral infections (TB, AIDS, SARS, Ebola...); inflammations; allergies; psychosis	Global warming
Weakened *Jing*: infertility, osteoporosis, tooth decay; increase in cancer; increase in dementia and mental diseases;	Depletion of fossil-fuel reserves (the *Jing* of the earth)
Yin deficiency patterns: insomnia; burn-out; menopausal syndrome; type-1 diabetes; diabetes insipidus...	Drinking water shortage
Yang-rising and internal Wind: hypertension; tinnitus; vertigo; stroke...	Unusual climatic extremes; Hurricanes and tornados
Weakened immune system; impoverishment of intestinal flora due to antibiotics...	Loss of bio-diversity through mono-culture and pesticides
Diseases of Phlegm and stagnation: obesity; type-2 diabetes; arteriosclerosis; arthrosis...	Sedentary life-style; processed foods; sugar addiction
Local accumulation and stagnation (lumps and tumours): Qi-Blood-Fluids-Phlegm-Food etc.	Conspicuous and inequitable accumulation of wealth
Respiratory diseases (especially in children)	Pollution; de-forestation
Auto-immune diseases	Genocide
Shen disturbances	Living proximity; sound and light pollution; life-style, in particular the loss of connection with nature and the natural cycles

It very much looks like, the technological development that was originally meant to free the humans from tedious daily chores, has had the opposite effect of actually enslaving them. And although science has been capable of increasing life expectancy, it has greatly contributed to a deterioration of life quality.

We are, at this time, faced with a stark fact; the exponential economic and population growth of our planet is not compatible with the limited supply of resources available and that there is a limit to growth (The limits of growth; Meadows et al).

The healing of our planet, desperately calls for a universal change of our collective values and belief systems

If we consider the history of the universe, according to the Big Bang theory, it has taken 15 billion years of evolution to reach this point in time and space. Earth is about 4.5 billion years old and life on earth is estimated to have appeared 3.5 billion years ago. If this time span is reduced to a scale of one year, the homo sapiens is only a few minutes old!

In this very short time, the human being has had an impact on this planet that will have far reaching consequences into the future.

Modern theories of evolution are primarily rooted on Darwinian notions of the "survival of the fittest" (1895) and Lamarck's 19th c. concept of orthogenesis "drive towards complexity", and adaptability to environmental factors (basis of modern epigenetics). All life forms follow the same fundamental laws of survival and continuation of the species. With the acquisition of consciousness, humans are now capable of better evaluating the consequences of their actions and better adapting to outer changes. But then humanity is only at its preliminary evolutionary stages.

Many ancient philosophical and metaphysical models have represented the human evolutionary process.

- The ancient Chinese ideogram representing the human being on three levels (▶ Fig. 7.1).
    - Earth level: mobility, life maintenance (survival) and reproduction (continuation of the species). At this level, the human being is identical to all other life forms.
    - The Human level: primarily consisting of emotions and passions.
    - The Heaven level: representing the mind and the spirit. The ideogram further symbolises the nine stages of evolution to attain the spiritual awakening

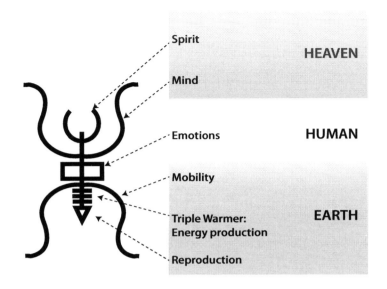

Fig. 7.1:   Heaven-Human-Earth levels and the Nine stages

- The ancient Hindu and Vedic traditions describe the human metaphysical evolution following five or seven stages or "Chakras": (▶Fig. 7.2):

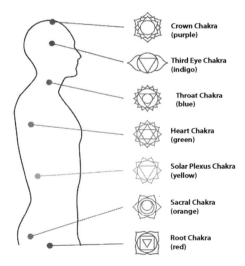

Fig. 7.2:   The Seven Chakras

- 1st chakra (Root/ pelvic): survival (basic needs and security)

- 2nd chakra (Sacral/ lower abdomen): sexuality, reproduction and creativity

- 3rd chakra (Solar plexus): personal power

- 4th chakra (Heart/ chest): humanity, love, interconnection, compassion; this is the bridge between the lower three chakras representing the material, and the upper three centres, corresponding to the spiritual realms)

- 5th chakra (Throat): expression(speech) and authenticity

- 6th chakra (Third eye): intuition

- 7th chakra (Crown/ apex): connection to the whole (to the divine); spiritual awakening

It seems that the human at this evolutionary stage, is at the level of the 3rd chakra, the centre of power and domination, reflected in the universal human beliefs and the source of human and ecological suffering.

Only an elevation of the global consciousness to the 4th chakra, the heart centre may bring the much-needed salvation.

Our planet, has been calling for help, but we humans have been ignoring this call, in the same way that the body-messages are often ignored or silenced until a serious disease is manifesting. At the time of writing of this text, the Covid-19 epidemic has forced the whole world to re-examine their options and positions. What all the thinkers, philosophers and scientists of our time did not manage to do, a tiny virus has achieved in a few months. We can only hope that this warning may be heard and heeded (▶ see also discussion about significance of cancer: 6.2.3).

By restoring the connection between humans (microcosm) and the earth (macrocosm), can we hope to heal both the humanity's mental and physical well-being and the planetary ecology.

"We have forgotten who we are.
We have alienated ourselves from the unfolding of the cosmos.
We have become estranged from the movements of the earth.
We have turned our backs on the cycles of life.
We have forgotten who we are."
(United Nations Environmental Sabbath Program, 1990, p. 70)

And when, Humanity, you will return to Nature,
on that day your eyes will open,
you will gaze straight into the eyes of Nature,
and in its mirror, you will see
your own image…
A.D. Gordon

APPENDIX

- **Zang-Fu disharmony patterns and the Psyche**

  - Heart disharmony patterns
  - Liver disharmony patterns
  - Spleen disharmony patterns
  - Lung disharmony patterns
  - Kidney disharmony patterns

- **Overview of the 8 Extraordinary Vessel symptoms and point indications**

  - *Chong Mai*
  - *Ren Mai*
  - *Du Mia*
  - *Dai Mai*
  - *Yin* and *Yang Wei Mai*
  - *Yin* and *Yang Qiao Mai*

- **Spirit of Acupuncture Points**

  - Symbolism of Heart-channel points
  - *Shen* and *Ling* points
  - *Gui* ≈ Ghost points
  - *Tian* ≈ Heaven points
  - The Five *Zhi* or *Shen* points: *Shen-Yi-Po-Zhi-Hun*

- **Specific exercises and meditation techniques**

  - The Central Axis
  - Psychology and Acupuncture Therapy (PAT) for Releasing the Body Armours and for changing the Beliefs
  - PAT exercises for changing the Belief mechanisms
  - PAT exercises for identifying and changing the subconscious programs
  - PAT exercises for transforming emotions
  - PAT exercises for restoring the brain connections

- **Case Studies**

Appendix

Appendix-I   Zang-Fu disharmony patterns and the Psyche

A.1.1 Heart disharmony patterns

A.1.1.1   Heart-Fire:

- Symptoms:

- Mental and emotional restlessness; overexcited, reckless character, loud, agitated, manic; possibility of sexual perversions
- Difficulty falling asleep through anxiety or worry; nightmares, dreams of flying,
- Bright eyes, loud voice, always feeling hot, thirsty, bitter taste
- Tachycardia; hypertension, heart diseases; bleeding problems
- Tongue: red, red tip, yellow coating; tongue ulcerations
- Pulse: rapid, overflowing

- Treatment: HE-7 *Shenmen*, HE-8 *Shaofu*, PE-7 *Daling*, PE-8 *Laogong*, BL-14 *Jueyinshu*, BL-15 *Xinshu*, RM-14 *Juque*, KI-23 *Shenfeng*, DU-19 *Houding*, RM-15 *Jiuwei* and PE-5 Jianshi, SP-6 *Sanyinjiao*.

A.1.1.2 Phlegm-Fire harassing the Mind

- Symptoms:

- Same as above; nightmares
- Snoring, chest oppression
- Nausea, lack of appetite
- Tongue: red, red tip, yellow coating

- Pulse: Rapid and slippery

- Treatment: PE-5 *Jianshi*, PE-8 *Laogong*, HE-8 *Shaofu*, BL-14 *Jueyinshu*, RM-12 *Zhongwan*, RM-9 *Shuifen*, ST-40 *Fenglong*.

A.1.1.3   Heart-Blood-Stasis:

- Symptoms:

- Anxiety when lying down, restless and dream disturbed sleep
- Palpitations; chest pains, angina pectoris
- Purple tongue, or purple spots
- Pulse: choppy

- Treatment: PE-6 *Neiguan*, HE-7 *Shenmen*, HE-5 *Tongli*, KI-23 *Shenfeng*, RM-17 *Shanzhong*, BL-14 *Jueyinshu*, BL-15 *Xinshu*, BL-17 *Geshu*, BL-15 *Xinshu*, BL-43 *Gaohuangshu*

A.1.1.4   Phlegm misting the mind

- Symptoms:

- Mental confusion, lack of concentration, disorientation; emotional numbness
- If more severe: psychosis, mania dementia or coma
- Reduced sensory functions
- Tongue: swollen, greasy coating
- Pulse: Slippery

- Treatment: PE-5 *Jianshi*, ST-40 *Fenglong*, DM-20 *Baihui,* DM-18 *Qiangjian;* also, *Jing Bie* of ST and SP: ST-30 *Qichong*, SP-12 *Chongmen*; RM-12 *Zhongwan*; ST-9 *Renying*; DM-20 *Baihui*

A.1.1.5   Heart-Blood-Xu/ vacuity:

- Symptoms:

- Anxiety, difficulty falling asleep, restless and light sleep, frequent waking, dreams, nightmares, dreams of flying

- Poor memory, concentration problems, feeling spaced out; easily tired

- Shyness, sadness; inhibition, trembling with emotions; regrets

- Palpitations, dizziness, blurred vision; low blood pressure

- Tongue: Pale

- Pulse: choppy or weak

- Treatment: HE-7 *Shenmen*, BL-14 *Jueyinshu*, BL-15 *Xinshu*, RM-14 *Juque*, KI-23 *Shenfeng*, KI-24 *Lingxu*, DU-19 *Houding*, RM-15 *Jiuwei* and PE-6 *Neiguan*, SP-6 *Sanyinjiao*, BL-20 *Pishu*, BL-17 *Geshu*, ST-36 *Zusanli*, *Yintang* (Extra).

A.1.1.6   Heart-Yin-Xu, often associated with KI-Yin-Xu: HE and KI out of harmony

- Symptoms:

- Anxiety and fear; sadness and melancholia; weak character, shyness; misanthropic

- Difficulty falling asleep, restless sleep, frequent waking; dreams of water, drowning or wounds

- Dry throat, palpitations, night sweats, "five palms" heat; tinnitus, lumbar pains

- Tongue: peeled, red tip, cracks; Heart crack

- Pulse: Floating and empty

- Treatment: same as above; for Heart and Kidney-Yin-Xu add: HE-6 *Yinxi*, KI-1 *Yongquan*, KI-3 *Taixi*, KI-6 *Zhaohai*, RM-4 *Guanyuan,* BL-23 *Shenshu*, BL-44 *Shentang* and BL-52 *Zhishi*.

A.1.1.7   Heart-Qi-Xu, (Often associated with GB-Xu)

- Symptoms:

- Superficial sleep, insomnia from anxiety; easily startled, timidity, indecisiveness easily tired and needing rest; difficulty in attaining sexual satisfaction

- Palpitations (arrhythmia); shortness of breath, fatigue, depression

- Tongue: Pale, swollen in the front, possibly Heart crack

- Pulse: Empty

- Treatment: HE-7 *Shenmen*, BL-14 *Jueyinshu*, BL-15 *Xinshu*, RM-14 *Juque*, KI-24 *Lingxu*, KI-25 *Shencang*, PE-6 *Neiguan*, GB-40 *Qiuxu*, REN-17 *Shanzhong*, RM-6 *Qihai* and ST-36 *Zusanli*.

A.1.1.8   Heart-Yang-Xu

- Symptoms:

- Same as above; often accompanies Kidney-Yang-Xu,
- Disliking the cold; cold with emotions; depression
- Tongue, Pale, bluish
- Pulse: Slow, deep

- Treatment: same as above, add DM-4 *Mingmen*, DM-14 *Dazhui*, DM-20 *Baihui*

A.1.2 Liver disharmony patterns

A.1.2.1   Liver- Fire:

- Symptoms:

- Anger, irritability, envy, jealousy; hysteria; fits of rage with loss of control
- Restless sleep, nightmares, insomnia between 1-3 am, waking early,
- Headaches, red eyes, red face; internal wind
- Bitter taste; dark urine, dry stools
- Tongue: red sides, dry-yellow coating
- Pulse: Rapid and wiry

- Treatment: LR-2 *Xingjian*, LR-3 *Taichong*, GB-44 *Zuqiaoyin*, GB-12 *Wangu* or *Anmien*, GB-20 *Fengchi*, BL-18 *Ganshu*, BL-47 *Hunmen*, DM-20 *Baihui*, GB-13 *Benshen*, or GB-15 *Toulinqi* and DU-24 Shenting; also treat the Kidney.

For hysteria or delirium add: HE-4 *Lingdao,* HE-5 *Tongli,* PE-4 *Ximen* and DM-26 *Renzhong*

A.1.2.2   Liver Qi stagnation

- Symptoms :

- Feeling stressed, moody, depressed, frustrated
- Chest oppression and flank pains; premenstrual pain and tension; neck and shoulder tension; throat plum pit
- Irregular periods and bowel movements
- Tongue: red sides
- Pulse: Wiry

- Treatment: LR-3 *Taichong,* LI-4 *Hegu,* PE-7 *Daling,* PE-6 *Neiguan,* LR-14 *Qimen,* BL-18 *Ganshu,* BL-47 *Hunmen,* DM-20 *Baihui*

A.1.2.3   Liver-Blood-Xu

- Symptoms:

- Restless sleep, *Fan* ≈ Restlessness, waking early, vivid dreams
- Amnesia; lack of ideas, no direction in life
- Internal wind symptoms; vision problems; muscle cramps
- Tongue: pale sides
- Pulse: Choppy

- Treatment: BL-18 *Ganshu,* BL-20 *Pishu,* BL-17 *Geshu,* BL-23 *Shenshu,* LR-8 *Ququan* and SP-6 *Sanyinjiao; Anmien.*

A.1.2.4   Liver-Yin-Xu

- Symptoms:

- Irritability; feeling of heat; dizziness
- Restless sleep, nightmares, excess dreaming, sleep walking or sleep talking waking early
- Dryness of throat, eyes, skin and hair
- Tongue: dry, peeled sides, maybe red
- Pulse: Floating and empty, or thin and rapid

- Treatment: BL-18 *Ganshu*, BL-47 *Hunmen*, LR-8 *Ququan*, SP-6 *Sanyinjiao*, GB-2 *Tinghui*; GB-13 *Benshen*, DU-24 *Shenting*; also treat Kidney-Yin.

A.1.2.5   Gall Bladder Qi-Xu (often associated with Heart-Qi-Xu)

- Symptoms:

- Easily startled, timid, lack of will and initiative, indecision
- Insomnia from insecurity, light sleep, excess dreaming, dreams of fights, struggles, suicide; waking early, difficulty to get up
- Palpitation, shortness of breath, fatigue, vertigo
- Tongue: Pale, swollen
- Pulse: Empty

- Treatment: add GB-40 *Qiuxu,* GB-43 *Xiaxi,* GB-15 *Toulinqi,* and GB-12 *Wangu* or *Anmien*.

A.1.3 Spleen and Stomach disharmony patterns

A.1.3.1   Stomach-Heat; Stomach-Fire

- Symptoms:

- Mental restlessness ≈ *Fan*, discontentment, moving and talking too fast; accusing and insulting; agitation, and in extreme conditions, the tendency to "climb to high places to sing" or to undress and run around (streaking);
- Restless sleep; frequent dreams, nightmares; needing to eat or drink in order to fall asleep
- Gastritis, thirst, bad breath, hunger; acne, red eyes,
- Tongue: Stomach crack, red, yellow-dry coating
- Pulse: Flooding

- Treatment: BL-21 *Weishu*, RM-7 *Yinjiao*, RM-12 *Zhongwan*, ST-41 *Jiexi*, ST-36 *Zusanli*, ST-21 *Liangmen*, ST-40 *Fenglong,* SP-1 *Yinbai* with ST-44 *Neiting*, DM-20 *Baihui*.

A.1.3.2   Spleen-Qi Xu

- Symptoms:

- Depression, melancholia; fixed ideas, obsessiveness, obsessed with the past

- Insomnia after 3 am, sleep walking, nightmares; general fatigue with daytime sleepiness,

- Bloating after meals, soft stools

- Tongue: Pale, swollen with teeth marks

- Pulse: Empty

- Treatment: BL-20 Pishu, BL-49 *Yishe,* LR-13 *Zhangmen*, RM-12 *Zhongwan,* KI-17 *Shangqu*, SP-2 *Dadu*, SP-3 *Taibai*; SP-1 Yinbai with ST-44 Neiting; DM-20 *Baihui*

A.1.3.3   Stomach-Qi Xu

- Symptoms:

- Similar to the above pattern;

- Obsessional neurosis; altruism or even masochism; phobia, pessimism, doubting, suicidal tendency; oversensitive to noise (hyperacousia)

- Treatment: add ST-42 *Chongyang,* ST-36 *Zusanli,* SP-4 *Gongsun,* SP-5 *Shangqiu*

A.1.4 Lung disharmony patterns

A.1.4.1   Lung-Heat

- Symptoms:

- Sadness, neurasthenia; obsessed and worrying about the future; self-sacrificing; schizophrenia (calm madness)

- Insomnia with agitation, waking at 3 a.m. (solar time); dreams of flying, fear or tears

- Asthma, cough with yellow sputum; hypertension

- Tongue: Red in the front part

- Pulse: Flooding and fast

- Treatment: BL-13 *Feishu*, LU-1 *Zhongfu*, LU-5 *Chize*, LU-6 *Kongzui*, LU-10 *Yuji*, KI-22 *Bulang*, BL-13 *Feishu,* BL-42 *Pohu,*   LI-4 Hegu, LI-11 *Quchi,* ST-40 *Fenglong,* PE-5 *Jianshi*.

A.1.4.2   Lung-Qi-Xu

- Symptoms:

- Antisocial behaviour, holding grudges, aggressivity, perversions, sadism,

- Insomnia, waking at 3 a.m. (solar time),

- Weak breathing, cough, asthma, frequent colds, dry skin, hair loss

- Tongue: Swollen in the front, pale

- Pulse: Empty, floating

- Treatment: BL-13 *Feishu*, BL-42 *Pohu*, LU-1 *Zhongfu*, LU-9 *Taiyuan*, LU-7 *Lieque,* KI-22 *Bulang,* KI-24 *Lingxu,* LI- 4. *Hegu*

A.1.5 Kidney disharmony patterns

A.1.5.1   Kidney-Yin-Xu accompanied by Heart-Yin-Xu: Heart and Kidney not in harmony

- Symptoms:

- Mental and emotional restlessness; overexcited, reckless character, loud, agitated, manic

- Difficulty falling asleep, restless sleep, frequent waking; dreams of water, drowning or wounds

- Dry throat, palpitations, night sweats, "five palm" heat; tinnitus, lumbar pains; dark urine

- Tongue: peeled, red tip, cracks; Heart crack

- Pulse: Floating and empty

- Treatment: same as for Heart Yin Xu add HE-6 *Yinxi,* KI-1 *Yongquan,* KI-3 *Taixi,* KI-6 *Zhaohai,* RM-4 *Guanyuan,* BL-23 *Shenshu,* BL-44 *Shentang* and BL-52 *Zhishi.*

If the *Shen* is very unsettled with persistent insomnia, use KI-21 *Youmen* if tired but cannot sleep, KI-23 *Shenfeng* for a restless mind, KI-25 *Shencang* for insomnia from worry, KI- 26 *Yuzhong* for waking in a bad mood, and KI-27 Shufu for persistent insomnia.

A.1.5.2 Kidney-Yang-Xu, accompanied by Heart-Yang-Xu

- Symptoms:

- Anxiety and fear, easily startled; sadness and melancholia; weak and introverted character, shyness and indecisiveness; misanthropic tendency; cold with emotions

- Superficial sleep, insomnia from anxiety

- Mental fatigue; yawning, sighing, tearful; dislike of cold,

- Lumbar pains, urinary frequency; palpitations (arrhythmia); shortness of breath, fatigue, depression

- Tongue, Pale, bluish

- Pulse: Slow, deep

- Treatment: HE-7 *Shenmen,* KI-3 *Taixi,* BL-15 *Xinshu,* BL-23 *Shenshu,* BL-52 *Zhishi,* BL-44 *Shentang,* RM-14 *Juque,* RM-4 *Guanyuan,* SI-3 *Houxi* with BL-62 *Shenmai,* KI-24 *Lingxu,* KI-25 *Shencang,* DM-4 *Mingmen,* DM-14 *Dazhui,* GB-39 *Xuanzhong,* DM-20 *Baihui*

Appendix-II   Overview of the 8 Extraordinary Vessel symptoms and point indications

A.2.1 *Chong Mai*

(▶ Fig. A.2.1)

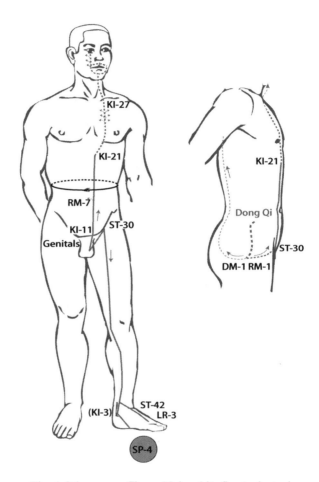

Fig. A.2.1:   *Chong Mai* and its five trajectories

Overview of Chong Mai Symptoms

- Counter-flow Qi: energy rushing up, internal Heat
- Hot head, cold feet
- Heart pains
- Digestive symptoms, abdominal heaviness

- Fatigue

- Depression; panic attacks

- Gynaecology: blood stasis, PMS, myoma, endometriosis

- Sterility, miscarriage

- Prolapse, ptosis, hernia

- Lumbar pains after lifting

Constituent point selection and treatment strategies

- KI-11 *Henggu* to KI-21 *Youmen* for supplementing the *Zang* organs and for the *Gaohuang*≈Protective and Vital membranes (KI-16 *Huangshu* and RM-6 *Qihai,* with BL-43 *Gaohuangshu,* BL-51 *Huangmen,* BL-53 *Baohuan*g*)*

- KI-22 *Bulang* to KI-27 *Shufu* for chest symptoms, Blood or Phlegm accumulations and for Heart and Kidney not communicating

- KI-11 *Henggu,* KI-10 *Yingu,* BL-40 *Weizhong* are added for prolapse, oedema, heaviness in the legs and osteoporosis

- ST-30 *Qichong,* ST-42 *Chongyang* for supplementing ST-Yin and SP-Qi

- *Dai Mai* and *Du Mai* for *Bi*≈Impediment syndromes

- KI-12 *Dahe* for astringing and, consolidating the Kidneys with BL-43 *Gaohuangshu* for leucorrhoea or spermatorrhoea.

- KI-13 *Qixue* (*Baomen*) for infertility from Blood-*Xu* ≈ *Vacuity* with KI-Qi-*Xu.*

- KI-14 *Siman:* drain to move stagnation of Blood, Qi, food or Water, supplement to help ovulation in women, and sexual arousal in men.

- KI-15 *Zhongzhu* nourishes *Jing,* to regulate the menses and move Qi and Blood and regulate Fluids.

- KI-16 *Huangshu* to support the *Huang* ≈ Vital membranes, regulate Spleen, Stomach and Intestines, descend the Qi and move Blood.

- KI-8 *Jiaoxin* regulates *Chong* and *Ren Mai,* helps to build trust and supports *Jing*

- KI-17 *Shangqu* fortifies Spleen, Stomach and Intestines, moves Qi and Blood and eliminates accumulations.

- KI-19 *Yindu* moves Qi, dispels Dampness, harmonises the middle Triple Warmer.

- KI-21 *Yaomen* regulates Liver, Spleen and Stomach, especially for Liver invading the Earth, subdues counterflow Qi.

- SP-4 *Gongsun,* ST-25 *Tianshu,* RM-9 *Shuifen,* ST-44 *Neiting.* For abdominal pain with boating

- For ST-Yin depletion, with dryness of the eyes, mouth or throat: add ST-42 *Chongyang,* RM-22 *Tiantu,* RM-23 *Lianquan,* ST-4 *Dicang,* ST-1 *Chengqi*

- For rebellious Qi and running piglet syndrome: SP-4 *Gongsun*, PE-6 *Neiguan,* LR-3 *Taichong,* PE-7 *Daling* or LI-4 *Hegu.* KI-14 *Siman,* KI-21 *Youmen,* possibly RM-18 *Yutang,* and in case of rapid and hoarse breathing, RM-17 *Tiantu* and for plum-pit throat ST-5 *Daying.*

- To release the abdominal rectus muscle: ST-25 *Tianshu,* or by a Japanese method, by needling LR-4 *Zhongfeng* and if not sufficient, followed by LU-5 *Chize.*

- For moving/ invigorating Blood in gynaecology: add KI-14 *Siman,* or KI-15 *Zhongzhu* for regulating menses, also KI-16 *Huangshu,* together with KI-5 *Shuiquan*, SP-6 *Sanyinjiao* and SP-10 *Xuehai.*

- Benefiting the breast: to move stasis, add *Yaomen* KI-21 or *Shenfeng* KI-23; to transform Phlegm add KI-27 *Shufu;* to nourish the breast milk after childbirth add KI-16 *Huangshu,* BL-43 *Gaohuangshu* and BL-51 *Huangmen.*

- In andrology: for prostatic adenoma add LR-3 *Taichong,* LI-4 *Hegu,* RM-2 *Qugu,* KI-11 *Henggu* and KI-14 *Siman,* as well as SP-*9 Yinlingquan*, BL-32 *Cilaio* and BL-34 *Xialiao.*

- For erectile problems add KI-12 *Dahe,* RM-4 *Guan-yuan*, RM-6 *Qihai,* SP-6 *Sanyinjiao,* BL-23 *Shenshu,* BL-15 *Xinshu* and BL-43 *Gaohuangshu.*

- For *Bi*≈Impediment syndromes due to Blood stagnation as in fractures, Raynaud's syndrome, discus hernia, or osteoporosis: invigorate Yang and move Blood: add DM-4 *Mingmen,* BL-17 *Geshu* and BL-11 *Dazhu.* For cold and numb feet, add ST-30 *Qichong,* ST-39 *Xiajuxu,* LR-3 *Taichong.* For heavy legs, add ST-42 *Chongyang,* LR-3 *Taichong.*

- In case of neuropathy (Polio) add *Dai Mai,* GB-41 *Zulinqi,* and *Du Mai* SI-3 *Houxi;* add for the upper limbs LI-15 *Jianyu,* and for the lower limbs GB-30 *Huantiao.*

- For lumbar pains with stress and anxiety: SP-4 *Gongsun,* RM-6 *Qihai,* KI-5 *Shuiquan,* BL-23 *Shenshu*

- For sinking SP-Qi with prolapse, oedema, heaviness in the lower limbs, water retention in the legs, or even osteoporosis: SP-4 *Gongsun,* KI-11 *Henggu,* DM-20 *Baihui,* KI-10 *Yingu,* BL-40

Weizhong, KI-6 *Zhaohui,* KI-3 *Taixi* and KI-1 *Yongquan.* Generally, Moxa is used.

- For nine kinds of Heart or chest pains:

  - Due to Cold add HE-7 *Shenmen,* RM-12 *Weizhong,* SP-1 *Dadu*

  - Stabbing pain add PE-6 *Neiguan,* PE-7 *Daling* and KI-26 *Yuzhong*

  - Angina pain with anxiety add HE-7 *Shenmen,* BL-15 *Xinshu,* "EP" *Bailao*

  - Kidney and Heart not communicating with restlessness and anxiety and fright, add KI-1 *Yongquan,* KI-6 *Zhaohai* and KI-9 *Zhubin*

  - Oesophageal spasms with hiccups add ST-36 *Zusanli,* SP-3 *Taibai,* RM-17 *Shanzhong*

  - From indigestion with abdominal fullness add ST-44 *Neiting,* ST-25 *Tianshu* and RM-9 *Shuifen;* or with vomiting add RM-12 *Zhongwan,* for Phlegm add KI-27 *Shufu,* ST-40 *Fenglong*

  - Fullness below the hypochondrium, add LR-3 *Taichong,* GB-34 *Yanglingquan* and GB-39 *Xuanzhong*

  - With jaundice add RM-12 *Zhongwan,* ST-36 *Zusanli,* RM-17 *Shanzhong,* DM-9 *Zhiyang*

  - For malaria with chest pains add PE-6 *Neiguan,* PE-7 *Daling,* RM-13 *Shangwan;* or LU-7 *Lieque,* RM-17 *Zhongwan,* LI-4 *Hegu*

- Treating the central axis: SP-4 *Gongsun* and PE-6 *Neiguan,* add according to pattern

  - Due to birth trauma: add KI-16 *Huangshu* and RM-6 *Qihai*

  - Due to gestational trauma: add RM-1 *Huiyin,* RM-4 *Guanyuan* and DM-20 *Baihui*

  - Due to post-natal trauma: add KI-16 *Huangshu,* BL-43 *Gaohuangshu,* BL-51 *Huangmen;* also to help release somatic memories treat separately ST-14 *Kufang,* HE-3 *Shaohai* and BL-62 *Shenmai*

  - If there is a loss of desire to live: add RM-14 *Juque* and ST-23 *Taiyi;* with loss of will to live, combine BL-23 *Shenshu* and BL-52 *Zhishi* with BL-15 *Xinshu* and BL-44 *Shentang*

  - For difficulty in moving in the world or taking a stand: add KI-1 *Yongquan* or BL-61 *Pucan* with BL-62 *Shenmai;* to help accept oneself add KI-6 *Zhaohai* and to help accept the different transitional periods in life add KI-9 *Zhubin*

A.2.2 *Ren Mai*

(▶ Fig. A.2.2)

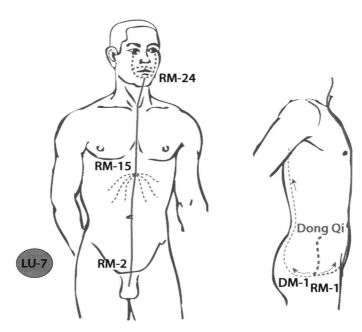

Fig. A.2.2:   *Ren Mai* **and its two trajectories**

Overview of *Ren Mai* symptoms

- Yin-*Xu* with empty Heat signs
- Yin-*Xu* with Yin-stasis
- *Shan* in men: hernia, varicocele, prostatitis
- *Zheng-Jia* in women: fibroid, ovarian cyst, endometriosis
- Vaginal discharge
- Sterility
- Lumbar pains
- Peri-umbilical pains
- Co-dependency, eating disorders, addictions

Constituent point selection and treatment strategies

- Lower *Sanjiao* area: RM-1 *Huiyin* to RM-8 *Shenque* are indicated for reproductive, urogenital and intestinal problems; as well as for group, gender or identity issues

- RM-1 *Huiyin:* supplements Yin, astringes Jing, benefits the lower orifices; genital pains

- RM-2 *Qugu:* supplements KI-Yang and *Jing*, regulates Bladder and uterus

- RM-3 *Zhongji*: supplements KI, regulates the lower TW; urogenital pathologies

- RM-4 *Guanyuan*: supplements KI and *Yuan* Qi, regulates the lower TW, astringes Jing; genito-urinary and intestinal pathologies

- RM-5 *Shimen*: supplements KI and *Yuan* Qi, astringes *Jing*, regulates the lower TW; urogenital pains and pathologies; rescues Yang

- RM-6 *Qihai*: supplements KI and *Yuan* Qi, regulates the lower TW

- RM-7 *Yinjiao*: for menstrual pains, or abdominal pains with bloating

- Middle *Sanjiao* area: RM-8 *Shenque* to RM-15 *Jiuwei,* are indicated for digestive problems, eating dysfunctions and issues pertaining to control:

  - RM-8 *Shenque*: regulates SP and ST, supplements KI and *Yuan Qi*, rescues Yang

  - RM-9 *Shuifen*: peri-umbilical or abdominal pains with diarrhoea or gastroenteritis

  - RM-10 *Xiawan*: command point of the second separation of solids

  - RM-11 *Jianli*: command point of the separation of solids

  - RM-12 *Zhongwan*: *Hui* of the *Fu* organs; *Mu* of the ST and the middle TW; command point of digestion, regulates SP and ST; all digestive problems

  - RM-13*Shangwan*: command point of the first separation

  - RM-14*Juque*: regulates Heart and Stomach Qi; indigestion, abdominal pains and bloating

- Upper *Sanjiao* area: RM-15 *Jiuwei* to RM-24 *Chengjiang,* for respiratory and cardiovascular problems, as well as issues to do with faith and trust

  - RM-15 *Jiuwei*: longitudinal *Luo* of *Ren Mai*; regulates Heart and Stomach Qi, opens the chest; command point of the sexual organs

  - RM-16 *Zhongting*: chest and gastric pains

  - RM-17 *Shanzhong*: supports *Zhong Qi* and Lung and Heart functions; chest and oesophageal pains; opens the chest

  - RM-18 Yutang and RM-19 Zigong: intercostal or thoracic pains

- RM-20 *Huagai*: chest pains with cough

- RM-21 Xuanji and RM-22 Tiantu: regulate Lung and chest Qi; asthma and cough

- RM-23 *Lian Quan*: mouth and throat pathologies, sore throats

- RM-24*Chengjiang*: facial paralysis, torticollis

- Yin *Xu* ≈ Vacuity: LU-7 *Lieque* with KI-6 *Zhaohui,* add:

  - RM-1 *Huiyin* for pelvic and urogenital and post-partum disorders

  - RM-4 *Guanyuan* for Kidney, uterus, Qi and Blood

  - RM-7 *Yinjiao* for uterine disorders

  - RM-12 *Zhongwan* for all eating and *Shen* disorders

  - RM-15 *Jiuwei* for *Shen* disorders; it descends the Qi

  - RM-17 *Shanzhong* supports *Zong* Qi, Heart and Lung, benefits the breasts, descends Qi

  - RM-22 *Tiantu* for throat and voice problems; it rectifies Lung Qi

  - RM-24 *Chengjiang* for mouth dryness and Heat

  - ST-1 *Chengqi* for dryness of the eyes

- Branch, knot and root treatment (*Gen Jie* ≈ Roots and Terminations):

  - For *Taiyin*: SP-3 *Taibai* or SP-1 *Yinbai,* RM-12 *Zhongwan,* LU-9 *Taiyuan* or LU-11 *Shaoshang*; or to help mobilise: SP-2 *Dadu* or SP-8 *Diji,* RM-12 *Zhongwan* and LU-10 *Yuji* or LU-6 *Kongzui*

  - For *Jueyin*: LR-3 *Taichong* or LR-1 *Dadun,* RM-18 *Yutang* and PE-7 *Daling* or PE-9 *Zhongchong*; to help mobilise: LR-2 *Xingjian* or LR-4 *Zhongfeng* **or** LR-6 *Zhongdu* and PE-8 *Laogong* or PE-4 *Ximen*

  - For *Shaoyin*: KI-3 *Taixi* or KI-1 *Yongquan,* RM-23 *Lianquan* and HE-7 *Shenmen* or HE-9 *Shaochong*; and to help mobilise: KI-2 *Rangu* or KI-5 *Shuiquan* and HE-8 *Shaofu* or HE-6 *Yinxi*

- To open a channel (temperaments) using the *Luo* and the Knot points:

  - To open *Taiyin* outward: SP-4 *Gongsun,* RM-12 *Zhongwan* and LU-7 *Lieque*

  - To connect *Jueyin* with *Shaoyang*: LR-5 *Ligou,* RM-18 *Yutang* and PE-6 *Neiguan*

  - To close *Shaoyin* inward: KI-4 *Dazhong,* RM-23 *Lianquan* and HE-5 *Tongli*

- For moving Yin

  - RM-5 *Shimen*: moves Fluids, benefits the uterus

- RM-7 *Yinjiao*: resolves Dampness, benefits the uterus

- RM-12 *Zhongwan* (Knot of *Taiyin*), moves *Taiyin*

- RM-17 *Shanzhong*: moves chest Qi and Fluids, descends the Qi

- For dispersing Yin

  - RM-3 Zhongji: dispels Dampness in the lower Triple Warmer

  - RM-4 *Guanyuan:* disperses accumulations

  - RM-9 *Shuifen*: disperses Fluid accumulation

  - RM-17 Shanzhong: benefits Lungs and breasts

  - RM-22 *Tiantu: dispels* Phlegm in the throat or chest

  - For moving Blood: RM-2 *Qugu*

- For supporting Spleen to manage Blood: RM-6 *Qihai*

- For neck nodules: LU-7 *Lieque* is combined with a Window of the Sky point: LI-18 *Futu,* ST-9 *Renying,* SI-16 *Tianchuang,* along with ST-12 *Quepen,* KI-27 *Shufu,* RM-17 *Shanzhong,* LI-4 *Hegu.*

- Supporting the three stages of digestion:

  - RM-15 *Jiuwei* and RM-13 *Shangwan,* help the descent of Lung and Stomach Qi

  - RM-12 *Zhongwan* and RM-11 *Jianli,* support the rotting and ripening

  - RM-11 *Jianli* and RM-10 *Xiawan,* support the second separation and excretion of solids

    - For all compensation problems "Three Worms", "Hungry ghosts": RM-12 *Zhongwan*

    - To harmonise the centre and regulate the production of *Ying* and *Wei* Qi (Li Dong Yuan): RM-12 *Zhongwan,* with ST-36 *Zusanli,* RM-13 *Shangwan,* with PE-6 *Neiguan,* RM-10 *Xiawan,* with ST-25 *Tianshu,* and RM-6 *Qihai.*

    - For Damp-Cold accumulation from dietary or emotional causes: LU-7 *Lieque* with RM-6 *Qihai,* RM-8 *Shenque* with Moxa, RM-9 *Shuifen* and RM-21 *Xuanji.*

A.2.3 *Du Mai*

(▶ Fig. A.2.3)

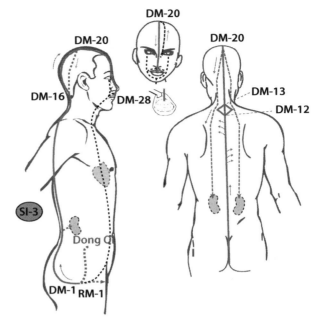

Fig. A.2.3:   *Du Mai* **and its four trajectories**

Overview of *Du Mai* symptoms

- Spinal pains, stiffness or deformation (scoliosis, kyphosis)
- Yang repletion
- Internal Wind
- Yang vacuity
- Weak character
- Chronic external pathogenic factors (EPF)
- Prolapse
- Amnesia

Constituent point selection and treatment strategies

In general: SI-3 *Houxi,* BL-62 *Shenmai,* and DM-1 *Changqiang*

- Lower Curvature: DM-1 to DM-4: For intestinal, reproductive and urogenital conditions
  - DM-3 *Yaoyangguan*: supports KI-Yang, moves Yang down, benefits the lower back and knees; indicated for spinal lesions or pains after surgery
  - DM-4 *Mingmen:* supports Kidney-Fire, strengthens individuality

- Middle Curvature (DM-5 to DM-6*)*: Deals with Digestive problems

    - DM-5 *Xuanshu* mobilises Yang up and downward, supplements Spleen and Stomach, the back and the legs

    - DM-6 *Jizhong* for dermatitis of the palms and soles of the feet.

- Upper Curvature (DM-9 to DM-16): For respiratory, cardiovascular, ear, nose, throat eye conditions as well as for psycho-spiritual issues

    - DM-9 Zhiyang: strengthens the spine; for spinal pains after surgery, or for depression

    - DM-10 *Lingtai* and DM-11 Shendao: affect the *Shen*

    - DM-12 *Shenzhu*, supports Lungs and *Zhong Qi*, Yang type psychological disorders

    - DM-14 *Dazhui:* strengthens Heart-Fire and supports individuality

    - Both DM-4 *Mingmen* and DM-9 *Zhiyang* help in making choices

- DM-17 *Naohu:* moves endocranial blood, dispels Wind and Heat

- DM-20 *Baihui:* lifts the mood and stimulates memory

- DM-19 *Houding:* for insomnia and restlessness

- DM-24 *Shenting:* calms the mind, manic behaviour

- For Yang repletion: SI-3 *Houxi,* DM-14 *Dazhui*; add for:

    - Head-Wind or hyperactivity: BL-1 *Jingming,* DM-20 *Baihui,* DM-16 *Fengfu,* DM-12 *Shenzhu*

    - External Wind: DM-16 *Fengfu*

    - Back pains: *Huatuojiaji* points of the area

    - Lumbar pains: BL-23 *Shenshu*

    - Pains all over the back: DM-8 *Jinsu*

    - For insomnia add BL-62 *Shenmai*

- Yang-*Xu* ≈ Vacuity: DM-4 *Mingmen* (Moxa), DM-20 *Baihui* (Moxa)

- For KI-Yang-*Xu*: add RM-4 *Guanyuan* with Moxa

- Spinal deformity: Treat Yang-*Shi* or Yang-*Xu* accordingly

- For a stiff and rigid back: add DM-9 *Zhiyang* (reduce)

- For kyphosis: supplement DM-9 *Zhiyang,* reduce RM-4 *Guanyuan,* RM-12 *Zhongwan* and RM-22 *Tiantu*

- For scoliosis: GB-27 *Wushu*≈Five axes add *Huatuo Jiaji*

- Menstrual irregularity, Infertility, frigidity, impotence: DM-4 *Mingmen,* BL-23 *Shenshu,* RM-4 *Guanyuan*

- Weak limbs: Bl-35 *Huiyang* (with Moxa), DM-14 *Dazhui*
  - Weak legs: add GB-34 *Yanglingquan*
  - Weak arms: add LI-11 *Quchi*

- Weak character: add DM-4 *Mingmen,* DM-20 *Baihui,* BL-23 *Shenshu,* BL-52 *Zhishi,* BL-11 *Dazhu,* also GB-39 *Xuanzhong*

- Nourishing the Sea of Marrow, amnesia: add DM-16 *Fengfu,* DM-17 *Naohu,* DM-20 *Baihui*

- Loss of voice, speech problems: add DM-15 *Yamen*

- Haemorrhoids or prolapse: add DM-20 *Baihui,* BL-57 *Chengshan*

- Chronic External pathogenic factors (EPF): add DM-16 *Fengfu,* DM-20 *Baihui,* BL-12 *Fengmen*

- For allergies add LU-7 *Lieque,* LR-3 *Taichong,* RM-12 *Zhongwan,* ST-42 *Chongyang,* also BL-13 *Feishu,* BL-18 *Ganshu,* BL-21 *Weishu*

A.2.4 *Dai Mai*

(▶ Fig. A.2.4)

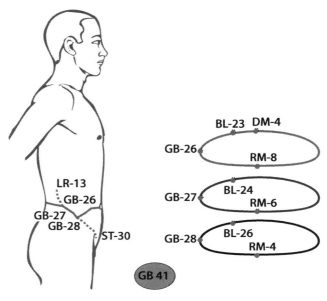

Fig. A.2.4:   *Dai Mai* **and the three belts**

Overview of *Dai Mai* symptoms

- Abdominal fullness, flaccidity of the waist
- Sensation of sitting in water

- Heavy legs, paralysis
- White and red discharge
- Feeling heavy with rain, afraid of the cold
- Excess above, deficiency below
- Breast or eye pains
- Belt-like lumbar pains
- Emotional suppression

Constituent point selection and treatment strategies

In general: GB-41 *Zulinqi,* coupled with TW-5 *Waiguan,* and GB-26 *Daimai* (starting point)

- To resolve Dampness: add LR-13 *Zhangmen*
    - For Damp-Heat add: GB-27 *Wushu*
    - For Damp-Cold add GB-28 *Weidao*
    - For lower TW Dampness add: LR-2 *Xingjian,* LR-3 *Taichong* (vaginal discharge, dysmenorrhoea, irregular menses), LR-4 *Zhongfeng*
    - For Dampness in the Bladder: add BL-60 *Kunlun*
    - For Dampness in the upper parts: add TW-5 *Waiguan,* GB-20 *Fengshi* and BL-60 *Kunlun*
- Belt-like lumbar pains: GB-41 Zulingqi with the most affected branch
    - If BL-23 is most reactive, add GB-26 *Daimai* and BL-40 *Weizhong*
    - If BL-24 is most reactive: add GB-27 *Wushu* and RM-6 *Qihai*
    - If BL-26 is most reactive: add GB-28 *Weidao* and RM-4 *Guanyuan*
    - For lumbar pains during sex: add LR-13 *Zhangmen,* GB-28 *Weidao,* ST-30 *Qichong* and Moxa on LR-1 *Dadun*
    - For lumbar pains and a sensation of coldness in the pelvis: add GB-29 *Juliao,* GB-31 *Fengshi*
- Relaxing the five major axes of the body: add GB-27 *Wushu.*
- Frequent ankle sprains: add GB-34 *Yanglingquan,* GB-40 *Qiuxu*
- To treat the *Bao Mai*: add SP-21 *Dabao,* RM-15 *Jiuwei,* SP-1 *Yinbai,* SP-1 *Diji,* GB-26 *Daimai* or GB-28 *Weidao,* RM-1 *Huiyin* or SP-1 *Diji* to affect the uterus.

A.2.5 *Yin Wei Mai*

(▶ Fig. A.2.5)

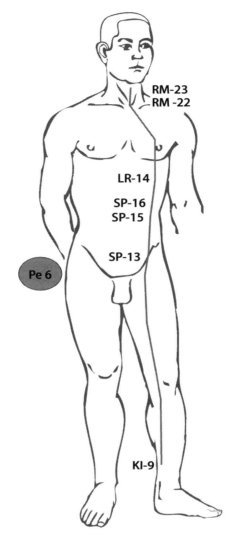

- *Taiyin*: SP-13, SP-15, SP-16
- *Jueyin*: LR-14
- *Shaoyin*: KI-9, RM-23

Fig. A.2.5: *Yin Wei Mai* **and its three segments**

Overview of *Yin Wei Mai* symptoms

- Chest oppression, palpitations
- Heart pains
- Intense headaches, hypertension;

- Energy shooting up; panic attacks
- Intestinal bloating and gas
- Lumbar pains after a psychological shock
- Insomnia from fear
- Depression; irritability; regrets
- Holding on to the past; Heartbreaks
- Dreaming about the future

Constituent point selection and treatment strategies

In general PE-6 *Neiguan,* with SP-4 *Gongsun,* and KI-9 *Zhubin.*

- To calm *Shen* and supplement Blood: add SP-15 *Daheng,* LR-14 *Qimen,* RM-17 *Shanzhong* (regulates Qi)
- To help talk about emotional pain, plum pit: add PE-7 *Daling,* RM-17 *Shanzhong*
- For amnesia or repressed emotions; shyness: add HE-5 *Tongli*
- For food compensations to repress emotions: add BL-20 *Pishu*
- Anxiety feeling in the Stomach: add BL-17 *Geshu*
- For holding emotions in the Intestines; constipation: add BL-57 *Chengshan*
- Heart pains
  - *Taiyin* type: add RM-17 *Shanzhong,* SP-15 *Daheng*
  - *Jueyin* type: add RM-17 *Shanzhong,* LR-14 *Qimen*
  - *Shaoyin* type: add RM-17 *Shanzhong,* RM-23 *Lianquan*
- In pregnancy: needle KI-9 *Zhubin* 3rd, 6th and 9th lunar months
- For morning sickness: add ST-21 *Liangmen*
- Insomnia: superficial and poor sleep quality: according to the night segment
  - Difficulty in the first segment of the night: *Taiyin*, add SP-6 Sanyinjiao, SP-13 *Fushe* or SP-15 *Daheng* or SP-16 *Fuai*
  - Difficulty in the middle of the night: *Jueyin,* add LR-14 *Qimen*
  - Difficulty in the terminal portion of the night: *Shaoyin*, add KI-9 *Zhubin,* RM-23 *Lianquan*

A.2.6 *Yang Wei Mai*

(► Fig. A.2.6)

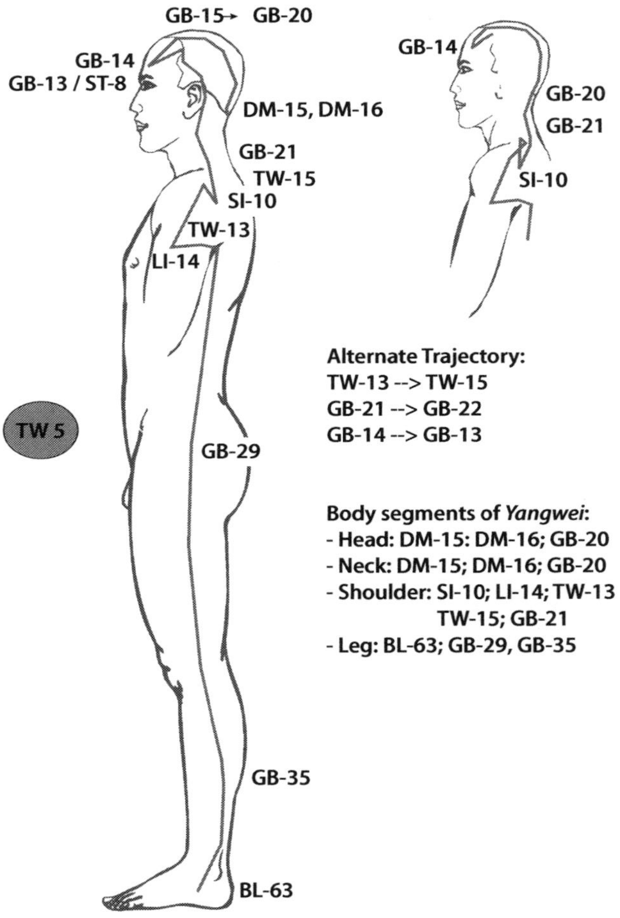

GB-15→ GB-20

GB-14
GB-13 / ST-8

DM-15, DM-16

GB-21
TW-15
SI-10

TW-13
LI-14

GB-14

GB-20
GB-21

SI-10

TW 5

GB-29

Alternate Trajectory:
TW-13 --> TW-15
GB-21 --> GB-22
GB-14 --> GB-13

Body segments of *Yangwei*:
- Head: DM-15: DM-16; GB-20
- Neck: DM-15; DM-16; GB-20
- Shoulder: SI-10; LI-14; TW-13
           TW-15; GB-21
- Leg: BL-63; GB-29, GB-35

GB-35

BL-63

Fig. A.2.6: *Yang Wei Mai* and its three segments

Overview of *Yang Wei Mai* symptoms

- Alternating fever and chills
- Sensitivity to weather change
- Chronic and frequent EPF conditions
- Headaches with Wind or storm or snow
- Superficial pains
- Unstable emotions

Constituent point selection and treatment strategies

In general TW-5 *Waiguan,* with GB-41 *Zulinqi,* and BL-63 *Jinmen,* GB-35 *Yangjiao*

- For weakness of the *Biao*≈Surface with chronic and frequent upper respiratory infections, head-Wind, headaches, neuralgia, loss of voice, throat-*Bi*, laryngitis, rhinitis, anosmia. Add DM-14 *Dazhui,* DM-12 *Shenzhu*

- Inability to support Yang, lumbar pains: add BL-58 *Feiyang* and SI-3 *Houxi*

- For Damp-Heat conditions add GB-41 *Zulingqi,* BL-63 *Jinmen,* GB-35 *Yangjiao*

- For Damp-*Bi* syndromes add LI-14 *Hegu* for the arm, GB-21 *Jianjing* for the shoulder and GB-13 *Benshen* for the head

- For Hot-Phlegm nodules around the neck or for tinnitus: add TW-17 *Yifeng*

- For oral infections, tooth decay, periodontitis: add LI-4 *Hegu*

- For Damp-Heat type *Wei*≈Wilting syndromes as in multiple sclerosis: add SI-4 *Wangu*

- For dysentery with blood or haemoptysis: add BL-17 *Geshu*

- For chest oppression, with chest knotting: add BL-15 *Xinshu*

- For mania or hysteria: add DM-27 *Duiduan*

- For obsessions with past events or future aspirations: add cupping on GB-29 *Juliao* and SI-10 *Naoshu*

- Helping transitional periods, dying process: add BL-63 *Jinmen*

A.2.7 *Yin Qiao Mai*

(▶ Fig. A.2.7)

Overview of *Yin Qiao Mai* symptoms

- Somnolence, fatigue
- Pelvic heaviness, fibroids, PMS
- Leucorrhoea
- Genital swellings pain or hernia,
- Urinary frequency, incontinence
- Loss of libido
- Lumbar pains radiating to the genitals
- Pain or flaccidity along the medial side of the leg
- Chest tightness, palpitations
- Throat dryness or tightness

- Eye dryness, redness
- Lack of self-acceptance
- Aggravation of symptoms at night

Constituent point selection and treatment strategies

In general: KI-6 *Zhaohai*, with LU-7 *Lieque* and KI-2 *Rangu*, KI-8 *Jiaoxin*.

- For Insomnia: supplement KI-6 *Zhaohai*, reduce BL-62 *Shenmai*, add BL-1 *Jingming*

- For unilateral *Bi* ≈ Impediment or *Wei*≈Wilting from Cold and Damp: add *Ahshi* points locally and GB-34 *Yanglingquan*, cupping on SI-10 *Naoshu* and GB-29 *Juliao*

- For all accumulations add SP-6 *Sanyinjiao*

- For throat tightness add ST-9 *Renying*

- For retention of placenta add SP-6 *Sanyinjiao* and LR-3 *Taichong*

- For pelvic accumulations or genital swellings add KI-2 *Rangu* with Moxa, and LR-2 *Xingjian*, RM-6 *Qihai*, RM-9 *Shuifen*, also SP-4 *Gongsun (Chong Mai)*, GB-41 *Zulingqi (Dai Mai)* may be used

- For *Xiao Ke* ≈ Wasting and thirsting (diabetes) add KI-3 *Taixi* and KI-1 *Yongquan*

- For lack of self-confidence add KI-8 *Jiaoxin*

- For lack of self-acceptance add LR-8 *Ququan*

- For excessive self-love, narcissism add KI-10 *Yingu*

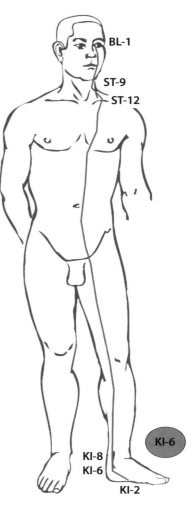

Fig. A.2.7: *Yin Qiao Mai*

A.2.8 *Yang Qiao Mai*

(▶ Fig. A.2.8)

Overview of *Yang Qiao Mai* symptoms

- Insomnia
- Pain or tightness along the lateral side of the leg
- Unilateral headaches
- Unilateral lumbo-sciatica
- Unilateral *Bi* ≈ Impediment or *Wei* ≈ Wilting
- Stroke, epilepsy, hyperthyroidism
- Symptoms aggravated during the day

Constituent point selection and treatment strategies

In general: BL-62 *Shenmai,* with SI-3 *Houxi,* BL-61 *Pucan* and BL-59 *Fuyang*

- Insomnia: reduce BL-62 *Shenmai,* supplement KI-6 *Zhaohai,* add BL-1 *Jingming*
- For unilateral *Bi* ≈ Impediment involving Wind-Heat, add BL-62 *Shenmai* on the opposite side, local *Ashi* points, and cupping on GB-29 *Juliao* and SI-10 *Naoshu*
- For Wind-stroke add BL-59 *Fuyang,* GB-39 *Xuanzhong,* BL-1 *Jingming,* LI-4 *Hegu* and *Guasha* on LI-15 *Jianyu*
- For unilateral headaches add LI-14 *Binao* or LI-15 *Jianyu*
- For conjunctivitis, exophthalmia, add DM-20 *Baihui*
- For facial paralysis (Bell's Palsy), add ST-4 *Dicang,* ST-6 *Jiache*
- For *Biao* Wind-Cold add DM-16 *Fengfu,* GB-20 *Fengchi*
- For Fire toxins, abscess, add BL-54 *Zhibian*
- To help adjust to external changes, accepting the outer world, add BL-60 *Kunlun*

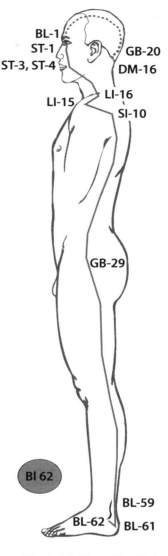

Fig. A.2.8: *Yang Qiao Mai*

Pulses for the 8 Extraordinary vessels according to *Li Shi Zhen*

Certain pulse qualities may also reveal the disturbances of the Extraordinary vessels:

Chong Mai	Deep, Wiry, Tight and Firm
Du Mai	Floating, Wiry and Long
Ren Mai	Deep, Long, Tight and Thin especially in the *Guan* and *Cun* positions
Yin Wei Mai	Deep, Big, Full that rolls to the thumb or to *Cun* (distal) position
Yang Wei Mai	Floating, Big, Full that rolls to *Chi* (proximal) position
Yin Qiao Mai	Left-right vibration and Tight on the *Chi* (proximal) position
Yang Qiao Mai	Left-right vibration and Tight on the *Cun* (distal) position
Dai Mai	Left-right vibration and Tight on the *Guan* (Barrier)

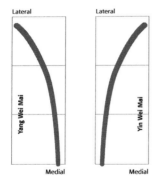

Fig. A.2.9: Yin and Yang Wei pulses (*Li Shi Zen*)

Pulses of the 8 Extraordinary vessels according to Master J. Yuen

Chong Mai	Deep, Wiry, Tight and Floating on the *Chi* position
Du Mai	Empty, Wiry, Tight and also Floating on the Chi position
Ren Mai	Moving (Bean) or Soft and Choppy, or Hollow and Tight
Yin Wei Mai	Thready, Choppy and Rapid

Yang Wei Mai	Floating, Slippery and Rapid
Yin Qiao Mai	Left-right vibration and Weak and Empty
Yang Qiao Mai	Left-right vibration and Full
Dai Mai	Left-right vibration and Tight and Slippery

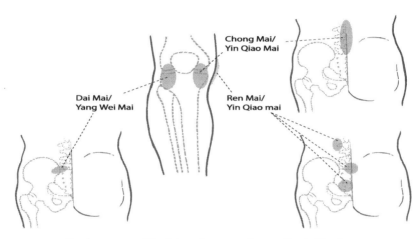

Tension zones and the Extraordinary vessels according to Manaka

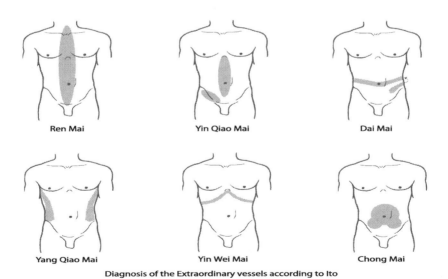

Diagnosis of the Extraordinary vessels according to Ito

Fig. A.2.10: Japanese abdominal Diagnosis according to Manaka and Ito

Appendix-III   Spirit of the Acupuncture Points

Generally speaking, most acupuncture points have a tri-dimensional impact: physical, energetic and psycho-spiritual.

Most point names emphasise one or another of these actions:

- *Shen* 神
- *Ling* 靈
- *Gui* 鬼 and *Bai* 白
- *Tian* 天
- and the Five Wills: *Shen* 神 - *Yi* 意 - *Po* 魄 - *Zhi* 志 - *Hun* 魂

A.3.1 Symbolism of the Heart-channel points

Although most of the *Shou Shaoyin* ≈ Heart channel points do not contain a particular reference to mental or spiritual functions, in the Daoist tradition, according to Master Yuen, the HE points represent the nine stages of our life towards redemption, recovery and sovereignty:

- HT-1: *Jiquan* ≈ Highest spring= endless possibilities
- HT-2: *Qingling* ≈ Green spirit= a young soul
- HT-3: *Shaohai* ≈ Lesser sea= ocean of life
- HT-4: *Lingdao* ≈ Spirit path= path for the soul
- HT-5: *Tongli* ≈ Connecting li= life challenges
- HT-6: *Yinxi* ≈ Yin cleft= theme of life (mid-life crisis)
- HT-7: *Shenmen* ≈ Spirit gate= entering the heart
- HT-8: *Shaofu* ≈ Lesser mansion= lesser roots (less attachment)
- HT-9: *Shaochong* ≈ Lesser surge= less blueprint (less karma)

A.3.2 *Shen* and *Ling* Points

In the Daoist tradition, it is believed that *Shen* ≈ Spirit (Fire) directs the *Ling* ≈ Soul (Metal). It is said, "When *Jing* ≈ Essence embodies the *Shen* ≈ Spirit, the *Ling* ≈ Soul appears".

Shen is Yang, intangible, whereas *Ling* is Yin, visible, and refers to the personality, identity and life passages.

Shen orchestrates life, the *Ling* is the representation of the different segments or phases of life, represented by cycles of 7 or 8 and it is believed to be influenced by memory.

The *Shen* and *Ling* points help regulate and calm the mind and adapt our energy to the various life mutations.

Ling points represent difficulties in certain periods of life, to help re-integrate the orchestra, this could also include difficulties with ageing.

The Shen points concern the loss of control of the entire life.

Shen also represents our Spiritual evolution. To become responsible for carrying out our *Ming≈* life curriculum, as stored in the Kidneys.

Shen Points and their indications:

Shen points are indicated in the presence of *Shen*-disturbances:

- To calm *Shen,* when it is overstimulated or unsettled,

- To supplement *Shen,* when it is depressed,

- To remove stagnation when it is obstructed, usually by Phlegm or by Blood.

As *Shen* is intimately related to Blood, all *Shen* treatments also require the harmonisation of *Xue* ≈ Blood by supplementing or by mobilising Blood.

- HE-7 *Shen Men* ≈ Spirit Door: Calms, Quiets and lifts *Shen* (depressions, insomnia, excess dreaming, hysteria, psychosis, hallucinations; amnesia mental retardation, mental anorexia); opens the Heart orifices (disorientation, amnesia, coma)

- DM-11 *Shen Dao* ≈ Spirit Path: For Yin type psychological disorders (amnesia, fear, emotivity, sadness, regrets)

- BL-44 *Shentang* ≈ Spirit Hall: Benefits and calms the *Shen* (depression, disorientation, insomnia, anxiety, mania)

- DM-24 *Shen Ting* ≈ Spirit Court: Helps to settle *Shen* (schizophrenia, severe anxiety, mania, hysteria)

- KI-23 *Shen Feng* ≈ Spirit Seal: Helps to quiet the mind (anxiety when lying down, mental restlessness)

- RM-8 *Shen Que* ≈ Spirit Gate: Rescues collapsed Yang (stroke, coma with chilled extremities, shock)

- KI-25 *Shen Cang* ≈ Spirit Storage: Relates to the "Self" (middle Cinnabar Chamber); calms the *Shen* (insomnia from worry, anxiety, mental restlessness, depression, disliking life, seeing the negative aspect of things)

- GB-13 *Ben Shen* ≈ Root of the Spirit: Clears and settles *Shen* (nightmares, anxiety, fixed ideas, paranoia, jealousy, schizophrenia); supports will power

Ling points and their indications

Ling points are indicated when there are difficulties with life passages or acceptance of changes in life (ageing): i.e.

- HE-4 *Ling Dao* ≈ Soul Path: difficulty or obsession with certain periods of one's life

- HE-2 *Qing Ling* ≈ Green Soul: lifts (livens) the soul

- KI-24 *Ling Shu* ≈ Soul Ruins: difficulty letting go or forgiving; difficulty burying the past

- GB-18 *Chen Ling* ≈ Soul Support: helps assume one's spirituality

- DM-10 *Ling Tai* ≈ Spirit Tower: helps introspection; strengthens the perception of danger; obsessions about the past; stuck at a life-stage

A.3.3 *Gui* ≈ Ghost Points

These points contain the word *Gui* ≈ Returning Spirit/Ghost, in their primary or secondary names. This is a definite reference to earlier time Shamanic view of harmful spirits causing disease. Their indication is not very clear in the tradition and seems to refer to psycho-emotional problems and diseases that were considered to be due to possession by spirits:

- LU-5 *Chi Ze* or *Gui Tang* ≈ Ghost palace or *Gui Shou* ≈ Ghost Reception

- LU-9 *Tai Yuan*, also called *Gui Xin* ≈ Ghost Heart

- LU-11 *Shao Shang*, also called *Gui Xin* ≈ Ghost Sincerity

- LI-10 *Shou San Li*, also called *Gui Xie* ≈ Ghost Evil

- LI-11 *Qu Chi*, also called *Gui Tui* ≈ Ghost Leg or *Gui Chen* ≈ Ghost Minister

- ST-6 *Jia Che*, also called *Gui Chuang* ≈ Ghost Bed or *Gui Lin* ≈ Ghost Forest

- ST-36 *Zu San Li*, also called *Gui Xie* ≈ Ghost Evil

- Sp-1 *Yin Bai*, also called *Gui Yan* ≈ Ghost eye or *Gui Lei* ≈ Ghost Pile

- BL-62 *Shen Mai*, also called *Gui Lu* ≈ Ghost Road

- PE-5 *Jian Shi*, also called *Gui Lu/* Ghost Road or *Gui Ying* ≈ Ghost Camp

- PE-7 *Da Ling*, also called *Gui Xin* ≈ Ghost Heart

- PE-8 *Lao Gong*, or *Gui Ying* ≈ Ghost Camp or *Gui Lu* ≈ Road or *Gui Ku* ≈ Cave

- RM-24 *Cheng Jiang*, also called *Gui Sh I* ≈ Ghost Market

- DM-16 *Feng Fu*, or *Gui Xue* ≈ Hole or *Gui Zhen* ≈ Pillow or *Gui Lin* ≈ Forest

- DM-22 *Xin Hui*, also called *Gui Men* ≈ Ghost Door

- DM-23 *Shang Xing*, also called *Gui Tang* ≈ Ghost Temple

- DM-26 *Shui Gou*, or *Gui Shi* ≈ Market or *Gong* ≈ Palace or *Ting* ≈ Reception

Sun Si Miao described a set of thirteen Ghost Points to treat "Possessions". There is no indication about the exact use and the therapeutic protocol for these points (▶ Section 4.4.2).

Some points containing the word *Bai* ≈ White have also been associated with the concept of *Gui* ≈ Ghost. Technically *Bai* ≈ White is a reference to Metal and possibly to Phlegm. As Phlegm pathologies are known to produce strange symptoms and behaviour, it may be understood their associations with the concept of *Gui*.

A.3.4 *Tian* ≈ Heaven Points

Tian ≈ Heaven is a reference to the Heaven part of the human being or to the Yang energies. The most relevant to the head energetics are the "Window of the Sky" or "Window of Heaven points". All, except two, are situated in the neck area, which represents the passage between the Body/Earth and the Head/Heaven. These are Windows through which Earth communicates with Heaven.

Other *Tian* ≈ Heaven points are not classified amongst the "Window" points: GB-9 *Tianchong*, TW-10 *Tianjing*, TW-15 *Tianliao*, ST-25 *Tianshu*, SP-18 *Tianxi* and SI-11 *Tianzong*. Some do have an action on the head energetics.

Of the heavenly windows, five points are mentioned in the *Ling Shu* chapter 21 with symptom indications, another five points are mentioned in chapter 2. They control the passage of Blood and Qi, to and from the head, and especially help carry clear Yang to the head.

There are Ten Heavenly Window points corresponding to the Ten Heavenly Stems:

- BL-10 *Tianzhu*: brings Yang down from the head

- ST-9 *Renying* or *Tianwuhui:* carries clear Yang up to the head

- TW-16 *Tianyu:* moves Yin and Blood in the head and the face

- SI-17 *Tianrong:* controls the ascent of Yin and Blood

- SI-16 *Tianchuang:* brings outer Yang inward, seems to complement BL-10 *Tianzhu*

- LI-18 *Futu* or LI-17 *Tianding*: moves Yang outward, complementing ST-9 *Renying*

- DM-16 *Fengfu:* mobilises Yin and Yang in the head

- RM-22 *Tiantu* : controls the exit of Qi from the chest

- PE-1 *Tianchi* and LU-3 *Tianfu:* control the passage of Qi and Blood to the head

The French school relates six of them to the six pairs of *Jingbie*-Divergent/Distinct channels. When these points are painful it would signify a disturbance of the corresponding *Jingbie:*

- BL-10 *Tianzhu*: BL and KI *Jingbie*

- SI-17 *Tianrong*: GB and LR *Jingbie*

- ST-9 *Renying*: ST and SP *Jingbie*

- SI-16 *Tianchuang*: SI and HE *Jingbie*

- TW-16 *Tianyou*: TW and PE *Jingbie*

- LI-18 *Futu* or LI-17 *Tianding*: LI and LU *Jingbie*

Three regulate the internal energies: BL-10 *Tianzhu*, ST-9 *Renying*, SI-17 *Tianrong*

Three are in charge of the interaction with the outer world: SI-16 *Tianchuang*, TW-16 *Tainyou*, LI-17 *Tianding* or LI-18 *Futu*

Four have a general action on Qi and Blood movements to and from the head: LU-3 *Tianfu*, PE-1 *Tainchi*, DM-16 *Fengu*, RM-22 *Tiantu*

These points may be used in various ways:

- As they all influence the energetics of the head, they will have a strong impact on the mind and the emotions

- They may be used together with the corresponding *Jingbie* ≈ Divergent channel to enhance their functions: i.e.

  - Using BL and KI *Jingbie* together with BL-10 *Tianzhu* to bring excess Yang down from the head to the legs;

  - Or GB and LR *Jingbie* with SI-17 *Tianrong* to carry Yin or Blood up to the head;

  - Or ST and SP *Jingbie* with ST-9 *Renying* to carry clear Yang to the portals

- Another method is using them in complementary groups: i.e.

  - BL-10 *Tianzhu* and SI-16 *Tianchuang* to bring Yang down: vertigo, hypertension

  - TW-16 *Tianyou* and SI-17 *Tianrong* (or GB-9 *Tianchong*) for one-sided headaches; unstable walk, blocked ear

  - ST-9 *Renying* and LI-18 *Futu* (or LI-17 *Tianding*) to move Yang up for clear Yang not ascending

- But also, for the treatment of the sensory organs affected by Pathogenic factors:

  - *Taiyang:* BL-10 *Tianzhu* and SI-16 *Tianchuang* for Wind-Cold

  - *Shaoyang:* TW-16 *Tianyou* and SI-17 *Tianrong* for Wind-Damp

  - ST-9 *Renying* and LI-18 *Futu* for Wind-Heat

- Points of opposite actions may be combined to harmonize a movement: i.e.

  - BL-10 *Tianzhu* and ST-9 *Renying*

  - Or LU-3 *Tianfu* with PE-1 *Tianchi* (to move Qi and Blood to and from the head)

Indications

Primarily for mental-emotional disorders:

- LU-3 *Tianfu:* depression, vulnerability, distraction, amnesia, disorientation, possession, hallucinations, "Ghost talk"; also helps to set priorities in life

- PE-1 *Tianchi:* possession

- DM-16 *Fengfu:* mania, running wild, suicidal, fear and fright, lack of coordination

- BL-10 *Tianzhu:* over-excitement (speech or sexual), seeing ghosts, lack of coordination (clumsiness)

- ST-9 *Renying:* energy shooting up and down (panic attack); modern use for pain
- TW-16 *Tianyou:* strange dreams, dreams of falling or of standing on the head
- SI-16 *Tianchuang:* mania, ghost talk, lack of coordination
- LI-17 *Tianding:* muteness, stammering
- LI-18 *Futu:* trembling lips

All affect the sensory organs:

- Eyes: BL-10 *Tianzhu*, ST-9 *Renying*, TW-16 *Tianyou*, DM-16 *Fengfu*, LU-3 *Tianfu*, PE-1 *Tianchi*
- Ears: SI-16 *Tianchuang*, SI-17 *Tianrong*, TW-16 *Tianyou*, DM-16 *Fengfu*. LU-3 *Tianfu*
- Nose: BL-10 *Tianzhu*, TW-16 *Tianyou*, DM-16 *Fengfu*, LU-3 *Tianfu*
- Speech: SI-16 *Tianchuang*, SI-17 *Tianrong*, TW-16 *Tianyou*, LI-17 *Tianding*, LI-18 *Futu*, DM-16 *Fengfu*, RM-22 *Tiantu*

A.3.5 The Five Wills or Spirit Points: *Shen - Yi - Po - Zhi - Hun*

Their indications have been covered in (▶ Section 1.1).

Appendix-IV   Specific exercises and Visualisation techniques

There are three main purposes in encouraging patients to undertake these exercises:

- To involve the subject in their healing process.

  Quite often patients bring their problems to the therapist with the expectation of, "you fix it"! The therapist alone can only do so much. When some symptoms may be alleviated, a profound healing may only take place when the person takes responsibility to "own" their problem. Accepting to deal with the problem also, helps to focus the intention ≈ *Yi* on to the issue; this conforms with the Chinese premise that *Shen* leads the *Qi*.

- To help engage the person in a dialogue between their conscious mind and the subconscious pre-established programs, beliefs and impulses. And to examine the consequences of these mindsets and to question the necessity of the older beliefs; …do I still need this program?

- Most importantly, to discover the "Higher Self".

  Previously we have explored the multi-segmented aspect of the psyche, with the conscious mind ≈ *Shen* coordinating the other parts. But *Shen* itself has two aspects, the more common earthly one concerned with the daily and worldly matters and involved with the habitual thoughts, value systems and emotions*. The other facet of *Shen* is its spiritual dimension, termed as the "Higher Self" or simply the higher intelligence. This is the *Shen* that is beyond duality, judgment and the matters of the world. Healing of the mind and the body can only take place through this higher self. For many of us, the concept of a "Higher Self" may take a religious dimension of "God" or a "Guardian Spirit". Relinquishing the personal will power to this higher self, is to re-locate the Emperor to its Heavenly palace*.

* As described in section 1.1.1, *Shen* has two residences: The Earthly residence is in the Heart (chest) and deals with the Earthly matters, in particular interpersonal issues and emotions), the Heavenly residence is behind the third eye and is in charge of mental and spiritual transformations (the three *Dan Tian* centres ► Fig. 1.4).

This is the process understood as the "Cultivation of the Mind". In modern terms it could be understood as "Spiritual Intelligence".

Spiritual intelligence (► Section 1.2.9) is about the ability to discern the positive aspect of any negative situation. For example, asking the question: what are this pain and suffering teaching me? Through this vision, life difficulties, become growth challenges. In this manner, adversity may be embraced, and accepted, rather than rejected. As we have seen earlier, healing can only happen, once there has been an acceptance of the suppressed parts of the psyche (▶ see exercise A.4.6.3 on Higher Self).

Many of the following exercises have been adapted from Buddhist practices and Chinese Qigong techniques.

As described in section 3.2, the Buddhist explanation for human suffering is mankind's general misconception of reality, hence their inappropriate psycho-emotional reactions. In Buddhist practices, numerous meditation techniques and exercises have been designed to help realise and to change this mental framework and to put an end to this suffering.

In the following section, these exercises have been adapted to the Chinese energetic concepts with an attempt to help release the hidden mental programs the *Gui* ≈ Ghosts (hidden memories), and to re-program the beliefs.

Four approaches are proposed:

- Through the physical stimulation of certain acupuncture points, involving the *Po* ≈ Corporeal soul. These exercises are ideal for releasing the body memories and the "Body Armours".

- Through mental affirmations, involving the *Hun* ≈ Ethereal soul. The affirmation of new concepts or words is very important in the process of changing old belief mechanisms, patterns and mindsets. Self-affirmations are a form of self-hypnosis. A major difference with hypnosis is that these exercises are done with full consciousness, allowing for the *Shen* ≈ Mind/ consciousness to take possession of the hidden segments of the psyche. These self-affirmations complement the other exercises.

- Mental exercises, helping to change mindsets, transform beliefs and emotions, and search for the hidden roots of a deeply established mental mechanism.

- Visualisation methods, involving the visualisation of shapes, colours and the breath in specific areas of the body. This kind of exercise helps the mind involve consciously with a specific organ or function.

In practice, quite often the above techniques may be combined to achieve a stronger impact. After each exercise it is very important to "integrate" any realisation or physical sensation by associating it with a symbol (word or image), so as to later recall the feeling simply by imagining the symbol.

A limiting aspect of many new-age mental developments and visualisation techniques is that most are utilizing the powers of the mind and the "Will" in particular. True healing, involves the acceptance and welcoming of a particular condition (very different from resignation), and to be able to forgive and to let go. To welcome the good as well as the bad, and to be able to forgive, and to trust, are the highest virtues of the *Shen* ≈ Spirit. Hence several of the following exercises aim at reconnecting with the Heart centre (▶ A.4.5.1 and A.4.5.2).

A.4.1   Psychology and Acupuncture Therapy PAT, for Releasing the Body Armours and for changing the Beliefs

The following exercises are given to the patient, to be performed daily. Specific affirmations are vocalised while stimulating the indicated areas.

Explanation: These exercises are based on the principle of associating physical and mental inputs. The stimulation of specific body areas and acupuncture points further helps the integration of the desired mental affirmations. The objective of this method is to replace existing subconscious mental structures and belief systems that have been harmful in the past, with positive and empowering concepts and affirmations. To further help the integration process it might be proposed to the patient to put the suggested affirmations in their own words.

It is recommended to clearly instruct the procedure and to supply a simple chart for the patient. Have the patient perform the whole procedure during each visit to verify and to correct their performance.

The tapping and the slapping should be strong enough to stimulate Qi, but not so vigorous as to provoke pain.

Usually, the points are stimulated several times, but when a particular Body Armour has been identified, the number of tapping stimulation may be increased.

It is very important, for the patient to self-evaluate their progression, by scoring the emotional or the psychological issue before and after the exercise.

Important note: The purpose of this exercise being the release of the trapped psycho-emotional issues, it is important to identify and to address the physical sensations, as they are perceived (naming). Then accepting the feeling or the pain as belonging to oneself (owning).

This process puts an end to the habitual rejection of a painful part perceived as foreign, hateful and unwanted. By repeating a sentence such as: …. Although, I have this pain (or symptom); I love and accept myself… The patient is, in fact, acknowledging their condition and allowing it to manifest fully in order to be released. Similar to facilitating the discharge of pus from an abscess, by not covering it up.

It is fundamental not to censure or repress the negative feelings associated with a given condition. It is quite alright for the patient to describe their situation in the following manner:

… although I hate this pain, …I love and fully accept myself…; etc.

Often, at first, patients feel reticent in exposing their negative feelings, openly. In this case, it is useful for the therapist to accompany the patient by doing the exercise together with them, and by suggesting the appropriate sentence. For example, …although, I don't trust in myself, I love and totally accept who I am…; or although I am fearful of…., I love and totally accept myself…; or although I always have to be perfect, … etc.

A.4.1.1   PAT-1: General PAT exercises for releasing the Sinew channels

Explanation: These exercises aim at releasing the energy retained in the defensive layers of the body, having initially been installed by *Po* ≈ Ethereal soul, in reaction to a perceived external aggression. Later the defensive response is activated below the conscious level of the subject, manifesting as, unexplained pains and tensions, many types of phobias, psycho-somatic reactions and inappropriate emotional responses.
The process calls on the activation of all the *Jingjin* ≈ Sinew channels

- Make tight fists squeeze, then release and extend the hands and the fingers fully (to stimulate the upper *Jing* ≈ Well the starting point of the Sinew channels). Repeat this procedure five to ten times while concentrating on or vocalising the affirmations below (▶ Fig. A.4.1).

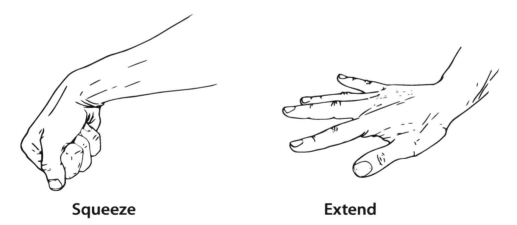

Squeeze   **Extend**

Fig. A.4.1: Squeeze the fist then let go and extend the fingers

- Raise on tiptoe, then drop back on your heel. Repeat five to ten times while maintaining the affirmations below (▶ Fig. A.4.2). This stimulates the lower *Jing* ≈ Well points.

- With the tips of the fingers, tap with average force the main confluent areas of the Sinew channels, repeat a dozen times (▶ Fig. A.4.4):

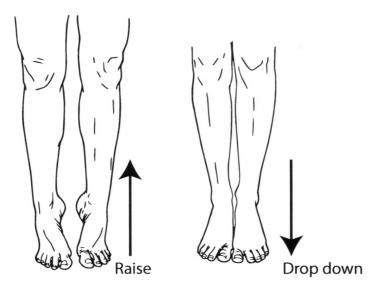

Fig. A.4.2: **Raise on tip-toe, then drop down on the heels**

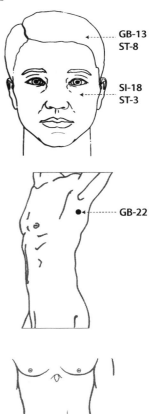

- Corner of the forehead (area of GB-13 *Benshen* and ST-8 *Touwei*)

- Below the cheek-bone (area of SI-18 *Quanliao* and ST-3 *Juliao*)

- Side of the chest, below the armpit (area of GB-22 *Yuanye*)

- Above the pubic bone (area of RM-3 *Zhongji* and RM-2 *Qugu*)

Affirmation to be repeated while performing the exercise:

…. Although, I have this pain (or symptom)…

I love and totally accept myself…

For example, for a patient suffering from a neck tension, the procedure is adapted in the following manner:

- First, evaluate the intensity of the discomfort or pain on a score of 1 to 10.

Fig. A.4.3: **The upper and lower Yang and Yin sinew confluent points**

- Proceed with the above stimulating sequence while repeating the phrase: "although, I have this neck tension, I love and accept myself".

- Evaluate the local symptom on the score of 1 to 10 once more. If there has been no notable improvement, start the whole procedure over, keep repeating until a positive result has been noted.

A.4.1.2   PAT-2: Specific exercises for releasing the Body Armours

The above procedure (PAT-1) may be followed by one or several of the following if a particular body armour has been identified:

- **For the Ocular segment:** add tapping with the finger tips on the head apex (area of DM-20 *Baihui* and GB-18 *Chengling; Yintang; Taiyang*; and the area around the eyes, as well as the area below the occiput: DM-16 *Fengfu* and GB-20 *Fengchi*); pinch and massage the nose bridge (between the eyes = BL-1). With closed eyes, rotate the eye-balls clock-wise and anti-clockwise 12 times (▶ Fig. A.4.4)

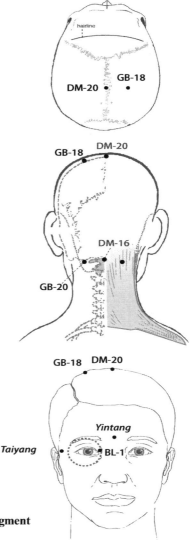

Affirmations for the Ocular segment: choose the most appropriate sentence or make your own;
  - I am guided by a higher power
  - I am guided by my inner vision/ .... by my higher self/....by my inner wisdom…
  - I see clearly
  - I can manifest my vision

Fig. A.4.4: Ocular Segment

For the Oral and Cervical segments:

- add tapping with the finger tips, on DM-26 *Renzhong* and the corner of the jaw the (area of ST-5 *Daying* and ST-6 *Jiache*); the sides of the neck (area of ST-9 *Renying*, LI-18 *Futu* and LI-17 *Tianding*) and the top of the clavicle (area of ST-12 *Quepen*); (▶ Fig. A.4.5).

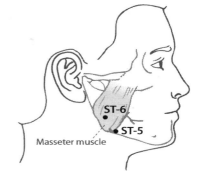

Affirmation for the Oral and Cervical segments: choose the most appropriate sentence or make your own;
- I express myself with authenticity
- I have the right to speak the truth

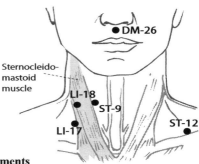

Fig. A.4.5: Oral and Cervical segments

- **For the Thoracic segment:** add slapping with the palm on top of the shoulder (area of GB-21 *Jianjing*) and simultaneously with the opposite backside of the hand slap the thoracic spine (area of 4th and 5th vertebrae); repeat the procedure by slapping the middle of the sternum (area of RM-17 *Shanzhong*) with one hand, and the thoracic spine with the other (▶ Fig. A.4.6 and Fig. A.4.7).

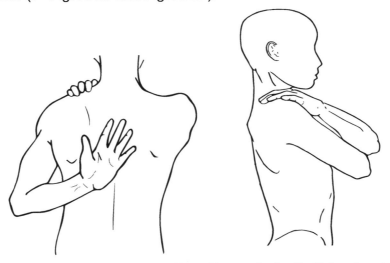

Fig. A.4.6: Slap simultaneously the top of the shoulder and between the shoulder blades; alternate sides

Thoracic segment
affirmation:

…I am loving to myself and
to others…

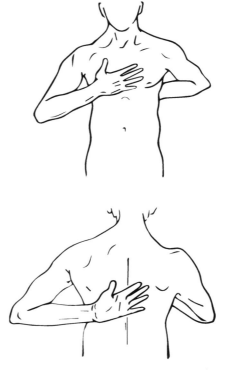

**Fig. A.4.7: Slap simultaneously the sternum and
the mid-back; alternating hands**

- **For the Diaphragmatic segment:** Tap gently the solar plexus area;
  then with open hands slap from front to back below the ribcage. (▶
  Fig. A.4.8)

Affirmation for the
Diaphragmatic
segment:
- I honour the power
  within me…;
- I respect others…

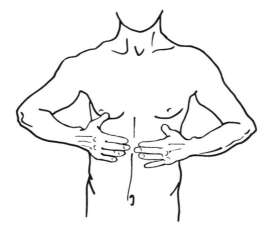

Fig. A.4.8: Slap from front to back below the ribcage

- **For the Abdominal and Pelvic segments:** Slap simultaneously the sacrum with one hand and the side of the waist with the other five to ten times; then with closed fists tap on the lumbar area, and above and in front of the iliac crest (area of GB-26 *Daimai*, GB-27 *Wushu* and GB-28 *Weidao*); (▶ Fig. A.4.9).

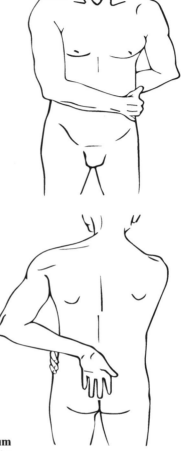

Affirmation for the Abdominal and Pelvic segments: choose the most appropriate:
- I move effortlessly
- I take pleasure in life
- I take pleasure in what I do
- It is safe for me to be here; I feel secure
- I feel grounded
- I am entitled to get what I need

Fig. A.4.9: **Slap simultaneously the sacrum and the side of the waist**

A.4.1.3   PAT-3: Exercises to change the beliefs, mindsets and mental images

(▶ Fig. A.4.10):

- Start by tapping the neck area (at the base of the occiput: DM-16 *Fengfu*; GB-20 *Fengchi*); repeat the following affirmations (or make your own): I am flexible…; I welcome change…;

- Pinch the base of the nose (Bl-1 Jingming); then gently tap around the eyes (area of BL-*2* Zanzhu; GB-14 *Yangbai;* TW-23 *Zhukong*; GB-1 *Tongziliao* and ST-1 *Chengqi*); repeat the following affirmations (or make your own): I see clearly…; I have an open vision…; I can see new options…;

- Now tap the area above the forehead (DM-24 *Shenting*; GB-13 *Benshen* and ST-8 *Touwei*): repeat the following affirmations (or make your own): I have an open mind...; I am free of judgement and prejudice...; I welcome new ideas...

- End by tapping the top of the head (area of DM-20 *Baihui* and GB-18 *Chengling*): repeat the following affirmations (or make your own): I welcome the challenges of my life...; I have the capacity to learn from my challenges...; I can be enriched by my experiences...; I am grateful to be alive...

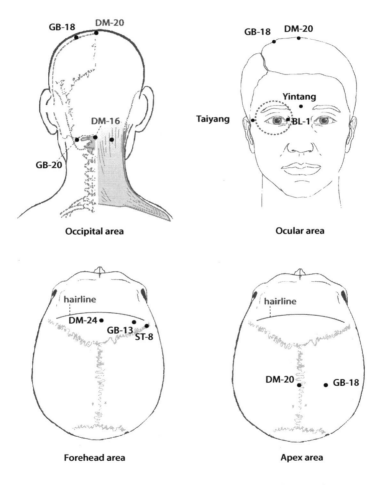

Fig. A.4.10: PAT exercises for changing beliefs and mind-sets

Explanations: The Wind points at the neck area correspond to change (confluence between *Yang Wei* and *Yang Qiao Mai*); the points around the eyes, help inner and non-dualistic vision; the forehead area helps to let go of fixed ideas and assumptions; and the head apex, helps to connect with the higher self and assume one's *Ming* ≈ Destiny.

A.4.2 Exercises for changing the "Belief Mechanisms"

The unconscious beliefs, especially about health, disease, life and death are the strongest building blocks of all our experiences, actions and attitudes. Habitual mindsets cannot just be replaced by new ones, this is a progressive procedure involving various stages of mental training and the change of perspective.

The way to work with the unconscious negative beliefs is first to bring them into the awareness and to recognise and identify them (i.e. I do not trust in myself…); next to challenge them through an opposite positive affirmation (i.e. I have total trust in myself…).

When the following exercises are being done alone, to check if the new affirmation has been integrated, it is best to use a mirror while vocalising the affirmation. Is the person in the mirror saying those words sound convincing to you, or are they repeating the sentence mentally?

If there is a doubt manifesting with …yes, but…, you will have to find the ramifications of the initial belief, like peeling an onion. Each root belief needs to be addressed separately. For example, I don't trust in myself because I was often told by my parents that I was wrong, that I had done it wrong… I don't trust in myself because it is hard to make decisions… I don't trust in myself because I am a fearful person… Life is full of dangers… I need help…

Each discovered disruptive belief has to be challenged and transformed until the initial statement of …I have total trust in myself… is readily accepted by the subconscious. If the resistances remain, perform the PAT-3 exercise to help change the mental images and beliefs and repeat the affirmations.

It is recommended to perform the appropriate exercises with the patient to help them understand and integrate the process. They can then practice the exercise at home. When a change or a positive transformation has been observed by the patient, they realise that all phenomena are not fixed and that everything can evolve. This understanding encourages them to continue with the practices. It is very important to have them write down their realisations.

The following procedures, follow the basic Chinese philosophical concepts, in particular, that of duality: opposition, complementarity, relativity etc.

- **Step-1   Relativity: Comparison**
    - Choose an object: describe and determine the dimensions, weight, texture etc. of this object.
    - Next, define this object: small, big, hard, soft, etc.
    - Now formulate an opinion: useful, useless, pretty, ugly, etc.

- Next, find out how you determined this opinion. For example, small compared to......, or soft compared to......, useful as compared to ..., etc.

- Ask the question: can the same object, have two opposite definitions at the same time? Repeat this exercise at home, taking various objects, until you have a clear conclusion, write it down.

- **Step-2   Evaluation and judgement concerning objects**

  - Choose an object or a plant: describe and determine the dimensions, weight, texture etc. of this object.

  - Now become one with it. Imagine that you have "become" the object, feel from inside what it feels like to be this object.

  - Next take a distance from this object and formulate an opinion of it: small, big, hard, soft, useful, useless etc.

  - Now become the object again, and try to feel how the object feels from inside now that you have put a judgement on it.

  - Next change your judgement of the object and feel how it feels with this new definition.

  - Repeat until you have a clear insight. Repeat at home, taking various objects, until you have a clear conclusion, write it down.

- **Step-3   Evaluation and judgement concerning the body**

  - Choose a part of your body, first describing it and then becoming one with it. Now create a value judgment of that part: small, big, hard, soft, beautiful, ugly, painful, relaxed etc.

  - Become one with this part of your body again and feel what it feels from inside.

  - Now change your judgment on that part of your body and again feel what it feels.

  - Repeat until you have a clear insight. Repeat this exercise at home, taking various body parts, in particular the parts that you do not like, until you have a clear conclusion, write it down.

- **Step-4   Evaluation and judgement concerning tension, pain or disease "Body oriented guided fantasy"**

Once the above exercise has been integrated, the same process may be applied to a particular tension, pain or disease by establishing a dialogue with it.

- Choose a pain or tension in your body. Describe it: shape, ramifications, colour density, intensity... Evaluate the intensity on a scale of 1 to 10.

- If this pain could speak, what would it say (express)? What aggravates it? Explore on all dimensions (physical, mental, emotional, etc...).

- Ask the pain, what it needs and what could help it? Is there a message that this pain has for you?

- Now re-evaluate the intensity on a scale of 1 to 10.

- Repeat this exercise at home, until you have a clear conclusion, write it down.

- **Step-5   Evaluation and judgement concerning a concept or a belief system**

    - Choose a concept or an idea:

    - Now create a judgment of this concept. Identify with it and feel what it feels to see the world through this concept.

    - Change your judgments on this concept and again feel what it feels to have this new point of view.

    - Repeat until you have a clear insight. Repeat this exercise at home, taking various belief systems, in particular, those that you have problems with, until you have a clear conclusion, write it down.

- **Step-6   Evaluation and judgement concerning an animal**

    - Choose an animal: describe them: big, small, thin, heavy, etc...

    - Next formulate an opinion of them: beautiful, ugly, powerful, scary, cuddly, etc.

    - Now become one with the animal. Imagine that you are the animal, and feel from inside what it feels like to embody one of the projected opinions.

    - Next, change to the opposite value or opinion, and feel from inside what it feels like now.

    - Repeat until you have a clear insight. Repeat this exercise at home, taking various animals, in particular if you have certain phobic issues (spiders, snakes, mice etc.) until you have a clear conclusion, write it down.

- **Step-7** **Evaluation and judgement concerning another person**

  Once the above exercise has been integrated, the same process may be applied to another person, in particular the ones that you may have an issue with.

- **Step-8** **Witnessing things just the way they are**

  At this stage contemplate things the way they are without any judgments or opinions. Become like a camera registering and witnessing all things the way they are with an open vision without choosing anything in particular.

  Repeat until you have a clear insight. Repeat this exercise at home, taking various examples, until you have a clear conclusion, write it down

Explanation:

The purpose of these exercises is to understand that how we perceive the outer world, as well as ourselves and other people, depends entirely on our constant scrutiny and evaluation. An object is simply an object, it only becomes beautiful or ugly based on our opinion.

The habitual Western mind is dualistic, good or bad, black or white, either, or… Understanding the "complementarity" of phenomena, that one aspect cannot exist without the opposite, helps to embrace both aspects of the so-called reality. This puts an end to rejection and exclusion, not only in our minds but also in our societies.

Outer events, are just what they are, neither good or bad. They only become harmful if I perceive them as such….

This line of reasoning is valid only for the conscious mind, the subconscious follows rather the reflexive and instinctual survival programs. As we have previously explored, survival instincts are genetically transmitted, but some programs have been incorporated based on our personal life experiences.

These instincts will by-pass the intellect and the conscious mind, manifesting as reactions to outer events, which may prove appropriate in some situations or inappropriate in others.

Here lies the hidden root of our suffering.

A.4.3 Exercises for identifying and changing the hidden roots of the "Belief Systems"

The next stage of exercises concerns the identification of these subconscious programs and their ramifications:

- **Identification of fixed images or concepts**
  - Choose an idea or a belief that is causing limitations in your life. For example, I am not good enough....; I am afraid of...; This is too much for me...; I cannot manage ... etc.
  - What was the situation that was at the root? Parents words and judgments: you did not do it well...; be careful you might hurt yourself...; you are not strong enough...; or you are not old enough...; etc.
  - What were the circumstances later in life that confirmed this idea? Teacher's comments; the failure in exams; rejection; criticism...
  - How has this concept affected you in your life? For example, choosing security...; always staying in a comfort zone...; not taking risks...; dependency on another person...; etc.

- **Getting rid of the old reality**
  - At this stage, you need to make a story, like a film scenario, and visualise yourself as the actor in this movie, playing out the scenes involving the limiting belief. For example, of the helpless person, failing in life and being criticised and put down. Give your film a title. Feel how it feels to be this person.
  - Next, become the spectator of this movie. Simply watch the movie without any feelings or judgments. Realise that this is only a film, it is not who you are.
  - Now destroy or erase this version of the scenario.

- **Changing the "story", re-creating a new reality**
  - Re-write the scenario; make a new story, in which you have been praised and supported. Choose the better memories in your past, or create (invent) new ones.
  - Become the actor of this new film; become identified with this personality.
  - Feel how it feels to play this new role.

- Stay with this new feeling. Create a symbol to represent this image of yourself (an object, a colour, a particular location…)

- During the coming days, regularly visualise this symbol and bring up the positive feelings that go with it.

- If you have difficulty re-creating this space, repeat the exercise, and watch the film once more

Some doubtful thoughts might surface hindering the new image. For example, in your new scenario, the actor is strong and powerful but you have difficulties in identifying with this personality. What are the limiting doubts? Find the life situations that contributed to this self-image (outer events, guilt, shame, self-blame…). Identify each limiting belief, and the scene in which it was re-enforced (failure, criticism…). Re-write the story and proceed as above.

- **Changing interpersonal, emotional or health issues**

  Once the above exercise has been understood and integrated, apply the same method to other interpersonal, emotional or health issues.

- **Exercise on Self-acceptance and forgiveness**

  - Make a list of what you dislike about yourself (physical, mental, emotional or interpersonal.) For example:

    - I don't like my nose…;

    - I hate this pain…;

    - I don't like my stress…;

    - I don't like my fear…;

    - I cannot stand my mother-in-law…;

    - I hate my job or work atmosphere…

  - For each item, find the antidote; For example:

    - In order to love my nose, I need to be kind with it; it is part of my special character…

    - In order to accept my pain, I need to welcome it and communicate with it and to understand what message it is bringing…;

    - In order to deal with my stress, I need to demand less of myself, to "Be" more and "Do" less…;

    - In order to deal with my fear, I need to first understand its roots, then to remember that I am not that fear, and have the wisdom to see the options and make choices and the power to move into action...

- In order to accept my mother-in-law, I need to recognise her positive traits, and also be thankful to her for showing me my reactivity and short-comings...

- In order to accept my work situation, I need to realise the importance of what I am doing...; to find creativity in my routine work...; to put my full attention into it...

- **The Higher Self**

Spiritual intelligence (▶ Section 1.2.9) is about the ability to discern the positive aspect of any negative situation. For example, asking the question: what are this pain and suffering teaching me? Through this vision, life difficulties, become growth challenges. In this manner, adversity may be embraced, and accepted, rather than rejected. As we have seen earlier, healing can only happen, once there has been an acceptance of the suppressed parts of the psyche.

A.4.4 Exercises for transforming Emotions

Working with emotions is different, in fact, there are two major difficulties:

- Naming the emotion: frequently the true emotion which is felt is not identified correctly due to socio-cultural conditioning. For example, most societies condemn anger, as a result a person who has a suppressed anger, will identify the feeling as sadness; or fear could be expressed as worry, etc. Some might even feel the emotion physically, for example, repressed anger could be expressed as an intense epigastric pain or a romantic rejection might be felt as an intense chest constriction and pain. Helping the patient identify correctly their emotion is very important at the onset.

- Owning the emotion: This point is very difficult to grasp by most. When angry, the cause of the anger is automatically related to and blamed on an outer event or another person; it is hard to recognise that the emotion actually belongs to us and that it is our response to the outer event. Without this realisation, the emotions cannot be transformed. It has to be further understood that "owning the emotion", does not imply holding on to the feeling (indulging), or rejecting, or denying, or suppressing the emotion.

- Letting go of emotions:

- The following exercise is helping to dissolve and let go of emotions. It is recommended to start with minor emotions and not tackle major issues of rage or panic or deep depression etc.

  - Choose any emotion, or simply get in touch with the emotion that you are feeling now: describe it as accurately as possible; where about in the body do you feel it; what are the words that best express and define this feeling? Name this emotion, recognise it...

  - Own this feeling; do not repress or reject it, rather accept and embrace it (do not reject, do not repress).

  - Now change your relation to this emotion: rather than saying "I am angry", say "anger is there".

  - Take note of how it feels not to be identified with the emotion.

  - Now imagine wrapping up this emotion into a bundle and mentally disposing of it by any means that you prefer: burn it, let it disappear like smoke or evaporate into space...

  - Repeat until you have a clear insight. Write up a short conclusion.

As emotions are the outcome of our belief mechanisms, they have often had deeper ramifications. Once an emotion has been cleared out, one may discover another layer, for example below the anger, there may be guilt, and below the guilt, maybe fear etc. What had been at the root of this outlook or mental framework may be dated back to early childhood events, later re-enforced by life experiences. In this case, it is useful to apply the previous exercises "getting rid of old reality" and "changing the story".

A.4.5   Visualisation Exercises

A.4.5.1   The Central Axis

Explanation: The central axis constitutes the inner core of the energetic body and it represents the universal principle of change and stability. According to Daoist principles, change is successful when combined with stability, as reflected in the image of the "great rooted tree" (stability), by the "flowing river" (activity/ change).

The central axis is a fundamental exercise for both therapists and patients.

Exercise to develop the "Central Axis"

- Keep in mind that throughout the exercise the axis should remain firm and yet flexible, solid without being rigid (▶ Fig. A.4.11).

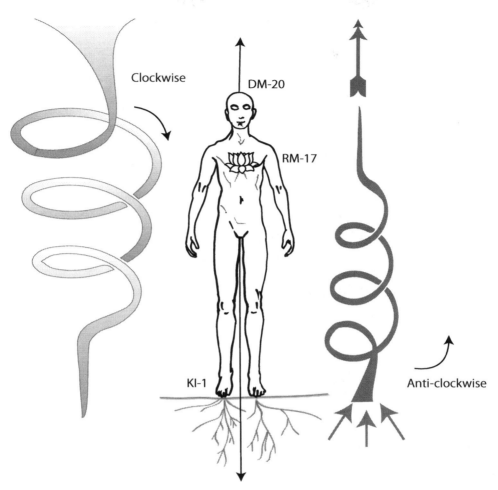

Fig. A.4.11: The Central Axis

- Starting position: feet parallel, shoulder wide. Knees slightly bent, arms hanging on the sides, hands open and relaxed. Back and head are held straight in the axis.

- The "Central Axis" has 2 poles, Heaven and Earth. From the sole of the feet (KI-1 *Yongquan*), visualise roots growing and reaching to the centre of the earth. Connect with the fire at the centre of the earth and visualise a red spiral moving anti-clockwise upwards and through your feet, surrounding the bones and the sinews in the legs. Then moving further up to the inside of the trunk to wrap around the internal organs and further up to reach the top of the head (DM-20 *Baihui*). Visualise this red spiral shooting out of the head towards the sky. Imagine this energy moving effortlessly upwards with an uplifting, supportive, and nourishing quality.

- This upward movement of Earth improves the stability and rooting, and further nourishes and supports the vitality of the physical body. (Supplementing the *Ying* ≈ Nourishing energy).

- Next, connect to the vast sky, the pure luminous white light taking the shape of a white spiral moving clockwise downwards to surround the outside of the body and further down, all the way into the earth. This downward white spiral movement, like a white waterfall from Heaven, enhances evolution and change. It cleanses and clears the subtle energetic body as well as protecting it from external aggressions. (Fortifying the *Wei* ≈ Defensive energy)

- Now, concentrate on the Heart centre and the chest. Visualise the red and white spirals meeting in the Heart, where the colours are mixing and creating the shape of a beautiful pink rose or lotus.

- This fusion of the celestial "Heaven" energy and the "Earth" movement, meeting in the Heart centre, stimulates the "Healing *Shen*" with its capacity to unify, to understand, to love and to respect life.

- After the completion of the exercise, choose one or more of the following affirmations to concentrate on and repeat a few times (whispered or spoken out). Allow the intention of the thought to resonate in your body. End by emitting the request that this vibration accompany and sustain you throughout your day.

Sample affirmations to help integrate the qualities of the "Central Axis": (you can also make your own affirmations)

- I enjoy the feeling of remaining centred while in movement.
- I accomplish things effortlessly and well.
- I am responsible for what I create.
- I am balanced and centred.
- I trust and have faith in the deep essence of who I am.
- I enjoy making important decisions.
- Through choice I can change my experience.
- I am nourished and protected by existence.

Sample affirmations to help open the Heart centre (Healing *Shen*):

- I love and accept myself as I am.
- I love and respect others as they are.

A.4.5.2 The Healing Shen exercise

Explanation: This exercise has been adapted from a Buddhist meditation as instructed by Atisha, one of Buddha's disciples, for "transforming darkness into light".

- With closed eyes, start a series of slow, gentle and long breaths into your chest and Heart centre. Observe, if any tight areas are preventing your chest from fully expanding. Breath into these areas gently until they dissolve. Next, take note of any emotions or thoughts that are disrupting your process. Do the same, gently breath into them and let them settle down.

- With each breath, let go of all limitations and feel your chest cavity and your heart expanding more and more.

- Now on the in-breath, imagine inhaling your most urgent personal issue (sickness, pain, emotion etc…). Imagine it as a dark smoke that you inhale into your chest area / the Heart centre.

- Let the Heart transform this dark cloud into a vibrant and pure light; then breath out this light.

- As you inhale, imagine breathing-in all your pains, sickness, conflicts, your negative thoughts, judgments and emotions. Again, imagine all of this as a dark cloud of smoke that you gather into your Heart.

- And on the out-breath; exhale a clear light of joy, of lightness, of well-being and love.

- Breath-in all the darkness and misery of the world, the suffering of all the people. Let all of this darkness be absorbed into your Heart.

- And on the out-breath, exhale joy and happiness into the world.

Please note: Quite often, a person might resist doing this exercise, believing that they may absorb and retain the darkness inside. It is important to stress the alchemical power of the Heart centre in transforming darkness into light.

A.4.5.3 The Hollow Bamboo

This exercise has been adapted from a Buddhist meditation:

- Adopt a comfortable sitting posture: spine straight, body relaxed.
- Inhale and bring the focus to the head; imagine breathing-in a luminous crystal mist that fills the head;

- On the out-breath, let go of all the density of the head; imagine the head completely open and filled with empty space;
- Breath in the luminous mist once again
- Now draw down this luminous mist into the neck and throat; as you breath-out, let go of the constrictions; fill out this open space with light.
- Repeat for each body part; bring this open space to the chest, abdomen, pelvis, arms and legs.
- Maintain this image of a hollow body filled with space and light.
- If thoughts arise, simply let them dissolve into this luminous space.
- With each breath, increase this inner empty space; allowing for this this inner calm and harmony to deepen;
- Breathing in feel the calmness within; smile when breathing out…

A.4.5.4   Colour and Breathing exercises

Specific breathing and colour visualisations have to accompany the above exercises for releasing the Body Armours.

Before starting it is imperative to activate the diaphragmatic (abdominal) breathing: during the in-breath expand the lower abdomen. Take care not to tighten the lower back while performing the abdominal breathing. During the in-breath, visualise and follow the breath and direct it to the concerned area (▶ Fig. A.4.12).

Explanation: Breath control is fundamental in all *Qigong* practices; it is said to open the *Shen* capacities and heighten the levels of consciousness. The in-breath has a supplementing (tonic) action; the out-breath allows to let-go and release accumulations. Before starting the visualisations, short and forceful out-breaths are recommended when an area feels obstructed.

By visually directing the breath to a specific area, we are in fact, combining the *Shen* ≈ Consciousness with *Yi* ≈ Mind/ Intention to accompany the Qi.

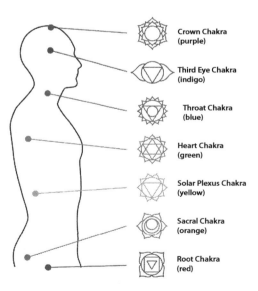

Fig. A.4.12: Chakras and colours

To help the colour visualisations, concentrate on DM-15 *Yamen and* DM-16 *Fengfu* area while looking on the tip of the nose. This will produce a heavy sensation in the area of the *Yintang*. Next look at a white surface before starting the colour visualisations.

- For the Apex, third-eye, oral and throat centres, accompany the breath by touching the area (to help concentrate the attention to that part). It might also be useful to intone a humming sound, and by modulating the sound to vibrate in that particular area.

- Apex: visualize the colour purple

- Third eye: visualize the colour indigo

- Throat: visualize the colour blue

- The Heart centre: breath and expand the chest in all directions: front, sides and back. Visualize the colour green.

- The Diaphragmatic centre: breath by lowering the diaphragm (abdominal breathing) and expand in all directions: front, sides and back. Visualize the colour yellow.

- The Abdominal segment: breath into the abdomen and expand in all directions: front, sides and back. Visualize the colour orange.

- The Pelvic/ Sacral segment: first tighten the perineal muscles, then breath-in and expand the pelvic area in all directions: front, sides and back and below. Visualize the colour red.

A.4.5.5   Focusing and Expanding the vision exercise

- Concentrate on the flame of a lit candle, placed 1.5-2 meters away for 2 minutes. Do not engage in any thought processes. Use the breathing described above.
- Now open your visual field and simply observe all that is around (without grasping or rejecting anything in this visual space) for 2 minutes
- Close your eyes and relax.
- Write a short conclusion

Explanation: The purpose of this exercise is to calm and expand the mind. The concentration on the flame, helps to focus the mind and restrain it from wandering. The second step, by observing without focusing on a particular object allows the mind to expand.

A.4.5.6 Exercises to help restore the connections in the brain

Many traumatic events may cause a momentary disconnection between the conscious mind and intellect ≈ *Shen* and *Yi* and the emotional brain. These exercises can help re-connect the fore-brain with the mid-brain and the left and right hemispheres:

Connecting left-right / front and back exercise:

Visualisation: With closed eyes, starting with the middle of the brain, imagine the infinity symbol "∞". First expanding horizontally between the front and the back of the brain. Mentally follow this shape and breath into it several times. Next visualise the same shape, but from left to right. While mentally following this shape, combine with a slight right and left swaying of the head and of the eyes (▶ Fig. A.4.13):

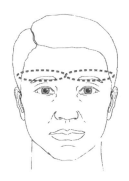

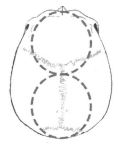

Connecting the brain areas:

Visualise an upside-down pyramid with a triangular base: with one corner of the triangle being at the third eye, and the other two corners at the ears. The tip of the pyramid is visualised at the throat area. Once the image of the pyramid is clearly visualised, start humming or intoning the *OM* sound. Bring the vibration into the brain. Maintain the visualisation and humming for a few minutes (▶ Fig. A.4.14).

Fig. A.4.13: Connecting left/right and front/back

Connecting the left and right brain:

With the right index finger touch the tip of the nose, with the left index touch the right ear.

On the in-breath slowly bend the knees and move to a squatting position. On the out-breath, slowly stand up. Change hands and sides (right index touching the left ear, right index touching the nose). Repeat 20 times, alternating sides.

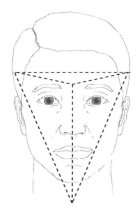

Fig. A.4.14: Connecting brain

A.4.6   Guided Reflections

The following exercises need to be guided by the therapist:

A.4.6.1   Self-Forgiveness

- Sit comfortably with closed eyes and a straight back. Allow the breath to gently flow in and out of your body.
- In life, we have been hard on ourselves in many ways and we need to forgive ourselves. To forgive ourselves, we need to soften the barriers around our hearts and let ourselves into our hearts.
- Gently get in touch with all the ways that you have hurt yourself, your body, your emotions, your mind. Reflect on the criticisms, judgments, and the many ways that you have put yourself down. Allow those times and those words to come into your awareness and realise how hard you have been on yourself.
- Now, acknowledge that it was out of your fears, ignorance, neglect, attachments and confusion that you have hurt yourself.
- It is now time to forgive yourself. You have suffered enough. You have now changed and are ready to open your heart.
- Open your heart to light and love and compassion towards yourself. Feel surrounded and filled by a special Spiritual energy, the universal love and light. Bring this light into your heart and touch those places where you hold the pains and judgments of the past. Touch those areas with kindness and forgiveness; it is time to let them go. Forgive yourself for all that you have done in the past. Open your heart and release all the judgments…
- It is time to open your heart and love yourself. To acknowledge your uniqueness and preciousness…
- Repeat this prayer:
  - May I be happy
  - May I be free from self-judgment
  - May I be free from my fears
  - May I know the joy of truly understanding myself
  - May I know the joy of accepting and loving myself unconditionally
  - May I be at peace

A.4.6.2   Forgiving others

- Sit comfortably with closed eyes and a straight back. Allow the breath to gently flow in and out of your body.
- In life, you have been hurt by others in many ways.
- Bring to mind those who have hurt you knowingly or unknowingly. Remember the words and the deeds. Picture in your mind how you

were hurt, harmed or even victimised. Feel it in your body and in your heart. See how you had to close your heart down to protect yourself.
- Now, acknowledge that it was out of their fear, their pain, ignorance, neglect, attachments and confusions that they have hurt you.
- With this new understanding, open your heart to forgiveness. To the extent that you are able, at this time, forgive them.
- Feel those areas that hold the past hurts, resentments and disappointments and touch them with kindness and forgiveness; it is time to let them go.
- Open your heart and forgive them and ask for forgiveness for what you may have done to hurt them. Forgive yourself.
- Your heart is now free…
- Repeat this prayer:
  - May you and I be happy
  - May you and I be free from suffering
  - May you and I come to know the joys of understanding one another
  - May we open our hearts and minds to each other
  - May we meet in harmony
  - May we be at peace
- Imagine that these messages have been received and accepted by the other. Acknowledge this feeling of healing, forgiveness and peace…

A.4.6.3   Higher Self

The importance of getting in touch and developing the higher-self was elaborated at the start of section A.4.
- Have the subject sit comfortably, with eyes closed, breathing gently and letting go of all thoughts.
- …You are a spiritual being…; within you is a vast reservoir of unlimited spiritual energy…; get in touch with this energy
- How does this spiritual energy feel like to you at this moment?
- Within this vast sea of energy, there is the voice of your Higher Self. Ask it to take form and be itself known…
- What is the energy of this Higher Self; what do you feel at this time?
- Your Higher Self is all-loving, all-knowing and all-powerful and wise. Be with it, welcome it and open your heart to it.
- Ask your Higher Self for a message. It could be a word, an image or a feeling. Sense the meaning of the message. Integrate this message into your life today.
- Ask your Higher Self for a tool, something that will help you in your life today. Receive the tool and sense its meaning.
- Be with your Higher Self
- Ask your Higher Self for advice, a teaching or to speak to you about a specific issue…

- Ask your Higher Self to touch your body in that place that needs healing. Feel the healing…
- Open your heart to your Higher Self. Draw your higher self into your heart (chest). Let this energy expand and flow throughout your body. Let every cell of your body feel and vibrate with this energy.
- Remember you are the Higher Self.
- Integrate this feeling.
- Make a symbol. Allow the symbol to bring you back to this same state whenever you need it.

A.4.6.4   For Accompanying a dying person

The following text has been inspired and adapted from the Tibetan Book of the Dead to help the passage for a dying person.

Beloved…

Now the time has come for you to seek a path…

You are dying, you are leaving your friends and family, your favourite surroundings will no longer be there, you are going to leave us…

Your friends and family know that you are going to die, but they are not frightened by it, they are really here for you, solid and grounded…

You can dissolve now, just like the snowflake dissolves into water…
Just like the drop of water becomes the ocean…

You are like an ocean, vast and endless…
Moving and changing constantly…
Each wave an individual form, and yet each wave made up of a multitude drops of water…

In this ocean of life, you are the drop of water, not separate from the ocean, not separate from each other…

You are part of the whole and deep down in your heart you know that you are part of everything else…

The time has come now for you to go…
Let go of all your worldly attachments, of the pain and sorrow, of the limitations of this body.
Let your essence leave this body and get ready to go back into the ocean, into the mystery of death and life…

Into the luminous void...

This mind of yours is an inseparable luminosity and emptiness in the form of a great mass of light, it has no birth or death, therefore it is of "Immortal light". (repeat 3 times and press on ST-9 *Renying* and TW-5 *Waiguan*)

Now, let what belongs to the earth go back to earth and what belongs to heaven go back to heaven...

Now the sign of Earth dissolving into Water is present...
Water into Fire...
Fire into Air...
Air into consciousness...
Let go of the identification and definitions of yourself...
Let go of the boundaries of your body...

Take space...
Open up to Existence...
Take space...

Let go of your limitations...
Expand...
Make yourself more and more vast, more and more empty, until you start extending in all directions. Until you are part of everything, until you are one with Existence.

When "You" are no more, the whole existence fills you up from every direction and every dimension...

Now remember and feel where you came from...

(Touch the head apex: DM-20 *Baihui* and GB-18 *Chengling*)

A.4.6.5   After Death

The following text on the Bardo* is to be vocalised after the Spirit has left the body:

Beloved....,

Listen carefully without distraction...

Now what is called death has arrived...

You are not alone in leaving this world, it happens to everyone, so, do not feel desire and yearning for this life...
Even if you feel desire and yearning you cannot stay, you can only wander in ignorance and suffering...
Do not desire, do not yearn...

O Beloved...

Whatever terrifying projections appear in the Bardo, do not forget these words, and go forward remembering their meaning; the essential is to recognise them:

"Now when the Bardo dawns upon me, I will abandon all thoughts of fear and terror,
I will recognise whatever appears as my projection and know it to be a vision of the Bardo..."

Witness and step out of your projection without judgement...

Realise that this is not me, this is my creation...
Let it dissolve into emptiness and luminosity...

This mind of yours is inseparable luminosity and emptiness in the form of a great mass of light, it has no birth nor death, therefore it is of Immortal light...

* Bardo: In Tibetan Buddhism, Bardo is a is an intermediate, transitional, or liminal state between death and rebirth during which the consciousness is not connected with the physical body. For the prepared and appropriately trained individuals, the bardo offers a state of great opportunity for liberation, since transcendental insight may arise with the direct experience of reality.

Appendix-V   Case Studies

Case 1   (Fear of Exams/ stage-fright)

A 23-year old medical student consulted for extreme nervousness before her exams. She described that for a week before each examination, she could not sleep or eat and would even have bouts of diarrhoea. This exam stress often caused her to forget what she had learned and to feel quite muddled during the examination, although generally she had a good memory.

Treatment: HE-7 *Shenmen*, HE-6 *Yinxi* and HE-5 *Tongli* were needled bilaterally for stage fright (with one needle, threading technique); and DM-20 *Baihui* was added to settle the mind and enhance memory and concentration. She regained her calm after the treatment, could sleep and eat and did very well at the exam. She came back regularly one week before each exam and send me many of her fellow students!

Case 2   (Aphasia after shock)

A young mother was brought by her husband for acute aphasia since 10 days following a traumatic incident. Their 4-year old son had managed to get himself electrocuted by sticking a nail into an electric outlet. She had succeeded in yanking him away but had consequently received the electrical shock. The medical treatment had not helped.

Treatment: HE-7 *Shenmen*, HE-5 *Tongli* and TW-17 *Yifeng* (sudden aphasia) were needled bilaterally with DM-21 *Qianding* (aphasia after shock). She had recovered her speech by the next day.

Case 3   (Nervous loss of voice)

A 25-year old woman consulted in an emergency for an acute aphonia having occurred the day before an important job interview for a position at the airport as a PA announcer.

Treatment: HE-7 *Shenmen*, HE-5 *Tongli* and LI-17 *Tianding* were needled bilaterally. She informed me that she had regained her voice and had secured the job.

Case 4   (Fear of Exams/ stage-fright)

A 35-year old female immigrant had been trying for the past two years to re-do her driving test. Although she had a driver's license from her home country and had actually been driving for over fifteen years and had even successfully passed her written tests, she kept failing the driving exam due to extreme nervousness. Her examiners considered her to be a public danger and had informed her that this would be her last chance.

Treatment: She was seen ten days before the exam: HE-7 *Shenmen*, HE-5 *Tongli* and BL-15 *Xinshu*; and again, the day before the exam: HE-6 *Yinxi* was added. She successfully passed her test.

Case 5   (Depression/ Blocked *Taiyin*/ Weakness of *Hun*)

A 47-year old patient consulted for depression. She was a school teacher, and complained of having lost her passion for teaching and having difficulties at home with her husband and children; she complained of easily feeling invaded. She had been consulting a psychiatrist with no improvement.

Analysis: The patient presented an Earth and Metal constitution, with a passive *Taiyin* blocked temperament that could explain the depressive mood. Her passivity and the feeling of being invaded pointed equally to an issue with *Hun* ≈ Ethereal soul. The palpation of BL-47 *Hunmen* confirmed the diagnosis, revealing a *Xu* ≈ Deficiency condition (pressure on the point felt good).

Treatment: The initial treatment aimed at strengthening the *Hun*: BL-18 *Ganshu* and BL-47 *Hunmen* with BL-23 *Shenshu* and BL-52 *Zhishe*. In the following sessions, the *Taiyin* level was treated with LU-7 *Lieque* with LI-4 *Hegu*; SP-4 *Gongsun* with ST-42 *Chongyang*; (*Luo-Yuan* points on alternate sides), with RM-12 *Zhongwan* (knot point of *Taiyin*). Although she felt slightly better, the progress was not satisfactory enough. In the follow up session I asked her to describe her living space set-up. Each of her two adolescent children had their own rooms, her husband had his office, and she shared the master bedroom and the wardrobe with him. She did her school chores on the kitchen table. In fact, she had no private or individual space to herself, hence the feeling of being invaded. I suggested for her to create a personal corner in her house, to install a small desk and to make it understood that it was her personal and private space. To take out private time for herself, fitness, culture, creativity, and not to insist on sharing it with her family. She was also given the "Central Axis" exercise to perform daily (▶ A.4.5.1). She was seen twice a month for three months and then once per month for another three months, and had regained her self-confidence and enthusiasm, and even had a much better relation with her family.

Case 6   (Depression/ Blocked *Taiyin*)

A 67-year old man in retirement for the past two years, was addressed to me by a colleague for depression, manifesting with a loss of motivation to do or to move, not at all in character for someone who had always been quite active. He also presented a lack of desire to communicate, although he had been known to have a good sense of humour, but had now become taciturn and aloof. He was often spending time alone in his room, and was reticent to participate in family gatherings. He arrived almost an hour before his appointment, saying: "just to be sure that I am not late"!

Analysis: He presented physically a typical Metal-type constitution, with a *Taiyin* Metal temperament, very precise and pre-occupied with the future-planning. The treatment aimed at opening the *Taiyin*.

Treatment: LU-7 *Lieque* with LI-4 *Hegu*; RM-12 *Zhongwan* (knot point of *Taiyin*); LU-2 *Yunmen* and SP-12 *Chongmen* were palpated for tenderness and needled to help open the *Taiyin* level. He was seen once a week for one month. After the second session he was cracking jokes with the secretary.

Case 7   (False depression/ suppressed rage)

A female patient consulted for depression after a difficult separation. Her psychiatrist had prescribed her an anti-depressant (Citalopram). She still had difficulties managing her emotions and managing her daily tasks and generally did not feel good.

Her pulses did not present the typical weak and empty qualities associated with a depressive state, they were rather tight and even wiry.

The six back points: BL-42, BL-43, BL-44, BL-47, BL-49 and BL-52 were palpated. The most reactive points were BL-43 *Gaohuangshu* and BL-47 *Hunmen*. Both were needled with a reducing method (bilateral). As well as GB-37 *Guangming* (bleeding technique) to help clear out the retained anger. I explained to her that she, in fact, was not depressed, but rather had a lot of retained anger that could be harmful to her.

In the follow-up session; the Liver-Qi was harmonised with LR-3 *Taichong* (right) and LR-14 *Qimen* (right); GB-37 *Guangming* (bilateral) was bled to help release the anger. PE-6 *Neiguan* (right) and SP-4 *Gongsun* (left), were added to help her come to terms with her suppressed emotions (see explanation for the *Luo)*. She was advised to take up a daily sport activity and to seek a cathartic psychotherapy group.

Case 8   (Fear of change)

A young woman in her last month of pregnancy had developed a severe case of Sciatalgia. Her obstetrician did not want to give her any anti-inflammatory or analgesic medication. The anamnesis revealed that she had an important position in a company, and that this was her first pregnancy. BL-52 *Zhishi* was the first point that was palpated. She strongly reacted to the pressure, describing that the pain actually started in that area.

Treatment: Three points were needled: BL-52 (reducing method), BL-23 *Shenshu* (supplementing) and BL-60 *Kunlun* (neutral). She was seen one week later; the pain had receded by 80%. BL-58 *Feiyang* was added (release fear). She was symptom free the following week, a set of points were needled to help with the up-coming birth (GB-34 *Yanglingchuan*, ST-36 *Zusanli* and SP-6 *Sanyinjiao*).

Explanation: the reactivity of BL-52 reveals retained fear concerning the future and change (obviously this information was not communicated to the patient). She was rather asked about how she saw the future in relation to her professional responsibilities and her new role of motherhood. She admitted having some concerns in managing both, that she did not wish to leave the child with a baby-sitter. I asked her to work-out a schedule with her husband and her parents in helping to keep the child. That it was important for her to have a clear strategy at this stage, rather than worrying about how things would work out.

Case 9   (Post-birth trauma/ *Chong Mai*)

A 28-year old woman had been diagnosed with colitis (irritable bowel syndrome) since her teens. She presented: abdominal distention with frequent abdominal pains and a bearing down sensation with frequent and soft stools; aggravated by stress. Generally, she was very easily stressed, had had several episodes of depression and felt often tired. She had regular cycles with a tendency to pre-menstrual abdominal pains. Her pulses were Firm and Wiry, the tongue was pale and slightly swollen. Another notable event in her history was the fact that she was born prematurely and had spent ten days in an incubator.

Analysis: The digestive symptoms and the tiredness in this patient were in favour of a Spleen-Qi-*Xu* ≈ Vacuity pattern. The bloating, distension and the wiry pulses indicated a pattern of Qi-stasis. The PMS also pointed to Qi and Blood-stasis. The chronicity of the symptoms, however, indicated the use of an Extraordinary Vessel. All the patterns and the fact that the condition had started during her adolescence, and especially the notion of post-birth trauma, were all suggestive of *Chong Mai*. In this case, as there were also psychological issues, the *Yin Wei Mai* was added to support the *Chong Mai*.

Treatment: SP-4 *Gongsun* on the right was coupled with PE-6 *Neiguan* on the left. LR-3 *Taichong* on the left was coupled with PE-7 *Daling* on the right, with the addition of RM-6 *Qihai* and KI-14 *Siman* (mobilise stasis). These points were alternated in the follow-up sessions with RM-4 *Guanyuan* with Moxa, and KI-17 *Shangqu* (to support the SP) and KI-11 *Henggu* (to uplift the Qi).

She was seen once a week for four weeks, then twice a month for four months. The needling of SP-4 *Gongsun* was alternated from right to left; once the Qi stasis had improved the LR-3 *Taichong* and PE-7 *Daling* were not needled replaced by ST-30 *Qichong*, ST-36 *Zusanli*, ST-37 *Shangjuxu*, ST-39 *Xiajuxu* to support the intestines.

In the third month two sessions were given to address the birth trauma and the *Gao Huang*: KI-16 *Huangshu*, BL-43 *Gaohuangshu*, BL-51 *Huangmen*, RM-6 *Qihai*.

Her condition improved rapidly and was stabilised. She was seen once every few months over the next year with no recurrence of colitis.

Case 10   (Death wish/ guilt)

A 46-year old woman was addressed to me by a colleague. She had been in a great state of despair since the suicide of her 21-year old daughter. She had stopped her work, had hardly slept and was barely nourishing herself. The daughter, who had been depressive and under psychiatric treatments, had gotten worse. The mother suspecting the possibility of her daughter committing suicide, had contacted the psychiatrist, who had reassured her, that the therapy was going very well, and that the daughter was under medication anyway. After the suicide of her daughter, the mother felt responsible for not having been more insistent with the doctor. She blamed herself and the psychiatrist for her daughter's death, and expressed immense rage for both herself and the therapist.

During the initial interview, it became apparent that she was letting herself die. Obviously, she did not want to hear about seeing a psychiatrist, and had even accepted, grudgingly, to have acupuncture.

Treatment:

- First session: to re-enforce her "desire for life" three points were needled: RM-14 *Jiuwei* (supplemented) and ST-23 *Taiyi*. To help change her perspective, I asked her to describe to me the degree of pain and despair and grief that the suicide of her daughter had caused her. After which I asked her if honestly, she was ready to cause the same degree of suffering for her husband and younger son? I could see that there had been a shift in her attitude.

- Second session: I saw her 3 days later. She had slept a few hours. BL-23 *Shenshu*, BL-52 *Zhishi* and BL-44 *Shentang* were all supplemented to restore the will to live. BL-42 *Pohu* and BL-47 *Hunmen* were extremely tight and reactive, they were both reduced to release grief and rage. Again, she was asked to remember her love for her son and her husband, that they both needed her.

- Third session: 1 week later: BL-42 *Pohu* (the point was still very reactive); LU-7 *Lieque* and KI-24 *Lingxu* (to let go and to forgive); RM-17 *Shanzhong* and BL-43 *Gaohuangshu*; (to help open the chest and release the grief)

- Fourth session: 1 week later: LU-7 *Lieque* and KI-24 *Lingxu* were repeated; LU-3 *Tianfu*, was added for helping to set priorities; LI-6 *Pianli* was bled to further release sadness.

- The following week: She was sleeping more and had started cooking for her family once again. PE-6 *Neiguan*; KI-9 *Zhubin* and RM-17 *Shanzhong* were needled to further help to release sorrow and regret.

- She was seen twice a month for another two months, and had resumed her work. I had some positive news of her a year later.

Case 11   (Panic attack)

A 43-year old man, had been having panic attacks in the last six months following an extramarital relationship that his wife had temporarily had. In spite of psychotherapy and anxiolytic medication he was still having several panic attacks per week that he more or less managed by going outside and taking deep breaths. He was prone to chest oppression, palpitations and claustrophobia. Constitutionally he presented as a Wood type with a *Jueyin* temperament. He admitted feeling insecure, lacking the desire even for sports, which he used to practice and greatly enjoy in the past.

Analysis: The *Chong Mai* was selected based on the symptoms, the lack of an axis, insecurity and the *Jueyin* temperament.

Treatment:

- First session: SP-4 *Gonsun* on the left coupled with PE-6 *Neiguan* (chest and emotional symptoms) on the right. LR-3 *Taichong* on the right, coupled with PE-7 *Daling* (relationship, jealousy issues) on the left, RM-4 *Guanyuan* and RM-18 *Yutang* (Knot of *Jueyin*).

- He was seen a week later and had had no attacks. The same protocol was applied, RM-18 *Yutang* was replaced by KI-21 *Youmen* (special Mu point for the LR to help express the subconscious).

- The back "*Zhi*" points were explored. BL-43 *Gaohuangshu* (self-respect; self-love) and BL-52 *Zhishi* (fear of change, fear of the future), were most reactive, they were needled with a reducing technique, BL-23 *Shenshu* and BL-14 *Jueyinshu* (to open the chest; rectify counterflow Qi) were supplemented, KI-8 *Jiaoxin* was added to strengthen self-trust and self-identity.   He was seen twice more during the following month with no recurrence of the symptoms.

Case 12   (Insomnia/ *Yin Wei Mai*)

A 54-year old woman was presenting insomnia and a menopausal syndrome for the past four years. Her sleep pattern was as follows: she fell asleep and slept deeply for 2–3 hours, then had hot flashes, and restless legs for several hours and finally would manage to have a deep sleep when it was time for her to get up. On weekends she could sleep another 2 hours peacefully. She had also been experiencing mood swings and some depression. The pulses were generally weak and thin, and the proximal (Kidney) pulses were quite deep and weak. The tongue was reddish, cracked with a peeled coating.

Analysis: The sleep was disturbed in its "quality" hence reflecting on the *Yin Wei Mai*, further confirmed by the reactivity of KI-9 *Zhubin* on the left side; as the middle section of the night was involved, it suggested a *Jueyin* disturbance (middle section of *Yin Wei*). The Liver-Blood and Yin vacuity was also manifesting in the restless leg syndrome.

Treatment: PE-6 *Neiguan* was needled on the left side as KI-9 was more reactive on this side, with SP-4 *Gongsun* on the right; LR-3 *Taichong* was needled on the left with PE-5 *Jianshi* (to draw Yin up) on the right and RM-18 *Yutang* the knot point of *Jueyin*. LR-8 *Ququan* was added on the right to supplement Liver-Blood, and SP-6 *Sanyinjiao* bilaterally to supplement Liver, Kidney, Yin and Blood. DM-20 *Baihui* was added to help ascend the Blood and Yin to the head, and help calm the mind. In the follow-up sessions PE-6 *Neiguan* and SP-4 *Gongsun* were combined with BL-18 *Ganshu*, BL-17 *Geshu*, BL-43 *Gaohuangshu*, and BL-23 *Shenshu* (all the back points were chosen according to reactivity). The patient was seen roughly once a month. Once the sleep had improved, the treatment was oriented more towards supplementing Kidney Yin and reducing Heat.

Case 13   (Facial tic/ smoker)

A heavy smoker (2 packs per day) was treated with a standard protocol to help him to stop smoking (GB-1, GB-8; *Bi Tong*, *Yintang* and Zero point in the ear), the points were all reduced every 10 minutes. The sessions were repeated every 3-4 days until the patient felt a metallic taste in the mouth. This treatment caused tobacco revulsion and helped the subject to stop smoking.

This 48-year old man stopped smoking after five sessions. After 10 days he came back because of a facial tic involving the eye muscle. He also complained of being very irritable and even easily flying into rage and sleeping very badly with nightmares.

Analysis: A tic in TCM, is considered an Internal Wind, from a Liver pattern: usually Liver Yang rising or Liver Heat. At the time, I should have analysed his condition better and done a more adapted treatment. In his case the need to smoke was an attempt to subdue an excessive Liver-Qi through the *Ke* ≈ Control cycle.

Treatment: Harmonising the Liver and extinguishing the Liver Wind: LR-2 *Xingjian*, LR-3 *Taichong*, LI-4 *Hegu*; GB-20 *Fengchi* and GB-1 *Tongziliao* (to move Yang away from the eye). Two treatments resolved the eye tic. I continued to see him twice a month to harmonise the Liver Qi.

Case 14   (Stuttering/ smoker)

A 42-year old man, very heavy smoker was treated with the same protocol as above to help him to stop smoking. During the second session the patient felt a metallic taste in the mouth. After which he not only developed a tobacco revulsion, but he could not even stand the smell of the ashtrays which would give him nausea. A month later he consulted again, complaining of stuttering, a difficulty that he had not experienced since his childhood. Although he did not relate the condition to his smoking withdrawal, the incidence was quite clear.

Analysis: Stuttering is a disturbance of the Heart *Luo* ≈ Connecting channel. In his case the bitter taste of the tobacco had been fortifying the Heart-Qi.

Treatment: HE-5 *Tongli* (*Luo* point) and HE-7 *Shenmen* and LI-18 *Futu* (Window of Heaven for speech difficulties), were needled three times to help stop the stuttering. He was still tobacco free 3 months later.

Case 15   (ADHD)

A young boy, aged six, has been diagnosed with ADHD by the school psychologist who has suggested starting a Ritalin treatment. The boy had been showing an aggressive behaviour and easily getting into fights with other children. His mother wanted a second opinion and brought the child for an acupuncture evaluation. The anamnesis did not reveal any particular pattern, except occasional nightmares. The tongue had red sides. He was evaluated as a Wood-type with a *Shaoyang* temperament. The most relevant information was the separation of the parents when the boy was two years old.

Analysis: The absence of the father, probably explains the hyperactivity of the *Du Mai* and the lack of social boundaries. The *Shaoyang* temperament which is not communicating with its complementary Yin level accounts for the aggressivity and hyperactivity, aggravated by the Liver-Fire (nightmares).

Treatment: A 50 mW infrared laser was used for the treatments: I proposed a trial treatment of weekly sessions for 2 months before attempting the Ritalin treatment.

-   First session: BL-47 *Hunmen,* with BL-18 *Ganshu*; HE-7 *Shenmen* (all reduced to calm *Shen* and *Hun*) and DM-5 *Xuanshu* (impulsiveness). He was taught to practice the simple form of reconnecting the brain (PAT-6.3), that we did together.

-   Next session: LR-2 *Xingjian*; LR-3 *Taichong*; DM-24 *Shenting* and GB-13 *Benshen* (reduced to clear Liver-Fire). I had the boy perform the exercises, making sure that he did them regularly. His mother mentioned that he actually looked forward to doing them.

-   The blocked *Shaoyang* level was treated with GB-37 *Guangming* TW-5 *Waiguan* (reduced) with LR-3 *Taichong* and PE-7 *Daling* (*Luo-Yuan* to re-connect *Shaoyang* with *Jueyin*) with RM-18 *Yutang* (knot of *Jueyin*)

-   The lack of concentration was managed with: BL-20 *Pishu*; BL-49 *Yishe* and SP-2 *Dadu* (supplemented)

- During the following sessions some other points were added for emotional over-reaction: HE-5 *Tongli* and restlessness: KI-23 *Shenfeng*; KI-25 *Shencang*; and *Yiming*

After two months his behaviour was sufficiently modified for the psychologist to change her diagnosis. I saw him once a month for another four months, and advised his mother to put him in a class of martial arts for children, to help channel his wood energy.

Case 16   (Depression/ weak character/ *Du Mai*)

A 52-year old man was having a depression following the separation from his wife. He had returned to live with his mother, who had called to make the appointment, and insisted in accompanying him for his session and to supply information on his medical background. His father had abandoned the family quite early, and very obviously the subject had grown up in an atmosphere of over protectiveness of the mother. His health was described as delicate, and in general he was sensitive to cold, with no other salient symptoms.

Analysis: The weakness of *Du Mai* and the character are in coherence with the feeling of insecurity that he was describing.

Treatment: SI-3 *Houxi* on the left, BL-62 *Shenmai* on the right, DM-1 *Changqiang*, DM-4 *Mingmen*, DM-20 *Baihui*.

In the following session, BL-11 *Dazhu* (*Hui* of bones) and GB-39 *Xuanzhong* (*Hui* of Marrow) were added to help strengthen the character. In the fourth session, the treatment was shifted to the *Yang Qiao Mai* to help him find his stance in the world: BL-62 *Shenmai* on the left, SI-3 *Houxi* on the right, BL-61 *Pucan* bilaterally. He was further seen once a month and had resumed his professional activity.

Case 17   (Sexual trauma/ *Dai Mai*)

A 25-year old woman complained of having a feeling of heavy legs. Although she was tall and thin, the examination revealed an accumulation of fat and cellulitis around her pelvis and hip areas. She also often felt coldness of the buttocks. The anamnesis did not reveal any important information, except the fact that she had no memory of her early years, before the age of eight.

Analysis: The physical symptoms were quite suggestive of a *Dai Mai* pattern. The lack of memory was in favour of a traumatic event that had been suppressed.

Treatment: The initial treatment aimed at opening the *Dai Mai* with GB-41 *Zulinqi,* GB-26 *Daimai*; GB-28 *Weidao* was added as it concerns the lower belt and the pelvic zone. Ten minutes after the needles were inserted, she started crying. I asked her what was going on? She explained that she had a vision of her father abusing her when she was a small child. She mentioned that at the first opportunity she would ask her father about this. I saw her two weeks later, she had confronted her father who had emphatically denied the facts and told her that she was crazy. She shared her suspicions with her younger sister who also confirmed having been molested by the father.

The follow-up treatments aimed at releasing the body memories (see Body Armours ▶ 4.2.7), and she was given some exercises and PAT exercises to help liberate the pelvic armour (▶ A.4.1.1 and A.4.1.2).

Case 18   (Sexual trauma/ *Dai Mai*)

A 26-year old woman consulted for paraplegia having occurred after an epidural anaesthesia given for a delivery, 18 months prior. She presented a hypertonic type paralysis, with muscular atrophy and cold and bluish legs. Her sphincter control was not affected. From a neurological point of view, the condition was quite puzzling for her doctors. Otherwise she was healthy and was adapting well to her condition, greatly helped by a very supportive husband. The pulses were rather weak in general, the tongue showed some paleness and especially a Heart crack. This prompted me to explore further her psychological past. She revealed having been hospitalised twice following attempted suicides. For the second session, I asked her husband to remain in the waiting room, so that she would feel more at ease to speak about her past. She had had a very traumatic childhood with numerous episodes of incest between the ages of eight until fourteen, when she had attempted her first suicide, since then she had been on and off under psychotherapy. Her life had been greatly stabilised after her marriage up until her labour and delivery. Although she had shared some of her past with her husband, there remained many un-resolved issues.

Analysis: The symptomatology and the psychological issues are both consistent with a *Dai Mai* pattern. The pain and trauma of labour had re-activated her body memory of the past pelvic trauma.

Treatment: The main treatment aimed at opening the *Dai Mai* (GB-41 *Zulinqi*, GB-26 *Daimai*) and helping release the holding patterns (ST-14 *Kufang*, HE-3 *Shaohai*, BL-62 *Shenmai*), mobilise the Yang downward (DM-3 *Yaoyangguan*, BL-36 *Chengfu,* GB-33 *Xiyangguan*, ST-39 *Xiajuxu*). The follow up treatments alternated between *Dai Mai* and the releasing of the pelvic armouring, and treating the *Yang Qiao* and *Du Mai* to give her back her strength and confidence to stand on her own feet again. After about a year of combined psychotherapy, physiotherapy and acupuncture, she had regained the use of her legs and was planning to start training as a therapist.

Case 19   (Anxiety/ Tinnitus/ fear of failure)

A 27-year old female patient consulted for acute high pitch tinnitus, extreme anxiety and panic preceding up-coming final engineering examinations.

The high pitch tinnitus was causing her severe insomnia. Medically a brain tumour was suspected, which had aggravated her anxiety state. Although the brain scans had revealed no tumour, she had remained in an extreme state of anxiety and panic.

She presented as a Fire and Water constitution, with a *Taiyang* temperament: wilful, ambitious, controlling, demanding, and expecting to always be the best in her studies; putting a great pressure on herself with a constant feeling of insecurity and of not performing well enough. Habitually, she was capable of studying 20 hours per day before her exams, which often resulted in a state of exhaustion and memory problems.

Physically she complained of neck tensions, lumbar pains, feeling easily cold and long cycles. The tongue was red with redder sides, with a peeled coating. Her pulses were rapid, wiry and weak on both Kidney positions.

Analysis: The anxiety background was a common pattern in her family (father, mother and sister). The psychological pressures were contributing to a disturbance of her sleep. The excessive worry and mental over-work, further disrupted the sleep and the memory and concentration (*Yi*). Her low confidence in her performance, despite excellent previous academic results, reflected on a lack of grounding and self-trust (*Yin Qiao*). The Kidney Qi and *Jing* were being constantly taxed.

- Treatment: The initial treatment was aimed at reducing the tinnitus. Extinguish Liver-Wind with LR-2 *Xingjiang* (left); LR-3 *Taichong* (right); GB-20 *Fengchi* (bilateral); and move Yang down from the head with BL-10 *Tianzhu*; GB-21 *Jianjing* (bilateral).

- The second session, one week later: the tinnitus was reduced by 50% and the pitch had changed from high to a low murmur (Liver-Wind from Yin deficiency): treatment was modified to LR-3 *Taichong* (left); LR-8 *Ququan* (right); BL-18 *Ganshu* (right); BL-10 and GB-21 were repeated; PE-6 *Neiguan* (right) was added to calm the mind and settle the panic.

- Third session: The tinnitus had almost disappeared completely; the sleep was better with some episodes of nightmares involving stress themes. Treatment was directed towards the *Yinwei*: PE-6 *Neiguan* (left, KI-9 was more reactive on this side); SP-4 *Gongsun* (right); LR-3 *Taichong* (left); PE-5 *Jianshi* (right); with DM-24 *Shenting* and GB-13 *Benshen* for the nightmares.

- Fourth session: The nightmares and tinnitus had disappeared, but she still was is a state of anxiety as her exams were due the following week. She complained of studying but unable to retain the information. BL-20 *Pishu* (supplemented), BL-49 *Yishe* (reduced); SP-2 *Dadu* (right) and SP-3 *Taibai* (left), DM-20 *Baihui*; HE-7 *Shenmen* (left) and HE-5 *Tongli* (right) were added to calm *Shen*. After the session, it was suggested to work on her belief systems.

  - Q: What is behind your stress and panic?

- A: I am afraid of failure; I am afraid of not being good enough; I lack confidence in myself.

- Q: Find an appropriate sentence that will help you in this context.

- A: "I trust in myself; I trust in my capabilities

- She was instructed to do the PAT exercises (A.4.1.1 and A.4.1.3) while repeating the above sentences, and to monitor her progress. The entire procedure was to be repeated until a concrete result was achieved. She was also instructed to change her learning patterns: to stop every hour, to go outside for ten minutes and consciously make note of all the sensory input by naming them (sounds, smells, sights etc…).

- Fifth session: She had successfully passed her finals with top grades; and she admitted that it was the first time in her life that she was passing an exam without stress. The treatment was shifted to *Chong Mai*: SP-4 *Gongsun* (right); PE-6 *Neiguan* (left); LR-3 *Taichong* (left); PE-7 *Daling* (right); DM-20 *Baihui*; RM-4 *Guanyuan*. She was also instructed to perform daily the Central Axis exercises (A.4.5.1), while repeating the self-affirmations above.

She was regularly seen once a month; *Yin Qiao* and KI-8 *Jiaoxin* were treated to help her "rooting" and self-confidence. Also, to harmonise Fire and Water: HE-7 *Shenmen*; KI-3 *Taixi*; KI-23 *Shenfeng*. She reported being much more relaxed and having slept very deeply, with no recurrence of panic. There still remained a background of tinnitus (buzzing): points were added to supplement the Kidney and relax the will: BL-23 *Shenshu* and BL-52 *Zhishi*; RM-4 *Guanyuan*; and to subdue the internal Wind: TW-17 *Yifeng* and TW-21 *Ermen* towards GB-2 *Tinghui* (with one needle).

Case 20   (Depression, anxiety, insomnia/ addiction/ *Ren Mai*)

A 35-year old man, a musician, consulted for recurrent episodes of depression, anxiety and insomnia; all getting worse in winter-time. The medical history revealed numerous addictive tendencies: tobacco, alcohol and drugs with multiple attempts at withdrawal and relapse. With a heavy family background of divorced parents at an early age, a victimised mother and an over controlling father. After the divorce, the children were abandoned by the father, with a non-functional and chronically depressive mother. Constitutionally, he is Water-Fire type and a *Shaoyin* temperament, with a tendency to isolate himself, and difficulty in assuming responsibility and engaging in relationships. The anamnesis further revealed a Kidney-Yin vacuity: night sweating, floating Yang, rapid pulses, red and peeled tongue. His insomnia pattern was coherent with a HE-KI (*Shaoyin*) pattern: difficulty falling asleep (*Yinqiao Mai*), with excessive mental agitation and waking in a state of anxiety.

Analysis: The psychological profile is that of a partially blocked *Shaoyin* temperament with difficulties communicating with his *Taiyang* level, although in public he could deceptively present a *Taiyang* behaviour. The co-dependence and oral compensations reflected on a *Ren Mai* issue consistent with his family background.

-   Initial treatment: Harmonising *Ren Mai* complemented by *Yin Qiao*: LU-7 *Lieque* (left), KI-6 *Zhaohai* (right); KI-8 *Jiaoxin* (right): to support the will and self-trust; KI-3 *Taixi* (left) and HE-7 *Shenmen* (right); RM-12 *Zhongwan*; RM-4 *Guanyuan*. He was encouraged to join an AA group, something he had resisted in doing for many years.

-   The following three weekly sessions were supporting his withdrawal process, including the diminishing of the anxiolytic dosage: GB-8 *Shuaigu* with GB-9 *Tianchong* (bilateral with one needle); BL-23 *Shenshu;* BL-52 *Zhishi;* KI-8 *Jiaoxin*; GB-6 *Xuanli* (To help strengthen the will power); and BL-58 *Feiyang* (addictive personality); were alternated with LR-3 *Taichong,* PE-7 *Daling* and LI-4 *Hegu* (to harmonise the Liver). The PAT protocolS (A.4.1.1 and A.4.1.3) for changing the mind-set were given to him to practice daily (besides the AA 12-step program).

After one month, he was alcohol and smoke free and on a very low dose of anxiolytic medication, the protocol was shifted to treating the roots:

-   *Chong Mai* (for the Central axis and to harmonise Water and Fire): SP-4 *Gongsun;* KI-14 *Siman* or KI-15 *Zhongzhu* (these are *Chong Mai* constitutional points to support the Kidney (selected according to palpational sensitivity); KI-23 *Shenfu* or KI-25 *Shencang* (to settle the mind and harmonise the Water and Fire axis); DM-20 *Baihui*

-   Harmonise *Shaoyin* with *Taiyang*: HE-5 *Tongli* with SI-4 *Wangu* and KI-4 *Dazhong* with BL-64 *Jinggu;* supplement *Shaoyin*: KI-3 *Taixi*; HE-7 *Shenmen*; and RM-23 *Lianquan* (knot point of *Shaoyin*).

-   For the *Ren Mai* and compensation issues (lack of maternal nourishment): LU-7 *Lieque*, KI-6 *Zhaohai*; RM-12 *Zhongwan*; RM-6 *Qihai*; BL-43 *Gaohuangshu* and according to palpational reactivity KI-16 *Huangshu* or BL-51 *Huangmen* or BL-53 *Baohuang.*

He was followed on and off for two years during which he had reported being stable and drug-free.

Case 21   (Infantile insomnia/ sexual trauma transmitted to the child/ *Chong Mai*)

A 25-year old woman, in her last month of pregnancy, consulted for birth-preparation treatments. The birth was evolving normally and the anamnesis did not reveal any notable dis-balance, except for the important fact that the pregnancy had been the consequence of a traumatic gang-rape while she had been hitchhiking through the middle east. At the time, she seemed to have well-adjusted to the trauma and had accepted and even welcomed the pregnancy. Two standard protocol sessions were given: first session: GB-34,

ST-36, KI-8 and KI-9; one week before the birth: GB-34, ST-36, KI-8 and SP-6.

She consulted 3 weeks later; the birth had gone very smoothly, but she was on the verge of a nervous breakdown. The infant was not sleeping and was crying all the time. She could calm him down for a short time while she carried him, but he would start wailing as soon as she put him in the crib. She had not slept in two weeks and was in a state of advanced exhaustion. The habitual causes of infantile crying such as pain, indigestion, milk intolerance, were discarded. I proposed to treat both the child and the mother.

Analysis: This is very unusual case of a transmitted trauma from mother to child, hence the *Chong Mai*, was selected for the infant. For the mother, certain aspects of the trauma had clearly not been dealt with and digested; and although there were no clinical indications, the *Jing* might also have been affected.

- First treatment: For the child, with an infra-red 50 mW Laser the following points were stimulated: SP-4 *Gongsun* (left); PE-6 *Neiguan* (right); PE-5 *Jianshi* (bilateral for infantile crying); KI-21 *Yaomen* (infants that need to be carried); and Moxa on DM-20 *Baihui*. For the mother: ST-14 *Kufang*; HE-3 *Shaohai* and BL-62 *Shenmai* (to help clear-out the shock). She was instructed to write in detail, what she could remember of the trauma.

- Second session: The infant had slept for six hours after the treatment, and it had been easier to calm him down since. BL-11 *Dazhu*; BL-14 *Jueyinshu*; (to regulate the autonomous nervous system); *Anmian*; and PE-5 *Jianshi* (bilateral). For the mother the same points were repeated with PE-4 *Ximen* added to help remember. She was instructed to write again in great detail, what she could remember of the traumatic event.

- Third session: The infant was treated with: SP-4 *Gongsun* (left); PE-6 *Neiguan* (right); PE-5 *Jianshi* (bilateral) and KI-9 *Zhubin* (bilateral). For the mother: BL-23 *Shenshu*; BL-52 *Zhishi*; DM-4 *Mingmen* and RM-4 *Guanyuan* to help consolidate *Jing*.

- Two more weekly sessions were given, to harmonise Water and Fire for the child (KI-3, HE-7, KI-9); and to help let go and to forgive for the mother (LU-7, KI-24, PE-6 and BL-43). Both were sleeping and recovering very well.

Case 22   (Addiction/ Blocked *Taiyang*)

A 30-year old female nurse, mother of three, consulted for anxiety, stress and insomnia with nightmares involving loss of control and powerlessness. Anamnesis revealed a pattern of Liver-Qi stagnation (PMS, Wood-type migraine headaches, frustration and anger producing tightness in the solar plexus and gastritis; hay-fever and occasional eczema). In her history: anorexia nervosa and bulimia between the ages of 18 and 20; several episodes of depression, requiring hospitalisation. She had been under an anxiolytic treatment (Lorazepam) for some time. The subject presented herself as a Fire-Water type with a blocked *Taiyang* temperament (inability to connect with her *Shaoyin* level; vulnerability and frequent feelings of injustice). She held herself in a very rigid posture, and an attitude of being in control and keeping her distance. She was accident prone, with a tendency to hurt herself with, cuts, bruises, burns and even multiple fractures in the past. A categorical refusal to speak about her past (not wanting to stir up bad memories); always pretending that she was capable of managing her life on her own (pride). After many sessions, she finally admitted with some difficulty, that she was an alcoholic (but refused to join the AA program); and that there was a lot of violence in her childhood. She was treated with acupuncture on and off for the above complaints, over two years, before she trusted enough to reveal her past traumas and her compulsive and addictive tendency.

Analysis: This was a very difficult case to treat; she was controlling the communication and refusing to "name" and "own" the problem. Furthermore, she consistently undermined the therapy, relapsing into her habitual addictive behaviour, and frequently missing her acupuncture or other therapy sessions. In the absence of her investment in the treatments, the protocol aimed at connecting *Taiyang* with *Shaoyin*; to help her assume her vulnerability; and to harmonise *Ren Mai* with *Du Mai*; for her addictive tendencies. And further attenuate her wilfulness and controlling attitude.

- Harmonise *Taiyang* with *Shaoyin*: SI-7 *Zhizheng* (left) with HE-7 *Shenmen* (right) and BL-58 *Feiyang* (left) with KI-3 *Taixi* (right) supplement *Shaoyin*: KI-7 *Fuliu* (right); HE-6 *Yinxi* (left); and RM-23 *Lianquan* (knot point of *Shaoyin*). In further sessions, the *Shaoyin* treatment was complemented by KI-8 *Jiaoxin* (bilateral for self-trust) and HE-5 *Tongli* (help remember and speak).

- To harmonise the *Ren* and *Du Mai* and address the compensation and addictive issues: LU-7 *Lieque* (right), KI-6 *Zhaohai* (left); RM-12 *Zhongwan*; RM-6 *Qihai*; SI-3 *Houxi* (left); BL-62 *Shenmai* (right) and DM-20 *Baihui*.

- Supplement Kidney (dreams of loss of control and power): BL-23 *Shenshu;* KI-3 *Taixi*; KI-6 Zhaohai; and to reduce the controlling and wilful attitude: BL-52 *Zhishi* and TW-10 *Tianjing* (reduced); KI-1 *Yongquan*.

- Other points: BL-11 *Dazhu* (feeling of being mistreated); KI-22 *Bulang* (feeling of injustice); KI-24 *Lingxu* (helps forgive and let go of the past; stress); BL-10 *Tianzhu* (lack of coordination).

- Although some small progress was being made, the overall results remained very average.

Case 23   (Agoraphobia/ Thoracic block)

A 36-year old woman consulted for agoraphobia. Her husband was a politician, and she had to accompany him to many social events and political rallies. After 10-15 minutes in a crowd, she would have the impression of suffocating and had to leave the room, which was obviously embarrassing for her husband. Otherwise, she had no problems in enclosed spaces or lifts, just with crowded areas. Anamnesis revealed a Wood-type constitution with a *Jueyin* temperament, quite coquettish, with some premenstrual symptoms (Liver-Qi stasis). The Five-element analysis further revealed a dislike of wind and in particular a strong dislike of the colour green.

Analysis: the condition was suggestive of a "thoracic block" (chest oppression, tight solar plexus and plum-pit), from Liver-Qi stasis. Her family history further supported the suspicion: she was weaned very early as the mother had to resume work. She was the eldest of four siblings and had to assume responsibility very early. Although the early weaning was more involving a *Ren Mai* issue, the *Yinwei* or *Chong Mai* were more indicated regarding the overall temperament and symptoms.

- First session: PE-6 *Neiguan* (right); SP-4 *Gongsun* (left); LR-3 *Taichong* (right); PE-7 *Daling* (left); RM-18 *Yutang* (knot of *Jueyin*); LR-14 *Qimen*

- Second session: SP-4 *Gongsun* (right); PE-6 *Neiguan* (left); LR-3 *Taichong* (right); BL-43 *Gaohuangshu* (bilateral), and the most reactive *Hoatojiaji* points in the area of the thoracic spine. She was instructed the PAT-2 exercise for releasing the thoracic segment.

- Third session: the chest points were palpated and needled superficially (ST-14; ST-15; KI-24; KI-25; RM-17; GB-22…).

- By the fourth session, she had attended several social events with no recurrence of the symptoms.

- She was seen once more, a month later to consolidate the treatment. She showed-up wearing an apple-green outfit!

Case 24   (Insomnia; panic and fear of death)

A 56-year old man had a CVA episode (aneurism) and had been saved in-extremis by emergency brain surgery. Since his operation, he had not been able to sleep more than one hour per night. He presented with a great state of panic, stress and fear. Trembling hands, blood-shot eyes, very red tongue with redder sides, wiry pulse, and a high blood-pressure (despite beta blocker medication). He was a heavy smoker (1-2 packs per day); drank 10 coffees per day and had a regular intake of alcohol.

Analysis: The CVA represents an extreme condition of Liver-Wind from Liver-Yang rising (hypertension) on a back-ground of Liver-Fire. The shock of near death and the recent death of a brother, had caused an extreme state of panic and fear of death. The insomnia was probably rooted in the belief that if he went to sleep, he would not wake up. The treatment aimed at clearing the shock; extinguishing Liver-Fire and re-establishing the sleep:

- First session: KI-1 *Yongquan* (bilateral)*;* LR-2 *Erjian* (right)*;* LR-8 *Ququan* (left); GB-20 *Fengchi* (bilateral)*;* KI-6 *Zhaohai* (left); HE-7 *Shenmen* (right); KI-27 *Shufu* (bilateral) for persistent insomnia

- Second session: He had managed to sleep twice, three hours per night, waking to eat. Generally felt much calmer. ST-14 *Kufang* (bilateral); HE-3 (right) *Shaohai* and BL-62 *Shenmai* (left), to help clear-out the shock; HE-7 *Shenmen* (right); KI-6 *Zhaohai* (right); ST-21 *Liangmen* (left), for waking to eat at night; *Yintang.*

- Third session: He had recovered his normal sleeping pattern (5 hours per night, without interruption. Treatment was shifted to *Chong Mai* to help mobilise Blood: SP-4 *Gongsun* (left); PE-6 *Neiguan* (right); BL-43 *Gaohuangshu* (left); GB-20 *Fengchi* (bilateral); DM-20 *Baihui;* BL-52 *Zhishi* (bilateral) for the fear of death; BL-18 *Ganshu* (right)

- He was seen on a weekly basis over two months; he had reduced his alcohol, coffee and tobacco consumption drastically.

Case 25   (PTSD)

A 32-year old woman had been involved in a pile-up car accident on the highway during a foggy day. Although she had not sustained any significant physical injury, she had no memory of the event. Since the accident, one year ago, she had not been able to go on the highway, even as a passenger. Daily she had to go to work in another city, obliging her to take the train and the bus, making a difference of one hour of travel time each way. She had sought out professional help, even hypnosis with no avail. She had become very jumpy, especially to the sound of honking and screeching brakes, that she associated with her accident. She also described a feeling of unexplained anxiety on cloudy and especially foggy days. She had recurring dreams involving accidents, from which she would wake up in a sweat.

Analysis: The post-traumatic shock with a loss of memory is suggestive of a disconnection between the *Shen* and the *Yi* (fore-brain and mid-brain). The suppressed memories involving impressions and sounds were retained by *Hun*.

- First session: to help release of the traumatic event: ST-14 *Kufang,* HE-3 *Shaohai,* BL-62 *Shenmai;*

- Second session*:* to help connect the fore-brain and the mid-brain: DM-24 *Shenting* and GB-13 *Benshen* with DM-17 *Naohu,* GB-18 *Chengling,* and DM-20 *Baihui*

- Third session: to fortify the Kidneys: BL-52 *Zhishi,* BL-23 *Xinshu,* DM-4 *Mingmen* and RM-4 *Guanyuan;* KI-2 *Rangu* and KI-27 *Shufu* were added for anxiety and apprehension. She was encouraged to revisit the day of the accident and to write down in detail what she could recall, and to repeat this exercise at least twice a week.

- Two more weekly sessions aimed at consolidating the Kidney; the *Jing*, and releasing the fear: BL-52 *Zhishi;* KI-4 *Dazhong;* KI-8 *Jiaoxin;* BL-58 *Feiyang;* HE-6 *Yinxi*

- By the sixth session, she had no more nightmares, felt much less apprehensive and could more clearly recall the accident. It was suggested that she try accompanying her friend for a short drive on the highway. He-5 *Tongli;* HE-6 *Yinxi* and HE-7 *Shenmen* were needled with one needle (threading technique); KI-3 *Taixi;* KI-27 *Shufu* and DM-20 *Baihui* to help stabilize the emotions.

She managed to remain calm during the drive on the highway, and one month later was back to driving herself to work.

Case 26   (Pain management)

A 32-year old man, very sportive and physically active, presented an inflammation of the pudendal nerve on the right side (main nerve of the perineum) after a long and arduous period of bicycling effort. With symptoms of intense perineal, sacral, genital, anal and lower abdominal burning pains with anal incontinence. The pain had caused a severe insomnia and depression, loss of appetite and 10 kg loss of weight. He had been treated for six months with a variety of anti-inflammatory, opiates, steroid infiltrations, anxiolytics and sleeping pills, with no avail. He consulted in an advanced state of despair, having tried a variety of other complementary therapies that had all aggravated the condition. Physically he appeared as a Fire-type constitution, tall and thin, with a very wilful character in conformity with a *Taiyang* temperament. Anamnesis revealed swollen and purplish sub-lingual veins (predominant on the right side); pulses were all deficient, except for wiry and thin Wood pulses. He also complained of chronic haemorrhoids.

Analysis: The intense and repetitive exercises had aggravated a pre-existent pelvic Blood stasis (haemorrhoids). The treatment aimed at mobilising pelvic Blood and upholding the Qi (incontinence).

- First session: SP-4 *Gongsun* (left); PE-6 *Neiguan* (right); DM-1 *Changqiang;* DM-20 *Baihui;* BL-53 *Baohuang* (bilateral to move pelvic Blood) and BL-54 *Zhibian*

- Second session: His pain had improved by 20%, he had no more incontinence and had reduced his medication by half. As the sacral pain seemed to radiate belt-like to the front on the right side, the *Daimai* was selected: with GB-41 *Zulinqi* (right); GB-26 *Daimai* (right); GB-27 *Wushu* (right); and other *Daimai* confluent points: RM-6 *Qihai;* RM-4 *Guanyuan;* LR-5 *Ligou* (bilateral for genital pains); RM-1 *Huiyin*

- Third session: He had stopped all medication, the pain had improved and changed from intense spasms to an electrical feeling. Local "Barrier" points were chosen to move the trapped Yang out of the pelvic area: BL-29 *Zhonglushu;* BL-36 *Chengfu; Chong Mai* was repeated with additional: ST-30 *Qichong* and DM-20 *Baihui.*

- By the fourth session, he was sleeping much better, had regained his appetite and had no more need of medication, although the pain level had remained at 40%. It was decided to explore further so as to better understand his psychological profile. He explained that he had started his carrier at 20, pushing himself without regard for his body. Later participating in extreme competitive sports, having the feeling that he had to be the best in order to be appreciated, and that nothing was good enough. This session aimed at reconnecting him with his deeper self (*Taiyang* with Shaoyin) to help relax his wilful attitude: SI-7 *Zhizheng* (right), with HE-7 *Shenmen* (left); BL-58 *Feiyang* (left) with KI-3 *Taixi* (right) and KI-1 *Yongquan* (right) with DM-20 *Baihui* to relax the will and KI-26 *Yuzhong* (impression of not being loved). During the session, a dialogue was established with the body:

  - Therapist: Get in touch in your body with the area that is calling for attention at this time; and describe it.

  - Patient: I feel a hard, dark disk-like mass, cold on the inside but electrified on the surface.

  - T.: What could help or relieve this feeling?

  - P.: A thick, oily orange coloured gel.

  - T.: If this area could speak, what would it say?

  - P.: Just relax and do nothing.

  - T.: Does this area need anything else? If not is there another place that needs attention?

  - P.: Yes, my hip and belly on the right side.

  - T.: Describe the feeling.

  - P.: I have the image of a blue fist pushing against a red elastic; that there is not enough space in there.

  - T.: What could help or relieve this condition?

  - P.: For the belly, the image of a cool mountain stream water, that is carrying a leaf. For the hip a blue coloured gel, with a flame that is melting it and helping it to penetrate the bones.

  - T.: How is the pain now?

  - P.: I still feel the compression and that the hip does not have enough space.

- T.: Start giving a lot of space to your hip. Imagine your hip dissolving into unlimited space. Do the same with your belly. Now how does it feel?

- P.: This feels very good; I do not feel the pain anymore.

- T.: Is there a message that this area has for you?

- P.: Just relax and be…

- T.: Is there anything you would like to tell your body

- P.: Yes, I would like to ask for forgiveness for having abused it to gain fame… (This acknowledgment brought up a great swell of emotion and tears).

He called two days later to report that he had been pain-free for the first time in six months, and sleeping very deeply and in peace.

Case 27 (Stress/ guided visualisation)

A 45-year old woman, mother of 3, whose husband has been unemployed for the past 6 months, was suffering from chest oppression with shoulder and neck pains, and pre-menstrual migraine headaches. She also had lumbar pains with cold feet. Her tongue was purplish with red sides. Her pulses were wiry, with a weak Kidney Yang.

I had treated her four times with acupuncture for liver-Qi stagnation and Kidney-Yang-Xu/ /vacuity over six weeks. She reported getting better for some time but the symptoms would recur.

She also mentioned that she had been having recurrent dreams of stress. In a dream she saw herself driving a heavy truck with a very heavy load. The truck could hardly move and she was worried not to be able to reach her destination. She also realised in her dream that she was very worried because she did not have a permit to drive a truck.

So, I took the opportunity this time to treat her only with "mind-body dialogue". I explained briefly the process to the patient that she should mainly be aware of her bodily sensations and welcome any thoughts, feelings, or images connected to the body impressions. The treatment session was structured to devote 20 to 30 minutes for the dream exploration, and a further 10 to 15 minutes to talk about the experience and bring the process to a conclusion. I usually take the pulses at the start and at the end of the session.

I started by suggesting to her to become aware of the most predominant feeling, or of any thought or issue that is present in her dream or and in her life now. I ask her to put words on these feelings.

- Patient: It just feels too much pressure on me to carry the whole family and the insecurity of my husband's situation.

- Therapist: Scan the body and relate this feeling to a place in your body. Describe what is going on there, in terms of sensations, shape, colour, landscape, quality.

- P.: I feel like a huge stone on my shoulders and neck, it weighs a ton. I feel like I could just collapse and be smashed by it. The setting is in a place where trucks go to discharge their loads, close to the evening with a sort of heavy atmosphere like before a rain. No one is there, and I feel a bit frightened. A strong wind is blowing and scattering the objects around.

- T.: what are you experiencing in your neck and shoulder area now?

- P.: I feel shaky and moved. My shoulders and neck are very tight.

- T.: if your shoulders and neck could talk and express emotions what would they say?

- P.: My shoulder and neck say: I have enough of this pressure, my arms are restless and they feel like pushing the pressure away. They feel angry.

- T.: Just be with it and recognise and accept that anger is there. Now, open up to the fact that your shoulder and neck feel pressure, and would like to push it away. What is happening now in your body?

- P.: As I focus on my neck and shoulders; I am aware of some pain in my lower back and feel tired, cold and sort of empty there.

- T.: If this area in your body could talk what would it say?

- P.: I am feeling sad and lonely as if my throat is tight and my lower back is missing something to warm it, to support it.

- Q.: Just be with it and acknowledge the sadness and loneliness, the lack of support and warmth. Now could you ask this area what qualities, colours, and sensations it would need?

- P.: I just see myself floating in a hot spring in a beautiful natural area with wild flowers and big trees. Nearby there is a powerful river with a sort of milky water that sends me a lot of vitality.

- T.: Are there any messages that you could receive from this environment?

- P.: The River is whispering in my ear: You can let me carry you to the sea; you can drink from my milky waters. I drink and feel the power coming into me. My whole body receives the warm and soothing waters.

- T.: if there is any other message or healing that you need to receive?

- And later, I ask her how is her neck and shoulders and the lower back pain now?

- P.: I just feel very good, relaxed and without pain.
- T.: Is it all right if we finish the process now?
- P.: I feel fine and we can end now.
- T.: Gently open your eyes bring your awareness back to your breathing, stretch if you need to.

After concluding this process, I take some time with the patient to take again her pulses and speak about the experience. This will help the person to integrate. I also ask the patient to write or paint some of the scenes of the story at home in the next days, and I will see her again the next week. In the following session the main focus is on the integration process of the mind-body dialogue into the everyday life.

During the next session the patient reported having had some new realisations. That she had re-sourced herself by going to a spa and also for a walk near a particular river that she liked. She had shared her dream with her husband, who had offered to take up some of the household tasks. She had also realised that she enjoyed painting and she would like to take up art classes. We talked together about her compulsion to be needed and her tendency to over-do. Through our discussion, it became clear to her that she had issues about loneliness and fear of being abandoned.

That will be the next topic to work with. I saw her occasionally after that, she had been free of her physical symptoms and had made some constructive changes in her life.

Case 28   (Loss of vitality / PTSD)

A 25-year old woman consulted for a condition of multiple distal joint pains, accompanied by generalised fatigue (physical and mental), a lack of vitality and coldness. She presented a sallow, a greyish complexion with a very dull *Shen* in her eyes. In her history, at age thirteen she had been in a major car accident, in which her parents and two siblings were killed. Anamnesis revealed general coldness, urinary frequency and night urination, long cycles, general fearfulness, with frequent nightmares involving fear, danger and dreams of falling, or dreams of vulnerability. Her pulses were deep, weak and slow.

Analysis: A pattern of Post-traumatic shock, depleted Kidney Qi and *Jing,* a loss of passion and will to live and residual feelings of guilt.

- First session aimed at rooting the *Shen* (Life principle): RM-14 *Juque* with ST-23 *Taiyi;*

- Second session addressed the release of the traumatic event: ST-14 *Kufang,* HE-3 *Shaohai,* BL-62 *Shenmai;*

- Third session consisted of reconnecting the subject with the "Central Axis" to help root her back in life: SP-4 *Gongsun* (unilateral); PE-6

Neiguan; RM-4 *Guanyuan;* RM-12 *Zhongwan*; RM-17 *Shanzhong; Yintang* and DM-20 *Baihui.*

- Fourth session was directed at fortifying the Kidneys: BL-52 *Zhishi,* BL-23 *Xinshu,* DM-4 *Mingmen* and RM-4 *Guanyuan; Yin Wei Mai* was added (traumatic event at puberty): PE-6 *Neiguan* and KI-9 *Zhubin*

- Fifth session: for connecting the fore-brain and the mid-brain (loss of memory of the traumatic event): DM-24 *Shenting* and GB-13 *Benshen* with DM-17 *Naohu,* GB-18 *Chengling,* and DM-20 *Baihui*

- After the initial weekly sessions, she was seen twice a month for six months the Kidney and *Zhi* fortification was supplemented by points to support *Shen* with BL-44 *Shentang*; to release sadness and guilt with BL-42 *Pohu* and BL-13 *Feishu;* and SP-21 *Dabao* for generalised pain. She was also encouraged to practice Qigong to further help fortify the Kidney *Jing.* She also joined a Salza dance class, where she met a young man and got married.

Case 29   (OCD)

A girl aged 13 had been diagnosed with OCD. She had the constant need to wash, having the impression of being dirty. This obsession had been causing multiple problems both at school and at home, where she was constantly locking herself up in the only family bathroom. She had been under psychiatric care for two months, with very little improvement. Her school-work had suffered a lot, and socially she had been somewhat outcast by her school friends.

Analysis: She presented as a shy and withdrawn girl with downcast eyes. The constitution was rather suggestive of Water with a *Shaoyin* temperament. Her parents had immigrated when she was six, and she had been trying to adapt and integrate since. The feeling of not being clean enough, was probably re-enforced by her sense of inadequacy and not belonging. The repetitive behaviour was probably giving her a sense of security.

- The initial two sessions: aimed at supplementing and opening *Shaoyin*: HE-7 *Shenmen;* KI-3 *Taixi* RM-23 *Lianquan* (Knot point), with RM-4 *Guanyuan and Luo/Yuan*: HE-5 *Tongli* with SI-4 *Wangu*; KI-4 *Dazhong* with BL-64 *Jinggu.* LI-6 *Pianli* was added for the need to be repetitive. The points were stimulated with a laser as she was too fearful of the needles.

- The following session: BL-23 *Shenshu*; BL-52 *Zhishi* (reduced for fear); BL-49 *Yishe* (reduced for obsessiveness); and KI-4 *Dazhong* (for the obsessive-compulsive behaviour); and GB-38 *Yangfu* for obsession with cleanliness and ST-40 *Fenglong* for phobia and obsession.

- Two more sessions were given, combining acupuncture: BL-1 Jingming; BL-2 *Zanzhu;* GB-1 *Tongziliao*; GB-13 *Benshen;* DM-24 *Shenting;* and DM-20 *Baihui* to help change her point of view and beliefs; KI-4 *Dazhong* was added for the OCD. After the session the PAT exercises for changing the beliefs: (▶ A.4.2) were performed. She was instructed to practice daily the (▶ A.4.2) (step-5) on changing a belief at home.

After seven weekly sessions, she had greatly improved; she was seen once a month for three more months to consolidate the treatment.

Case 30   (Arachnophobia)

A 29-year old woman consulted for a severe case of arachnophobia. What had encouraged her to seek acupuncture was the fact that recently, she had been in the car, with her husband driving, she had seen a small spider on the dashboard of the car, had opened the door and thrown herself out of the car! Fortunately for her, they had been in the city and driving very slowly. There were no outstanding TCM patterns

Analysis: The phobia could not be related to any remembered event. This is a manifestation of a hidden "*Gui*". The treatment aimed at releasing the hidden *Gui* and changing the belief system.

-   First session: Worsley 7 Dragon protocol (▶ 4.4.2); she was instructed to perform daily the PAT-1 exercise to release any body memories (▶ A.4.1.1), with the affirmation: ...although I am scared of spiders, I love and accept myself. She had to score her sense of fear on a scale of 1-10 after each process and to keep a written track.

-   Second session, one week later: Before the acupuncture treatment, the exercise A.4.2 (step-5) on changing a belief was performed with the patient:

Therapist: Choose a concept or an idea that you would like to work on

Patient: I would like to explore my fear of spiders

-   T.: Create a negative judgment about spiders

-   P.: Spiders are big, black, hairy with many legs, and moving very fast

-   T.: Identify with this idea and feel what it feels to see the world through this concept.

-   P.: I feel small, spiders are huge, I am paralysed with fear...

-   T.: Now let go of this belief and this identification, breath-out and come back to yourself. Change your judgments on this belief; emit a positive judgment.

-   P.: Spiders are small insects and harmless and useful to nature ...

-   T.: Identify with this new image and again feel what it feels to have this new point of view.

- P.: I feel big, spiders are small, they are useful, I feel strong and free,…

- T.: Now visualise a spider in your vicinity, evaluate your fear on a scale of 1-10.

The acupuncture treatment consisted of GB-8 *Shuaigu;* GB-13 *Benshen;* GB-35 *Yangjiao;* GB-20 *Fengchi* and DM-16 *Fengfu.* To help change her perception and release the phobia. After the session her fear os spiders was again evaluated on the scale of 1-10. She noted that the fear had been reduced by half. She was instructed to perform the PAT-3 exercise to help with changing beliefs, mindsets and mental images (▶ A.4.1.3).

- Third session, one week later: Before the acupuncture treatment, the exercise A.4.2 (step-6) on changing a belief concerning an animal was performed with the patient:

    - T.: Choose an animal: describe it: big, small, thin, heavy, etc…

    - P.: Spiders are big, black, hairy with many legs, and moving very fast

    - T.: Now formulate an opinion of them

    - P.: They are big, ugly, scary and dangerous…

    - T.: Now become one with the spider. Imagine that you are the spider, and feel from inside what it feels like to be big, ugly, scary…

    - P.: I feel like a monster…

    - T.: Change your image and opinion about spiders, find some positive qualities

    - P.: Spiders are small insects, part of nature and useful for catching mosquitos and other bugs. They are even quite pretty…

    - T.: Now become one with this new image and feel how it feels to be that way…

    - P.: I feel lighter… I see the spiders as small I see myself as big, and they are very small and they do not present any danger to me.

    - T.: Which of the two images of spiders do you choose to keep?

    - P.: I prefer to keep the second image.

    - T.: Stay with this new feeling. Repeat this last step at home every day.

The acupuncture treatment consisted of GB-13 *Benshen* with GB-24 *Shenting* (to let go of fixed ideas); ST-40 *Fenglong* (fixations); BL-58 *Feiyang* (release fear); KI-8 *Jiaoxin* (self-trust). She was instructed to continue with the PAT-3 exercises and affirmations (▶ A.4.1.3).

- Fourth session, two weeks later: She came in with a huge smile saying, "there is a huge spider outside the entrance making a web and it did not bother me a bit…"

Case 31 (Anxiety/ PTSD)

A 38-year old woman was consulted for anxiety and a tendency to palpitations and chest oppression. She admitted being very scared of needles and had only accepted to have acupuncture with laser, she even disliked being touched or even massaged. She presented with a Water constitution and a *Shaoyin* temperament, fearful and anxious in general with a tendency to see the dark side of things. In her history, there had been a major heart operation at the age of 4 for a congenital defect.

Analysis: The early physical trauma is retained in the body by Po ≈ Corporeal Soul producing a somatic Gui (dislike to be touched, fear of needles) and a Thoracic Body armour (chronic anxiety).

- First session: ST-14 *Kufang* (reduce), stimulate HE-3 *Shaohai* and BL-62 *Shenmai* (to help release the retained trauma), and ST-15 *Wuyi* (dislike to be touched), were stimulated with the Laser.

- Second session: *Chong Mai* for early infancy trauma. SP-4 *Gongsun*; PE-6 *Neiguan*, KI-9 *Zhubin* and DM-20 *Baihui* with BL-43 *Gaohuangshu*; all stimulated with the Laser. She was also instructed the PAT-1 general exercise for releasing the sinews (▶ A.4.1.1) to be followed by PAT-2 Specific exercise for releasing the thoracic segment (▶ A.4.1.2 Thoracic segment).

- Third session: she accepted being needled! *Yinwei Mai* to open the chest and release anxiety with PE-6 *Neiguan* SP-4 *Gongsun*; KI-9 *Zhubin* and DM-20 *Baihui*; to help BL-43 *Gaohuangshu*; ST-15 *Wuyi* was repeated.

- Fourth session: concentrated on releasing the chest segment: superficial needling of BL-43 *Gaohuang,* ST-14 *Kufang*, ST-15 *Wuyi*, KI-24 *Lingxu* (letting go), KI-25 *Shencang* (pessimism), RM-17 *Shanzhong* and plum-blossom on the *Huatuojiaji* area of T4–5. She was encouraged to continue the PAT exercises.

- Fifth session (2 weeks later): She had felt generally much better, with almost no anxiety or oppression. Treatment aimed at consolidating the Water: BL-23 *Shenshu*, BL-52 *Zhishi*; KI-7 *Fuliu*(right); KI-8 *Jiaoxin* (left); PE-6 *Neiguan*(right), SP-4 *Gongsun* (left) and BL-43 *Gaohuangshu*.

- She was seen twice more, one month apart and had been free of anxiety. She was instructed to take-up the PAT exercises in case of a relapse.

Case 32 (Insomnia; nightmares; fear)

A 45-year old woman, school teacher, had been plagued by the same recurring nightmare since many years. Lately their frequency had been increasing, almost weekly. They occurred in the middle of the night, causing her to wake up in a sweat, with fear and palpitations, and it would take her a long time to go back to sleep. Consequently, she was feeling exhausted from lack of sufficient sleep. Anamnesis revealed a pattern of Liver-Heat and Fire, confirmed by very red sides of the tongue, red eyes, a thin, wiry and rapid pulse. She also had occasional hot flashes at night. The themes of the nightmares invariably involved the attack by a horned animal, bull or cow, with a great sense of danger.

Analysis: The nightmares are consistent with a Liver-Fire pattern probably from Liver-Blood vacuity (clear image of an animal with horns), with a background of Kidney-Yin vacuity. The sleep quality is disturbed in the mid-section of the night: *Yin Wei Mai* and the *Jueyin* level.

- First session; KI-9 was palpated and was more reactive on the left: PE-6 *Neiguan* (left); KI-9 *Zhubin* (left); LR-14 *Qimen* (right) for the *Yinwei* and the *Jueyin* section; GB-13 *Benshen* and DM-24 *Shenting* (nightmares). KI-1 *Yongquan* (right) with KI-10 *Yingu* (right) and LR-8 *Ququan* (right) to supplement Kidney and Liver-Yin.

- Second session: She had the nightmare once in which a bull was attacking her and a group of children. In her dream, she had managed to save the children by having them climb a rock.

  - Therapist: How old were the children?

  - Patient: They were small, maybe 5 or 6 years old.

  - T.: Tell me about your early childhood, what was the situation at home?

  - P.: Not nice; my father was an alcoholic and very aggressive; I was always scared of him when he would get angry. He would often beat us for the of smallest reasons.

  - T.: Is he still alive?

  - P.: No, he died 15 years ago.

  - T.: Had you been in contact with him before he died?

  - P.: No, I had avoided seeing him as much as possible.

  - T.: When did the nightmares start?

  - P.: I already had them in adolescence, but they have become regular in the past 10 years now.

  - T.: Do you maybe see a relation between the fear and aggression in your dreams and your childhood situation? It feels like you have unfinished issues with your father, we will try and help you to bring them out.

    Treatment: (The fact that she had found a recourse in her dream for saving the children indicates an improvement of the Kidney Qi). PE-6 *Neiguan* (right); KI-9 *Zhubin* (right); LR-14 *Qimen* (left); KI-21 *Youmen* (to help remember); KI-24 *Lingxu* and LU-7 *Lieque* (to help forgive and let go); KI-22 *Bulang* (feeling of injustice) and KI-7 *Fuliu*.

- Third session: She had no more nightmares and her sleep was much deeper. BL-23 *Shenshu* and BL-18 *Ganshu* (supplemented)*;* BL-52 *Zhishi*; BL-47 *Hunmen;* BL-43 *Gaohuangshu;* BL-42 *Pohu* were all reduced on the reactive sides to help release the retained emotions. She was asked to write a letter to her father and express all that she would have liked to tell him when he was alive; and then burn the letter. She was instructed to practice the exercises on Self-forgiveness and forgiving others (▶ A.4.6.1 and A.4.6.2).

She was seen twice, over the following three months, and had no more nightmares.

Case 33   (Insomnia; *Gui*)

A 38-year old female patient had been consulting 2-3 times per year for various reasons. The motif of her last visit had been disturbed sleep, having difficulty falling asleep through the impression of something lurking around, that she described as an evil presence.

- First session: The Worsley Seven External Dragons was selected (▶ Section 4.4.2): DM-20 *Baihui*; BL-11 *Dazhu*; BL-23 *Shenshu*; BL-61 *Pucan*

- Second session: She had no more this impression: treatment aimed at consolidating the Water: BL-23 *Shenshu* and BL-52 *Zhishi*; BL-47 *Hunmen* was reduced (vague feeling of fear at night); KI-1 *Yongquan* with KI-10 *Yingu* to help the rooting.

Case 34   (Anxiety / Insomnia / Working with dreams)

A female patient, aged 49, was going through a very difficult period in her life involving sentimental issues as well as work insecurity. She described her situation as being on quicksand and slowly sinking; with a lot of confusion, great difficulty in deciding and a feeling of losing control. She had been having insomnia from anxiety, palpitations, night sweating and restlessness. She had also been having some nightmares involving an evil monster with a huge aggressive red head. She would wake up with a great feeling of fear and had difficulty going back to sleep.

Analysis: The pattern is suggestive of a disturbance of *Shen* through a pattern of Heart and Gallbladder Qi vacuity (insecurity and indecision); the theme of the nightmare is indicative of Phlegm (unknown monster), and a weakness of Lung (Red *Gui* ▶ Section 4.4.2).

- First session: PE-5 *Jianshi;* GB-43 *Xiaxi* and GB-12 *Wangu* (insomnia from insecurity); LI-4 *Hegu* and BL-13 *Feishu* (Red *Gui*). LU-3 *Tianfu* (set priorities)

- Second session: BL-23 *Shenshu* and BL-52 *Zhishi*; KI-7 *Fuliu* and HE-6 *Yinxi* and SI-5 *Yanggu* (lack of clarity) and DM-20 *Baihui*.

- Third session: She had the dream with the monster gain, but this time she had been able to confront it with the statement "you are unreal and have no power over me". She woke up from this dream feeling strong and liberated. The dream was clearly indicating that the Kidney had regained its power. The treatment aimed at reconnecting the subject with her centre (▶ Section 5.2.1): SP-4 *Gongsun* (unilateral); PE-6 *Neiguan*; RM-4 *Guanyuan;* RM-12 *Zhongwan*; RM-17 *Shanzhong; Yintang* and DM-20 *Baihui*. She was instructed to practice the "Central Axis" exercise (▶ A. 4.5.1), with the following affirmations: "I enjoy making important decisions…"; and "I trust in myself…"

INDICES

- **Index of Symptoms**

- **Glossary of Terms**
  - Pinyin-English-Chinese
  - English-Pinyin-Chinese

- **Bibliography**
  - Classical Chinese Texts
  - Modern Chinese References
  - Western References

- **Guide to Pinyin pronunciation**

- **General Index**

Index of Symptoms

Disorientation → BL-15, BL-44, BL-62, BL-65, KI-4

Eating → (see also Anorexia)
- anorexia, hunger but cannot eat → ST-41, BL-21
- appetite but loosing weight → BL-20, BL-21
- bulimia → ST-45
- eating but loosing weight → BL-25
- eating fast → GB-2
- excess appetite → ST-19
- excessive holding and obesity → BL-25
- food retention → ST-45
- hunger but cannot digest → LI-10, ST-36
- loss of appetite → ST-19, ST-21, ST-22, SP-3, SP-6, BL-13, BL-66, LR-13, RM-9, RM-11
- loss of appetite and vomiting with diarrhoea and undigested food in the stools → ST-21, BL-21,
- BL-22
- loss of desire to eat or to live → ST-41
- malnutrition → LI-4, PE-9
- no desire to eat → KI-21
- over eating → ST-19, SP-17
- over eating in compensation for sadness → SP-17
- stress related eating disorders → ST-23
- sudden weight gain → GB-20
- thinking about food all the time → BL-57

Emotions → (see also Fear)
- acute despair → LI-8
- addiction (tobacco) → ST-9
- addiction (alcohol) → RM-6
- aggressiveness → SP-20
- anger → BL-47, GB-39, LR-2
- angry or moody but better with movement → KI-21
- all dependencies → GB-8, GB-9
- alternating joy and aggression → ST-14
- alternating joy and sadness → GB-24
- altruism → SP-5
- always in a hurry → DM-5 attachment to the past → BL-47
- audacity → GB-38
- bereavement → LI-18
- boredom → SP-14, BL-13, RM-15
- broken heart → LI-16, BL-43
- claustrophobia → LU-3
- contemptuousness → SP-14, KI-14
- deceptions and rejections → BL-43
- deep sadness → KI-17
- delusions → KI-20
- difficulty with introspection → DM-10

- difficulty to move in to action → BL-52
- discontentment → ST-15, BL-18, BL-60, KI-9, PE-7, PE-8, GB-38
- discouragement → LU-7, HE-9, DM-9
- doubts → KI-24, BL-43
- dullness → BL-15
- easily angry → KI-26
- easily discouraged → GB-28
- easily frightened → GB-15
- easily hurt → GB-38
- tearfulness → LR-2, DM-14
- emotional consequences of trauma → ST-14
- everything seems too much → KI-10
- excessive crying → DM-20, DM-26
- excessive fright → ST-45
- excessive pride → SP-14, KI-14
- excessive sexual desire → LR-4
- excess sexuality (nymphomania) → BL-10
- excess thinking → ST-42
- excessive will power → KI-1, KI-2
- expecting a misfortune → KI-27
- excess worry → HE-4
- excessive worry → LR-5
- excessive yawning → SP-6, SP-7
- extremely emotional → LI-3
- false ideas → GB-2, DM-11, DM-20
- feeling of being mistreated → BL-11
- feeling of doom → RM-15
- feeling of injustice → KI-22
- feeling of fever and chills from shock → TW-2
- feeling worst at 11 am and 4-6 pm → KI-26
- fever from emotions → GB-13, GB-17
- fixed ideas → GB-13
- friendly but egotistical → SP-2
- frustration → BL-47
- grief → LU-5, LU-7, LU-10, ST-41, SP-15, BL-42, GB-9
- grief and crying → ST-41, SP-15, GB-9
- grief with chest pains → LU-10
- hating life → KI-17
- hating light → KI-18
- helping to detach (dying or mourning) → PE-7
- helping to "digest" bad news → ST-44
- helping to let go → LU-7, LI-18, KI-24
- helping to let go of the past, to forgive → KI-24, BL-47
- helps to release and express emotions → LU-7
- helps to surrender in the dying person → BL-60
- impatience → KI-17
- impression of not being loved → KI-26
- impulsiveness → DM-5
- inability to express → HE-4

- vulnerability from guilt or embarrassment
  →
- LU-9
- weak character → KI-7
- weeping → PE-7, GB-41
- worry → LU-7, LI-13, ST-14, ST-27, SP-2, SP-5, HE-4, BL-42, BL-49, KI-25, TW-10, GB-18, GB-43, LR-5
- worry about the future → SP-5, BL-42

Emotiveness → (see also Nervousness); LU-9, LI-3, ST-14, ST-27, SP-2, HE-5, HE-8, HE-9, BL-40, KI-20, KI-27, TW-10, LR-5, DM-11
- emotional outburst → LU-9
- emotional over-reactions → HE-5
- emotional skin rashes → TW-10
- emotional trembling → KI-20
- over emotionality → KI-1
- stage fright → HE-5, BL-15

Fear → LU-4, LI-11, LI-13, ST-27, ST-41, SP-1, HE-4, HE-5, HE-6, HE-8, BL-10, BL-15, BL-19, BL-30,
BL-47, BL-52, BL-60, BL-66, KI-2, KI-3, KI-4, KI-9, KI-20, PE-3, PE-4, PE-5, PE-6, PE-9, TW-18, TW-19, TW-23, GB-4, GB-8, GB-9, GB-34, GB-35, GB-43, LR-2, LR-5, LR-13, RM-13, RM-17,
DM-11
- apprehension → KI-2, KI-27
- apprehension: fear of being seized → KI-2
- fear with palpitation → ST-41, GB-35
- fearful children → LI-16
- fearfulness → KI-1
- fearful spirit → KI-26
- fear of being seized → KI-2, GB-34
- fear of change → TW-18
- fear of darkness → PE-9
- fear of heights → BL-10
- fear of people → HE-8, KI-4, PE-4
- fever and chills from shock → TW-2
- frequent fears → HE-6
- fright → LI-2, LI-16, ST-27, ST-45, HE-5, BL-15, PE-6, PE-7, TW-2, TW-18, GB-23, LR-3, DM-8, DM-16, DM-21, DM-22
- fright causing convulsions → DM-21
- fright in children → DM-8
- fright-Wind in children → LR-3
- phobia → ST-40, BL-1, BL-2, GB-1, DM-12, DM-14, DM-24
- phobia (animals, germs, heights etc.) → GB-8, GB-13, GB-35
- sensation of something sitting on the chest: SP-1 with BL-43
- terror → SI-7
- vague feeling of fear at night → BL-47

Hallucinations → LU-7, ST-40, HE-7, SI-19, BL-2, BL-15, BL-30, BL-61, PE-5, TW-17, DM-12, DM-14
- auditory hallucinations → SI-19, TW-17
- seeing ghosts → LI-5, LI-7, PE-5, LR-2, DM-26
- hallucinations: possessed by a demon → BL-2
- hallucinations: seeing ghosts → PE-5

Hysteria → (see also "Psychiatry"); ST-23, SP-5, SP-7, HE-4, HE-5, HE-7, HE-8, HE-9, SI-5, SI-7,
BL-15, BL-18, BL-43, BL-65, KI-1, KI-4, KI-6, KI-9,
PE-4, PE-5, PE-6, PE-8, PE-9, TW-2, GB-21, GB-24,
GB-35, LR-5, RM-1, RM-14, RM-15, DM-1, DM-12, DM-14, DM-15, DM-16, DM-17, DM-18, DM-19, DM-20, DM-23, DM-24, DM-26, *Zhongquan, Shixuan*
- hysteria with excessive talking → GB-24
- hysterical paralysis → *Yinwei*
- hysterical speech → LU-9, LI-5, LI-8
- hysteric laughter → PE-7, PE-8

Memory
- concentration and memory problems → BL-10, BL-49, KI-26
- forgetfulness → LI-11, HE-3, KI-1
- forgetting words → PE-6
- loss of memory → LU-3, LU-7, BL-15, BL-43, BL-62, GB-19, GB-23, RM-13, RM-14, KI-21, PE-4, PE-9, DM-11, DM-20, Sishencong
- helps to remember → PE-4
- poor memory → BL-23, KI-3, GB-20
- poor memory and concentration → BL-23
- reduced memory HE-7, BL-10, BL-49, KI-24

Mental retardation → HE-7, BL-15, DM-15
- mental retardation in children → HE-7, BL-15

Nervousness → (see also "Anxiety"); LU-7, ST-27,
BL-30, PE-3, LR-3, Anmien
- nervous agitation → BL-11
- nervous insomnia → ST-12
- nervous jerks at night → TW-23
- nervousness and fear → PE-3
- nervous pains → LU-9
- nervous palpitations → LR-2
- nervous spasms → TW-14
- nervous trembling → LU-7, LU-10

- insomnia from worry → ST-27, KI-25
- insomnia from worry with palpitations → ST-27
- insomnia with agitation → KI-6
- insomnia with excess dreaming → GB-44
- insomnia with restlessness → SP-6
- likes to lie down → LI-3, LI-13, LR-1
- needing to eat to fall asleep → ST-21
- nightmares → ST-44, ST-45, SP-1, SP-5, BL-2, BL-10, GB-13, GB-44
- nightmares or dream-disturbed sleep → ST-45
- nightmares involving predators → PE-4, HE-8
- night terrors → PE-5, RM-4
- palpitations at night → RM-18
- persistent insomnia → KI-27
- restless sleep → SP-1
- restless extremities at night → ST-44
- restless legs → TW-2, TW-19
- sensation of something sitting on the chest: SP-1 with BL-43
- sleepiness → ST-45, SP-5, BL-1, BL-23, KI-6
- sleepiness after eating → SP-5
- sleep walking → LI-8, *Anmian*
- sleep quality → LI-4
- somnolence → LI-2, LI-3, ST-45, BL-12, BL-18, BL-62, KI-3, TW-10, GB-24, LR-1, LR-10, DM-20, DM-22
- somnolence after eating → SP-5
- somnolence and dull spirit → BL-62
- somnolence with no desire to move → LR-10
- superficial sleep → BL-20
- tired but cannot sleep → KI-21
- tiredness upon waking → SP-3
- vague feeling of fear at night → BL-47
- waking up at 3 a.m. → LU-1
- wanting to lie down → KI-4

Speech
- aphasia → *Shanglianquan*
- aphonia → LU-6, LI-4, LI-10, ST-6, PE-5, TW-6, TW-8, RM-20, DM-13, *Hongyin, Jinjin, Yuye*
- aphonia or stammering → LI-17, PE-5
- difficulty finding words → RM-15
- incoherent speech → SI-7, LR-5, DM-26
- deaf-mutism → TW-17, TW-21, DM-15
- mutism → LI-17, KI-20, TW-8, TW-17, TW-21,
- DM-15, *Shanglianquan, Hongyin*
- speech difficulties → HE-7, SI-17, KI-1, KI-10, PE-5, *Shanglianquan*

- speech problems → ST-4, GB-6, DM-15, DM-16
- slurred speech → RM-23
- stuttering → HE-4, HE-5, PE-4, RM-20
- sudden aphasia → HE-5, DM-21
- sudden aphonia → LU-6
- sudden mutism → LI-17, KI-20

Stage fright → HE-5, BL-15

Glossary of Terms

Pinyin-English-Chinese

Ai Si	Grief	哀
Ān	Calm/quiet	安
Ān	Peaceful sleep	安
Bā	Eight	八
Bā	Eight principles	八
Bāo	Uterus (*Bao Mai* ≈ Uterin Vessel)	胞
Baihe Bing	Lilium syndrome (depression)	百合病
Bēi	Sadness	悲
Ben Tun	Panic attack (Running piglet) syndrome)	奔豚
Bí	Nose	鼻
Bì	Impediment/ obstruction (painful obstruction of Qi and Blood) from External Wind, Damp, or Cold)	痹
Biǎo	Exterior, surface	表
Biǎo-Lǐ	Exterior-interior	表
Bǔ	Supplement, tonify	补
Bu Yu Shi	Anorexia Nervosa	不欲食
Cháo Rè	Tidal fever (recurrent afternoon or evening fevers)	潮熱
Chéng	Over-act (*Xiang Cheng* / over-acting cycle)	乘
Chōng Mài	Penetrating vessel	衝脉
Còu Lǐ	Interstice (space between skin and sinews)	腠理
Dà Cháng	Large intestine	大肠
Dài Mài	Belt/girdle vessel	带
Dān	Gallbladder	胆

Dān / Dan Tian	Cinnabar, elixir (*Dantian* ≈ Cinnabar chamber)	丹 / 丹田
Dì	Earth/soil	地
Diān	Depression	癲
Diān/ Diān Kuáng	Withdrawal (*Dian Kuang* ≈ Withdrawal mania)	癲狂
Dìng	Settle/stabilize (*Ding Chuan* ≈ Settle wheezing)	定
Dū Mài	Governing vessel	督
Duo	Excessive dreaming	多
Èr	Two	二
Ěr	Ear	耳
Fán	Agitation/restlessness / vexation	烦
Fán Zào	Agitation and restlessness: mental agitation with physical restlessness/ fidgetiness	烦躁
Fèi	Lung	肺
Fēng	Wind	风
Fú	Hidden	伏
Fú	Superficial, to float	浮
Fù	Abdomen	腹
Fǔ	Bowel (*Zang-Fu* ≈ Organs and bowels)	腑
Fú Luò	Superficial connecting-network vessels	浮络
Gān	Liver	肝
Gāo	Fatty tissue, protective membrane *Gao Huang* ≈ Protective and vital/ nourishing membrane	膏
Gé	Diaphragm	膈
Gù	Consolidate, secure, strengthen	固
Gǔ	Bone	骨
Gǔ Qì	Food energy	谷
Guǐ	Ghost / unnamed spirit / demonic	鬼

Hán	Cold	寒
Hàn	Sweat	汗
Hé	Harmonize (*He Zhong* ≈ Harmonize centre)	和
Hé	Sea	合
Hòu Tiān	Later, post-heaven/ post-natal	后 天
Huà	Transform (*Hua Duo* ≈ Transform turbidity)	化
Huāng	Vital membranes	肓
Huì	Meeting (*Hui Xue* ≈ Meeting points)	会 (會、
Hui	Regret	悔
Hún	Ethereal soul	魂
Huó	Invigorate	活
Huǒ	Fire phase	火
Huò Luàn	Sudden turmoil disorder: sudden, severe diarrhoea, vomiting & abdominal pain; gastro-enteritis)	霍 亂
Jī	Accumulation, clumping (Ji Re ≈ Accumulated Heat)	积
Jiàn	Strengthen, fortify (*Jian Pi* ≈ Fortify the Spleen)	健
Jiān	Shoulder	肩
Jian	Amnesia	健
Jiàng	Descend, down-bear (*Jiang Ni* ≈ Down-bear counterflow)	降
Jiāo	Exchange, confluence, intersection	交
Jiǎo Qì	Leg Qi (leg and foot numbness, pain and weakness)	脚 气
Jiě	Release, resolve (*Jie Biao* ≈ Resolve the exterior)	解
Jīn	Sinews, muscles	筋
Jīn	Metal phase	金

Jīn Yè	Body fluids	津
Jǐng	Well	井
Jīng	River/channel	经
Jīng	Divergent channels	经
Jīng	Sinew/ Tendino-	经
Jīn	muscular channels	筋
Jīng Qì	Channel energy	经
Jǐng	Alertness	警
Jīng / Jīng Qì	Essence/ essential Qi	精 气
Jiǔ	Nine	九
Jù	Concentration, gathering (mass)	聚
Jué	Terminal yin	厥
Jué Zhèng	Reversal/ collapse syndrome (coma with coldness)	厥 证
Kè	Control (*Xiang Ke* ≈ Controlling cycle)	克
Kǒng	Fear	恐
Kǒu	Mouth	口
Kuān	Loosen, unbind (*Kuan Xiong* ≈ Unbind the chest)	宽
Kuáng	Mania / *Dian Kuang* ≈ Depression-madness	狂
Kuáng Zǒu	Mad walking	狂 走
Láo	Taxation/ consumption/ Labour	劳
Lì	Pestilence	沥
Lǐ	Interior (*Biao-Li* ≈ Exterior-interior)	裏 (里、
Lǐ	Rectify	理
Lǐ Jí	Abdominal urgency (cramping pain, urgency; dysentery)	裡 急
Liáng	Cool	凉
Lìn	Strangury (painful urination syndrome)	淋
Líng	Soul, spirit	靈
Liù	Six	六

Luàn	Confusion, mental confusion	乱
Luò	Connecting	絡
Lŭo Lì	Small & large nodules scrofula (neck, axilla, and groin)	瘰 歷
Luò Mài	Connecting/network channels/ vessels	絡 脈
Mài	Vessel	脈
Máo	Body hair/ wool	毛
Méi Hé	Plum-pit (feeling of a lump in the throat)	梅 核
Meng	Nightmares	梦
Meng	Sleep-talking	梦
Meng	Sleep-walking	梦
Mìng	Destiny, life, mandate	命
Mìng	Life, vitality gate	命
Mù	Collecting point	募
Mù	Wood phase	木
Nào	Shoulder, arm, deltoid	臑
Năo	Brain	脑
Nèi	Internal	内
Ni Qì	Counterflow/ rebellious/ inverse Qi (abnormal Qi flow)	逆 氣
Nù	Anger	怒
Páng Guāng	Bladder	膀 胱
Pí	Spleen	脾
Pí	Skin	皮
Pĭ	Glomus, focal	痞
Pí Bù	Skin, cutaneous	皮
Pò	Corporeal/animal soul	魄
Qì	Energy	气
Qī	Seven	七
Qí Jīng Bā Mài	Eight extraordinary vessels	奇 经
Qiào	Orifice, portal,	窍
Qiāo	Springing, stepping (*Qiao Mai* ≈ Stepping Vessel)	跷 / 蹺
Qíng	Emotion	情
Qīng	Clear/quiet (*Qing Re* ≈ Clear Heat); *Qing Shen* ≈ Quiet the mind	清 清
Qīng	Clear, pure energy	清
Rè	Heat	热
Rèn	Conception vessel	任
Ròu	Flesh	肉
Rùn	Moisten (*Run Fei* ≈ Moisten the Lung)	润
Sàn	Dissipate	散
Sān	Three	三
Sān	Three treasures	三
Sān Jiāo	Triple warmer/burner/heater	三 焦
Shàn	Hernia; acute urinary and bowel retention; disease of the external genitalia	疝
Shan Shi Yi Ji	Bulimia Nervosa	善 食 易 饥
Shào	Lesser yang	少
Shào	Lesser yin	少
Shé	Tongue	舌
Shén	Spirit, consciousness, intelligence, mind, emotions	神
Shèn	Kidney	肾
Shēng	Generate (*Xiang Sheng* ≈ Generating cycle)	生
Shí	Repletion, excess	实
Shī	Dampness	湿
Shi	Hypersomnia*	嗜
Shŏu	Hand, arm	手
Shū	Course, relax (Shu Gan ≈ Course the Liver)	疏
Shū	Stream	俞
Shù/ Bèi shū	Transport point/ back transport	俞 / 背
Shuĭ	Water phase	水

Shùn	Normalize, favourable (*Shun Qi* ≈ Normalize Qi)	順
Sì	Four	四
Sī	Pensiveness, worry	思
Suǐ	Marrow	髓
Sūn luò	Deep connecting, network vessels	孫 絡
Tài	Supreme yang	太
Tài Yīn	Supreme yin	太
Tán	Phlegm	痰
Tí	Raise, lift	提
Tiān	Heaven	天
Tiān chuān	Window of heaven / sky	天 窗
Tiān Gǔi	Growth promoting and reproductive substance; menstruation	天 癸
Tiáo	Regulate	调
Tòng	Pain	痛
Tōng	Free, open, unstop	通
Tóu	Head	頭
Tóu fēng	Head-Wind (severe recurrent headaches; or EPF headaches with vertigo and facial paralysis)	頭 风
Tǔ	Earth phase	土
Wài	External, outer	外
Wéi	Bind, preserve (*Wei Mai* ≈ Binding Vessel)	維
Wèi	Stomach	胃
Wěi (Wěi Zhèng)	Wilting/ atrophy; (*Weizheng* ≈ Wilting syndrome: atrophy, flaccidity & weakness)	痿 证
Wèi Qì	Defensive energy	卫
Wēn	Warm (*Wen Bing* ≈ Warm disease)	温
Wǔ	Insult (*Xiang Wu* ≈ Insulting cycle)	侮
Wǔ	Five	五

Wǔ Jī	Five accumulations (five types of mass)	五 积
Wǔ Láo	Five taxations (excessive use of the eyes → Blood; sitting → flesh; standing → bones; walking → sinews; lying → Qi)	五 劳
Wǔ	Five moving	五
Xī	Extinguish, pacify	熄
Xī	Joy	喜
Xī	Cleft/ Accumulation	郗
Xī	Knee	膝
Xiān Tiān	Pre-heaven, earlier heaven / pre-natal	郗 郗
Xiào	Wheezing (*Re Xiao* ≈ Heat wheezing)	哮
Xiào	Disperse, regulate	消
Xiâo Cháng	Small intestine	小 肠
Xiāo Kě	Dispersion/wasting and thirsting (thirst, hunger, polyuria and loss of weight;	消 渴
Xiè	Discharge, drain, vent	泄
Xiè	Discharge, release	泄
Xié Qì	Pathogenic, perverse, aggressive energy (External Wind, Heat, Damp, Dryness or Cold, causing a disease)	邪 气
Xīn	Heart	心
Xīn Bāo	Pericard / Heart protector/ envelop	心 包
Xū	Vacuity, deficiency	虚
Xuān	Diffuse, effuse (*Xuan Fei* ≈ Diffuse Lung)	宣
Xué	Hole, cavity, acupuncture point	穴
Xuè	Blood	血
Yǎn	Eyes	眼
Yáng	Yang brightness	陽
Yáng Qiāo Mài	Yang motility/ stepping Vessel	蹻 脉

Yáng Wéi Mài	Yang binding/ linking Vessel	陽維脈
Yao	Oppression	憂
Yè	Thick fluids, humour	液
Ye Jing	Night terror (Ghost-fright)	夜惊
Yì	Intellect, thought, reflection, intention	意
Yī	One	一
Yīn Qiāo	Yin motility/ Stepping Vessel	陰蹻
Yīn Wéi Mài	Yin binding/ Linking Vessel	陰維脈
Yíng	Spring	榮
Yíng Qì	Nourishing energy	營气
Yù	Jade	玉
Yuán	Source, original	原
Zàng-Fǔ	Viscera and bowels/ Yin and Yang organs	脏腑
Zào	Mental agitation/ irritability	躁
Zào	Dryness	燥
Zhēn	True energy	真
Zhèng	Syndrome / pattern	证 /
Zhèng	Symptom	症
Zheng Chong	Palpitations (fearful throbbing)	怔忡
Zhēng Gǔ	Steaming bone syndrome (tidal fever, from Yin-Xu with night sweats)	蒸骨
Zhèng Jīng	Primary channels	正经
Zhèng	Upright, correct	正
Zhēng-Jiǎ-Jī-Jù	Concretions and gatherings (masses; *Zheng* and *Ji* ≈ Hard masses with fixed pain; *Jia* and *Ju* ≈ Mobile masses)	癥瘕积聚
Zhì	Will power (mind)	志

Zhǐ	Suppress, relieve (*Zhi Tong* ≈ Relieve pain)	止
Zhōng	Central, middle	中
Zhú	Expel, dispel (*Zhu Tan* ≈ Expel Phlegm)	逐
Zhuàng	Invigorate / *Zhuang Yang* ≈ Invigorate Yang	壮
Zī	Nourish	滋
Zī Gōng / Bāo	Uterus	子宫胞
Zōng Qì	Ancestral/ Gathering energy	宗气

English-Pinyin-Chinese

English	Pinyin	Chinese
Abdomen	Fù	腹
Abdominal urgency (cramping pain, urgency; dysentery)	Lǐ Jí	裡急
Accumulation, clumping (Ji Re ≈ Accumulated Heat)	Jī	积
Agitation and restlessness (mental agitation and physical restlessness/ fidgetiness)	Fán Zào	烦躁
Agitation/restlessness/ vexation	Fán	烦
Alertness	Jǐng Shén	警神
Ancestral, gathering energy	Zōng Qì	宗气
Amnesia	Jian Wang	健忘
Anger	Nù	怒
Anorexia nervosa	Bu Yu Shi	不欲食
Belt/ Girdle vessel	Dài Mài	带脉
Bind, preserve (Wei Mai ≈ Binding Vessel)	Wéi	維
Bladder	Páng Guāng	膀胱
Blood	Xuè	血
Body fluids	Jīn Yè	津液
Body hair/wool	Máo	毛
Bone	Gǔ	骨
Bowel (Zang-Fu ≈ Organs and bowels)	Fǔ	腑
Brain	Nǎo	脑
Bulimia Nervosa	Shan Shi Yi Ji	善食易饥

English	Pinyin	Chinese
Calm/ Quiet	Ān	安
Central, middle energy	Zhōng Qì	中气
Channel energy	Jīng Qì	经气
Cinnabar, elixir (Dantian ≈ Cinnabar chamber)	Dān / Dantian	丹/丹田
Clear, pure energy	Qīng Qì	清气
Clear/quiet (Qing Re ≈ Clear Heat)	Qīng	清清
Cleft/accumulation	Xī	郄郗
Cold	Hán	寒
Collecting point	Mù	募
Concentration, gathering (mass)	Jù	聚
Conception vessel	Rèn Mài	任脉
Concretions and gatherings (masses; Zheng and Ji ≈ Hard masses with fixed pain; Jia and Ju ≈ Mobile masses)	Zhēng-Jiǎ-Jī-Jù	癥瘕积聚
Confusion, mental confusion	Luàn	乱
Connecting	Luò	絡
Connecting/network channels/vessels	Luò Mài	絡脈
Consolidate, secure, strengthen	Gù	固
Control (Xiang Ke ≈ Controlling cycle)	Kè	克
Cool	Liáng	凉
Corporeal/animal soul	Pò	魄
Counterflow/ rebellious/ reverse Qi: abnormal Qi flow	Nì Qì	逆
Course, relax (Shu Gan ≈ Course the Liver)	Shū	疏
Dampness	Shī	湿濕

Growth promoting and reproductive substance; menstruation	*Tiān Gǔi*	天 癸
Hand, arm	*Shǒu*	手
Harmonise (*He Zhong* ≈ Harmonise the centre)	*Hé*	和
Head	*Tóu*	頭
Head-Wind: severe recurrent headaches; or EPF headaches, vertigo and facial paralysis	*Tóu fēng*	頭 风
Heart	*Xīn*	心
Heat	*Rè*	热
Heaven	*Tiān*	天
Hernia; acute urinary and bowel retention; disease of the external genitalia	*Shàn*	疝
Hidden	*Fú*	伏
Hole, cavity, acupuncture point	*Xué*	穴
Hypersomnia (narcolepsy)	*Shi Shui*	嗜 睡
Impediment/ obstruction: painful obstruction of Qi and Blood from External Wind, Damp, or Cold	*Bì*	痹
Insult (*Xiang Wu* ≈ Insulting cycle)	*Wǔ*	侮
Intellect, thought, reflection, intention	*Yì*	意
Interior (*Biao-Li* ≈ Exterior-interior)	*Lǐ*	裏 里
Internal	*Nèi*	内
Interstice (space) between skin and sinews	*Còu Lǐ*	腠 理
Invigorate	*Huó*	活
Invigorate (*Zhuang Yang* ≈ Invigorate Yang)	*Zhuàng*	壮
Jade	*Yù*	玉
Joy	*Xī*	喜
Kidney	*Shèn*	肾

Knee	*Xī*	膝
Large intestine	*Dà Cháng*	大 肠
Later, post-heaven / post-natal	*Hòu Tiān*	后 天
Leg Qi: leg and foot numbness, pain and weakness	*Jiǎo Qì*	脚 气
Lesser yang	*Shào Yáng*	少 陽
Lesser yin	*Shào Yīn*	少 陰
Life, vitality gate	*Mìng Mén*	命 门
Lilium syndrome	*Baihe Bing*	百 合 病
Liver	*Gān*	肝
Loosen, unbind / *Kuan Xiong* ≈ unbind the chest	*Kuān*	宽
Lung	*Fèi*	肺
Mad walking	*Kuáng Zǒu*	狂 走
Mania (*Dian Kuang* ≈ Depression-madness)	*Kuáng*	狂
Marrow	*Suǐ*	髓
Meeting (*Hui Xue* ≈ Meeting points)	*Huì*	会 會
Mental agitation/ irritability	*Zào*	躁
Metal phase	*Jīn*	金
Moisten (*Run Fei* ≈ Moisten the Lung)	*Rùn*	润
Mouth	*Kǒu*	口
Nightmare	*Meng Yan*	梦 魇
Night-Fright / Ghost fright	*Ye Jing*	夜 惊
Nine	*Jiǔ*	九
Normalize, favourable (*Shun Qi* ≈ Normalize Qi)	*Shùn*	顺
Nose	*Bí*	鼻
Nourish	*Zī*	滋

Superficial, to float	*Fú*	浮
Supplement, tonify	*Bǔ*	补
Suppress, relieve (*Zhi Tong* ≈ Relieve pain)	*Zhǐ*	止
Supreme yang	*Tài Yáng*	太陽
Supreme yin	*Tài Yīn*	太陰
Sweat	*Hàn*	汗
Symptom	*Zhèng*	症
Syndrome / pattern	*Zhèng*	证證
Taxation / consumption	*Láo*	劳
Terminal yin	*Jué Yīn*	厥陰
Thick fluids, humour	*Yè*	液
Three	*Sān*	三
Three treasures	*Sān Bǎo*	三宝
Tidal fever (recurrent afternoon fevers)	*Cháo Rè*	潮熱
Tongue	*Shé*	舌
Transform (*Hua Duo* ≈ Transform turbidity)	*Huà*	化
Transport point/back transport	*Shū* / *Bèi Shū*	俞背俞
Triple warmer/burner/heater	*Sān Jiāo*	三焦
True energy	*Zhēn Qì*	真气
Two	*Èr*	二
Upright, correct energy	*Zhèng Qì*	正气
Uterus	*Zǐ Gōng* / *Bāo*	子宫胞
Uterus (*Bao Mai* ≈ Uterine Vessel)	*Bāo*	胞
Vacuity, deficiency	*Xū*	虚
Vessel	*Mài*	脈脉

Viscera and bowels/ Yin and Yang organs	*Zàng-Fǔ*	脏腑
Vital membranes	*Huāng*	肓
Warm (*Wen Bing* ≈ Warm disease)	*Wēn*	温
Water phase	*Shuǐ*	水
Well	*Jǐng*	井
Wheezing (*Re Xiao* ≈ Heat wheezing)	*Xiào*	哮
Will power (mind)	*Zhì*	志
Wilting/atrophy; (*Wei Zheng* ≈ Wilting syndrome: atrophy, flaccidity and weakness)	*Wěi* (*Wěi Zhèng*)	痿证
Wind	*Fēng*	风
Window of heaven / sky	*Tiān Chuāng*	天窗
Withdrawal (*Dian Kuang* ≈ Withdrawal mania)	*Diān* / *Diān Kuáng*	癲狂
Wood phase	*Mù*	木
Yang binding/linking vessel	*Yáng Wéi Mài*	陽維脉
Yang brightness	*Yáng Míng*	陽明
Yang motility/ Stepping Vessel	*Yáng Qiāo Mài*	陽蹻脉
Yin binding/ Linking Vessel	*Yīn Wéi Mài*	陰維脉
Yin motility/ Stepping Vessel	*Yīn Qiāo Mài*	陰蹻脉

Bibliography

Classical Chinese Texts

In chronological order

Huang Di Nei Jing Su Wen (黄帝内经素问) *Yellow Emperor's Classic of Internal Medicine*: The oldest text on Chinese Medicine, attributed to Huang Di, compiled around 100 BC from medical texts dating between 400-200 BC. It is composed of two parts: *Su Wen- Simple Questions*, covering the fundamentals of Chinese medical concepts, and *Ling Shu* (灵枢) *Spiritual Axis (Pivot)*, concerning more specifically the practice of acupuncture. Tradition has it that two other books also existed, but have been lost since: Tai Shu, describing the Mu-accumulation and Xi-cleft points, and the Ming Tang, on the location of the acupuncture points.

Nan Jing Jiao Shi (难经校释) *(Explanation of) Classic of difficulties*: published around 1st-2nd century AD and generally attributed to Bian Que. Contains 81 chapters attempting to explain the difficulties of the Nei Jing.

Zhong Zang Jing (中藏经) *Classic of the Central Organ*, by Hoa To circa 198 AD, discusses mainly pulse diagnosis and warming herbal remedies.

Shang Han Lun (伤寒论) *Cold-induced Diseases*, by Zhang Zhong Jing 220 AD, one of the four most important classics, discussing the diagnosis and herbal treatment of feverish diseases from external cold, as well as prognosis and medical errors.

Jin Gui Yao Lue Fang Lun- 金匱要略方論 – Prescriptions of the Golden Cabinet by Zhang Zhong Jing, circa 220 AD, later modified by Wang Shu He, indicating herbal prescriptions for internal, surgical and gynecological conditions

Zhen Jiu Jia Yi Jing (针灸甲乙经) *Systemic Classic*: ABC of Acupuncture and Moxibustion, by Huang Fumi (215–281), published in 282 AD, discussing and complementing the Su Wen, the Ling Shu as well as the Ming Tang (the lost text). It remains the reference book for acupuncturists covering the treatment of various diseases.

Mai Jing (脉经) *The Classic of the Pulse* by Wang Shu He (210–286); describing 24 pulse qualities and their significance. This text had a great influence later on Asian and middle-eastern medicine.

Zhou Hou Bei Ji Fang (肘後備急方) *Emergency Prescriptions* by Ge Hong (284–364), offering herbal prescriptions and moxa for emergencies.

Qian Jin Yao Fang (千金要方) *Prescriptions Worth a Thousand Ducats* by Sun Si Miao (581-682), published around 652, it is a compilation of herbal, acupuncture and moxibustion treatments for external, internal, gynecological and pediatric conditions. He also covers the 13 Gui-ghost points, previously cited by Bian Que, for the treatment of 100 diseases.

Qian Jin Yi Fang (千金翼方) *Supplement to the Thousand Ducats*, in which Sun Si Miao complements the previous text.

Zhen Jiu Zi Sheng Jin (針灸資生經) *Supplementing life with Acupuncture and Moxibustion* by Wang Zhi Zhong, (1220). Elaborating on acupuncture points, methods of treatment for various diseases.

Biao You Fu (標幽賦) *Ode to Elucidate mysteries* attributed to Dou Mai (1196–1280)

Ma Dan Yang Tian Xing Shi Er Xue Ge (馬丹陽天星十二穴歌) *Song of Ma Dan Yang's Twelve Celestial Star points*, cited in the Zhen Jiu Da Quan by Xu Feng, 15th century; describes the coupling of the main 12 acupuncture points: LU-7, LI-11, LI-4, ST-36, ST-44, HE-5, BL-40, BL-57, BL-60, GB-30, GB-34 and LR-3.

Yu Long Jing (玉龍經) *Classic of the Jade Dragon*: Bian Que's Spiritual Guide to cupuncture and Moxibustion by Wan Guo Rui, 1329; includes the Yu Long Ge

Yu Long Ge (玉龍歌) - Song of the Jade dragon by Wang Guo Rui, 1329, included in the You Long Jing, on 120 acupuncture points.

Zhen Jiu Da Quan (鍼灸大全) *Complete Collection of Acupuncture and Moxibustion* in six volumes by Xu Feng (1439); describing more over needling techniques and choice of points according to the Stems and Branches.

Ling Guang Fu (靈光賦) Ode of Spiritual Brightness, cited in the Zhen Jiu Da Quan by Xu Feng (1439)

Xi Hong Fu (席弘賦) *Ode of Xihong*, cited in the Zhen Jiu Da Quan by Xu Feng (1439)

Zhen Jiu Ju Ying (針灸聚英) *Glorious Anthology of Acupuncture and Moxibustion*, by Gao Wu (1529). This is a compilation of ancient texts by eminent acupuncturists, commented and complemented by Gao Wu.

Bai Zheng Fu (百症賦) *Ode of One Hundred symptoms*; by an unknown author, cited in the Zhen Jiu Ju Ying by Gao Wu (1529).

Yu Long Fu (玉龍賦) *Ode of the Jade Dragon*, cited in the Zhen Jiu Ju Ying by Gao Wu (1529), is a digest of the main points of the earlier Yu Long Ge.

Za Bing Xue Fa Ge (雜病穴法歌) *Song of Points for Miscellaneous Diseases*, recorded in the Zhen Jiu Ju Ying by Gao Wu (1529).

Yi Xue Gang Mu (醫學綱目) *Outline of Medicine* by Lou Ying (1565); a compilation and commentaries of ancient texts.

Zhen Jiu Da Cheng (針灸大成) *Great Compendium of Acupuncture and Moxibustion* by Yang Ji Zhou (1601); is the most complete text on acupuncture, compiling over 30 ancient texts with commentaries and additions.

Sheng Yu Ge (胜玉歌) *Song more precious than Jade*, cited in the Zhen Jiu Da Cheng by Yang Ji Zhou (1601).

Xun Jing Kao Xue Bian (循經考穴編) *Investigation into Points of the Channels*, attributed to Yan Zhen, referring to Ming Wan Li (1573–1620), with commentaries on the points of the 14 channels.

Dong Yi Bao Jian (東醫寶鑑) *Precious Mirror of Oriental Medicine*, by the Korean author Xu Sun (1611).

Jing Yue Quan Sh (景岳全書) *Complete Works of Jing Yue*; Zhang Jie Bin (1624); in which he analyses various diagnostic and therapeutic methods, states that there is no

Yang exuberance but only *Yin* vacuity, and moreover indicates supplementing and warming techniques.

Lei Jing Tu Yi (類經圖翼) *Illustrated Supplement to the Classic of Categories*, by Zhang Jie Bin (1624), is an illustrated adaptation of the Nei Jing.

Shen Jiu Jing Lu (神灸经論) *Divine Moxibustion*; Wu Yang Cheng (1853). He states that during his time only about 2 out of 100 doctors practice acupuncture and only 1 out of 10 use Moxibustion.

Zhen Jiu Ji Cheng (針灸集成) *Compilation of Acupuncture and Moxibustion* by Liao Run Hong (1874)

Shi Si Jing Yao Xue Zhu Zhi Ge (十四經要穴主治歌) *Song of the Points of the Primary Fourteen Channels*, unknown author.

Yi Zong Jin Jian (醫宗金鑑) *Golden Mirror of Medicine*, by Wu Qian (1742), on methods of Acupuncture and Moxibustion.

Zhen Jiu Feng Yuan (針灸逢源) by Li Xue Chan, 1815, in 4 volumes, discusses the principles of acupuncture with a description of 361 main and 96 extra points.

Classical Chinese texts in *Pin Yin* alphabetical order

Bai Zheng Fu (百症賦) Ode of One Hundred symptoms; by Gao Wu (1529).

Biao You Fu (標幽賦) *Ode to Elucidate mysteries* attributed to Dou Mai (1196–1280)

Dong Yi Bao Jian (東醫寶鑑) *Precious Mirror of Oriental Medicine*, by Xu Sun (1611).

Huang Di Nei Jing Su Wen (黄帝内经素问) *Yellow Emperor's Classic of Internal Medicine*:

Jin Gui Yao Lue Fang Lun 金匱要略方論 − Prescriptions of the Golden Cabinet by Zhang Zhong Jing, circa 220 AD

Jing Yue Quan Sh (景岳全書) *Complete Works of Jing Yue*; Zhang Jie Bin (1624

Modern Chinese References

Zhong Hua Zhen Jiu Xue (中華鍼灸學) *Contemporary Acupuncture*, by Zhao Erkang (1953).

Zhen Jiu Xue Shou Ce (針灸學手册) *Origin and Development of Acupuncture and Moxibustion*, edited by Wang Xue Tai (1956).

Zhen Jiu Xue Jian Bian (針灸學簡編) edited by the TCM Institute of research in 1957, covers methods and pathologies as well as acupuncture analgesia.

Shanghai Zhen Jiu Xue (上海针灸学) *A Study of Acupuncture*, edited by TCM Institute of Shanghai in 1974

Zhong Guo Zhen Xue Jiu Gai Yao (中國針灸學) edited by Qi Ye in Taipei (1979).

Western References

Andrès G.: *Proposition pour une méthodologie d'étude des points d'acupuncture*. Revue Française d'acupuncture, No55, 1988, pp.5-11

Andrès G., Berger G., Guillaume G., Kespi J.M., Chieu M., B. Teboul-Wang: *Les méridiens extraordinaires*; (1997), La Tisserande, Paris

Autroche B., Navailh P.: *Le Diagnostic en Médecine Chinoise*; (1983) Maloine

Autroche B. et al: *Pratique des Aiguilles et de la Moxibustion;* (1989) Maloine

Barrey J-F., Deporte P.: *Vivre en Cinq Mouvements;* (1994) Ed. du Prieuré

Beinfield H., Korngold E.: *Between Heaven and Earth;* (1991); Ballantine Books

Bensky D., O'Connor J. (1996). *Acupuncture A Comprehensive Text Shanghai College of Traditional Medicine.* Eastland Press.

Bertschinger R.,
• *Golden Needle; Yang Jizhou's Great Compendium.* (1991). Churchill Livingston.
• *The Great Intent (2013); Singing Dragon*

Borsarello J.F.:

• *Cahiers d'Acupuncture* (1987), Masson

• *Acupuncture Pratique* (1998), Masson

Bossy J., Maurel J.C.: *Acupuncture*; (1976), Masson Paris

Bridges, L.: *Face Reading in Chinese Medicine;* (2004); Churchill Livingston

Brown S.G.: *The Practical art of Face Reading*; (2000); Carroll & Brown limited

Campbell, J.: *Acupuncture Channels and Points; (2008)* By (author) Joan Campbell, Churchill Livingston

Chamfrault A.: Editions Coquemard; Angoulème,
• Tome 1: *Traité de médecine chinoise. Acupuncture, moxas, massages, saignées* (1954)

- *Tome 2: Traité de médecine chinoise d'après les textes chinois anciens et modernes.*

- *Tome 3: Traité de médecine chinoise. Pharmacopée* (1959)

- *Tome 4: Traité de médecine chinoise d'après les textes anciens et modernes, formules magistrales* (1961)

- *Tome 5: Traité de médecine chinoise - de l'astronomie à la médecine chinoise*

- *Tome 6: Traité de médecine chinoise - l'énergétique humaine en médecine chinoise* (1996)

Chang Po-Tuan: *The Inner Tachings of Daoism;* (1986); Shambhala

Chmielnicki B.: *Pulse Qualities;* Compleo

Clavey S.: *Fluid Physiology and Pathology in TCM;* (1995); Churchill Livingstone

Connelly D.: *All Sickness is Home Sickness* (1994); Wisdom Well Press

Coste M., Paugam J.Y.: *Acupuncture, Tradition et Recherche Moderne* (2006); FLETC, PALAJA.

Darras J.C.: *Zhen Jiu Da Cheng*, translated by Leung Kwok Po; 1981, Darras editions, Paris (F)

Deadman, P., Al-Khafaji, M., & Baker, K. *A Manual of Acupuncture.* (2007). Journal of Chinese Medicine pub., East Sussex (GB).

Deng T.: *Practical Diagnosis in TCM;* (1999); Churchill Livingston

Desoutter, B.: *Merveilleux Vaisseaux.:* (1996); Sauramps medical, Montpellier

Dispenza J.: *You Are the Placebo.* (1991). Hay House

Pert C.: *Molecules of Emotion* (1997); Pocket Books

Di Villadorata M, Côté B.: *Acupuncture en Médecine Clinique;* (1989); Maloine, Paris.

Duron A., Laville-Mery Ch., Borsarello J.: *Bioénergétique et médecine chinoise;* 1973, Maisonneuve, Paris

Eckman, P.: *In the Footsteps of the Yellow Emperor*, (1996); Cypress Book, San Francisco.

Ellis, A., Wiseman, N., & Boss, K. *Fundamentals of Chinese Acupuncture (Paradigm Title).* (1991). Paradigm Publications (MA).

Emoto M. *Messages from Water* (2005) HADO

Eyssalet J-M: (1990); Guy Trédaniel

- *Shen ou l'Instant Créateur*;

- *Le Secret de la Maison des Ancêtres*

Farrell Y., Chan D.: *Psycho-Emotional Pain and the Eight Extraordinary Vessels* (2016) Singing Dragon

Faubert, A.: Guy Tredaniel.

- *Traité didactique d'Acupuncture Traditionnelle* (1977)

- *Le Sceau du Destin (1988).*

Faubert G., Crepon P.: *La Chronobiologie Chinoise*; (1983) Albin Michel

Fisch G.: *La Médecine Traditionelle Chinoise*; (1993); LEP

Frey M.: *l'Acupuncture, comprendre cette médecine;* (2007); You Feng

Füye de la R.: *Traité d'acupuncture* (1956). Editions Le François, Paris.

Gardner-Abbate S.: *Palpatory Diagnosis in Oriental Medicine*; (2001); Churchill Livingston

Garvey M., Lifang Q.: *Chinese Medicine Psychology*; (2020); Singing Dragon

Gaurier T.: *Acupuncture Traditionelle*; (1985); Encre

Gaurier T.: *Bioclimatopathologie en Acupuncture*; (1980); T. Gaurier

Geng J. & Su Z. *Acupuncture and Moxibustion* (Practical Traditional Chinese Medicine & Pharmacology). (1998). New World Library.

Hammer L. I.: *Chinese Pulse Diagnosis*; (2001); Eastland Press

Hammer L. I.: *Dragon Rises, Red Bird Flies*; (2005); Eastland Press

Harper D.: *Early Chinese Medical Literature*, (1998), KPI London

Helms J.M.: *Acupuncture Energetics: Clinical Approach for Physicians* (1995); Thieme

Hempen C.H.: *dtv-Atlas Akupunktur*, (1995); Deutschert Taschenbuch Verlag, München.

Holman CT.: Singing Dragon.
- *Treating Emotional Trauma with Chinese Medicine* (2017);
- *Treating Emotional Trauma with Chinese Medicine: Integrated Diagnostic and Treatment Strategies (pp. 8-9). Kindle Edition.*

Hseuh C. C.: *Acupuncture A Comprehensive Text. (*1981). Eastland Press.

Hua-Ching Ni: *I Ching* (1983). Tao of Wellness

Keown D. *The Spark in the* Machine (2014); Singing Dragon

Kespi J.-M.: *Acupuncture* (1982). Maisonneuve, Moulin-les-Metz, France.

Kespi J.-M :. *Cliniques: Acupuncture* (1995). De la Tisserande, Paris.

Kirschbaum, B.: *Atlas of Chinese Tongue Diagnosis*; (1998). Eastland press

Lade, A. *Acypuncture Points: Images & Functions* (1989). Eastland Press.

Larre C.: *Les Chinois*; 1981, Lidis-Brepols, Paris

Larre C., Schatz J, Rochat de la Vallée E*.: Survey of Traditional Chinese Medicine* (1976); Institut Ricci, Paris

Larre C., Rochat de la Vallée E.:
- *The Seven Emotions;* (1996); Monkey Press
- *Les Mouvements du Coeur;* (1992), Desclée de Brouwer, Paris

Laurent Ph. *L'esprit des points: étude des trajets des méridiens et de la signification du nom des points.* (2000). Librairie You-Feng.

Lavier, J. A. *Médecine chinoise médecine totale.* (1973); Grasset.

Lawson-Wood O. & J.: *Acupuncture Vitality and Revival Points*, (1960); Health Science Press, Devon.

Leung Kwok-Po: *Points d'acupuncture*; Revue Française d'acupuncture, No12, 1977, pp. 7-17

Legge D. *Acupuncture Points and Meridians*, (1999); Sydney College Press, Australia

Li Ding: *Acupuncture, Meridian Theory and Acupuncture Points*, (1991); Foreign Language Press, Beijing.

Li Shi Zhen: *Pulse Diagnosis;* (1985) Paradigm

Li Tian, Lachner A.: *Wortschatz Chinesische Medizin*,;(2005); Elsevier, München

Li X., Zhao, J. Acupuncture Patterns & Practice; (1993); Eastland Press

Lipton B.: *Biology of Belief* (2015); Hay House

Low R.: *The Celestial Stems;* (1985); Thorsons

Lu H. C.: *Tongue Diagnosis in Color;* (1977) The Academy of Oriental Heritage, Canada

Maciocia, G.: Churchill Livingstone
- *Tongue Diagnosis in Chinese Medicine;* (1987); Eastland Press
- *The Foundations of Chinese Medicine;* (1989)
- *Diagnosis in Chinese Medicine; (2004);*
- *The Channels of Acupuncture* (2006)*;*
- *The Psyche in Chinese Medicine*

Matsumoto, K. & Birch, S.:
- *Extraordinary Vessels;* (1993), Churchill Livingstone.
- *Hara Diagnosis; (1987); Paradigm*

Medicine, T. A. o. T. C.: *An Outline of Chinese Acupuncture.* (1975). Foreign Languages Press.

Mi, H. *Zhenjiu Jiayi Jing (2 Volumes).* (2004). Editeur Guy Tredaniel.

Mitchel, S. *Tao Te Ching*, (1943). Harper & Row

Montakab H.:
- *Acupuncture for Insomnia* (2012); Thieme

- *Acupuncture Point and Channel Energetics* (2014); Kiener

- *Chinese Medicine Revisited* (2015); Homaya

- *Acupuncture for Headaches, Eyes and other ENT Pathologies* (2019), Singing Dragon

Mussat M.: *Physique de l'Acupuncture*: Hypotheses et Approches. Experimentales. (1972); Le Francois

Nguyen Van Nghi: Don Bosco. Marseille
- *Pathognie et pathologie énergtiques en médecine chinoise: Traitement par acupuncture et massages;* (1971)

- *Topography énergtiques en médecine chinoise, (1971); Zhen Jiu Da Cheng. (1982); NVN Marseille*

Nguyen Van Nghi, Tran Viet Dzung, Recours Nguyen C.: *Lingshu.* (1972); NVN. Marseille

Nguyen Van Nghi Niboyet J. E.H.:
- *Essai sur l'Acupuncture Chinoise Pratique,* (1951); Dominique Wapler. Paris

- *Traitement des algies par l'acupuncture et massages chinois* (1959). Jacques Lafitte.

- *Pratique de la médecine manuelle* (1968). Maisonneuve et Larose.

- *Nouveau traité d'acupuncture* (1998). Maisonneuve et Larose.

Noll A. et al.: *Stresskrankheiten* (2006); Elsevier

O'Conner J., Bensky D.: *Acupuncture – A Comprehensive Text* (1981); Eastland Press

Oury C. : *Les Points fenêtres du Ciel*; Institut Ricci, Paris

Pan, A. *Océan d'énergie: étymologie des noms des points d'acupuncture* (1998). Maloine, Paris.

Paugam J-Y, Coste M. (2006). *Acupuncture Tradition et Recherche Moderne - Compendium de Recherche.* Fletc.

Pert C.: *Molecules of Emotion* (1997); Pocket Books

Quaglia-Senta A.: *Système Sympathique en Acupuncture Chinoise;* (1976), Maisonneuve, St.-Ruffine

Quirico P. E., Pedrali T.: *Teaching Atlas of Acupuncture* (2007); Thieme Stuttgart.

Reuben A., Babey-Brooke A.M.: *The Pulse in Occident and Orient;* (1966) Aurora

Réquéna, Y.: (1996), Maloine, Paris.
- *Terrains & pathologie en acupuncture -I*

- *Terrains & pathologie en acupuncture-II*

- *Terrains & pathologie en acupunct.-III*

Réquéna Y.: *Acupuncture et Psychologie;* (1982), Maloine, Paris.

Réquéna Y.:
- *Morphotypological Hand Diagnosis in Acupuncture;* (1986); Solal

- *Character and Health* (1989); Paradigm

Rochat de la Vallée E.: *Cahiers préparatoires à une meilleure comprehension des points d'acupuncture Tome-1.* Paris: Institut Ricci

Rochat de la Vallée E. ; Larre C.:
- *La Bannière* (1995); Desclée Brouver

- *The Seven Emotions* (1996); Redwing

Rochat de la Vallée E. et al: *Jing Shen (Huainzi chapter 7);* (2010) Monkey Press

Rochat de la Vallée E.:
- *Rooted in the Spirit* (1995); Station Hill Press

- *The Eight Extraordinary Meridians* (1997); Monkey Press

- *Yin Yang* (2006); Monkey Press

- *Aspects of Spirit* (2013); Monkey Press

- *Five Elements* (2016); Monkey Press

- *Symbolism of Numbers in Classical China* (2018); Monkey Press

Rosen R. I.: *Heart Shock* (2018); Singing Dragon

Ross J.: Churchill Livingstone.

- *Acupuncture Point Combinations: Key to Clinical Success.* (1995).

- *Zang Fu, The Organ System of TCM;* (1994)

Rossbach S.: *Interior Design with Feng Shui;* (1987) Rider

Roustan C.: *Traité d'Acupuncture, Médecine Traditionelle Chinoise*, 3 vol. (1979); Editions, Masson, France

Rozeg J.: *Vaisseaux Merveilleux* (1983); Maisonneuve, Moulin-lès-Metz

Schatz J., Larre C., Rochat de la Vallée E.: *Aperçus de médecine traditionelle chinoise* (1979), éd Maisonneuve, Paris.

Seem M.: *Bodymind Energetics;* (1987); Healing Arts

Shima, M. & Chace, C.: *The Channel Divergences: Deeper Pathways of the Web* (2000). Blue Poppy

Shima M.: *The Medical I Ching;* (1992); Blue Poppy

Sionneau, P.:
- *Troubles Psychiques en Médecine Chinoise* (1996). Guy Trédaniel,
- *Acupuncture: Les points essentiels* (2000). Guy Trédaniel, Paris.

Simons R.: *Feng Shui step by step;* (1996); Rider

Song T.B.: *Atlas of Tongues and Lingual Coating in Chinese Medicine;* (1986); Sinomedic

Soulié de Morant, G.: Maloine 1972
- *l'Acuponcture Chinoise, Atlas.*

- *l'Acuponcture Chinoise, Texte.*

Spears J. A.: *Meridian Circuit Systems*, (2010); Integrative Healing Society

Stercks P., Jun C.:
- *Diagnostic des Symptomes;* (2002)

- *Diagnostic des Syndromes;* (2002)

Stercks P., Jun C.: *Organes et Entrailles;* (2002), Presses Universitaires Guang Ming

Taylor K.: *Chinese Medicine in Early Communist China* (2005); Routledge Curzon, Oxon.

Tchao Ming-Te: *l'Acupuncture et la Moxibustion.* (1967); Tcha Ming Te, Paris

Twicken D. *Eight Extraordinary Channels;* (2013); Singing Dragon

Veith, I. *The Yellow Emperor's classic of internal medicine;* chapters 1-34 translated from the Chinese with an introductory study by Ilza Veith. (1966). *New ed. Uni Cal press, Berkley*

Wang D.: *Manual of International Standardization of Acupuncture Point Names.* (1987).

Wang Ju-Yi & Robertson J.: *Applied Channel Theory* (2008); Eastland Press, WA, USA

Wangyal T.: *The Tibetan Yogas of Dream and Sleep* (1998); Snow Lion

Walters D.: Aquarian

- *Chinese Astrology;* (1992)

- *Feng Shui handbook;* (1991)

Wilhelm R., Perrot, E.:
- *Tao Te King (Lao Tseu)* (1974); Librairie Médicis

- *The Secret of the Golden Flower* (2013); Routledge

Wiseman, N. *Glossary of Chinese Medical Terms and Acupuncture Points.* (1991). Paradigm

Wiseman, N. & Feng, Y.: *A Practical Dictionary of Chinese Medicine* (1998); Paradigm Publications

Wolynn M.: *It Didn't Start With You* (2016); Pinguin

Wu Wei Ping: *Chinese Acupuncture.* (1962). Health Sci. P.

Wühr E.: *Chinesische Syndromdiagnostik;* (2010) Verlag für Ganzheitliche Medizin

Yan, L. *New Chinese-English Dictionary of Traditional Chinese Medicine.* (2003). China Medical Science and Technology Press.

Yan Zhenguo: *Anatomical Atlas of Acupuncture Points* (2003); Donnica publishing

Yu Lin Lian, Chen C.-Y., Hammes, M. *Seirin-Bildatlas der Akupunktur. Darstellung der Akupunkturpunkte.* (1999); Könemann, Köln

Yuan-Kuang: *Méthode Pratique de Divination Chinoise par le Yi-King;* (1977) Guy Trédaniel

Yuen J. C.: *Extract of lectures between 2000 and 2013*, Academy of Chinese Healing Arts, Winterthur

Zhang Y. I.: *Transforming Emotions with Chinese Medicine;* (2007); State Uni. of New York

Zhenguo, Y. (2003). *Anatomical Atlas of Acupucture Points.* Donica Publishing.

Guide to *Pinyin* pronunciation

Pinyin is the official phonetic system for transcribing the Mandarin pronunciations of Chinese characters into Latin alphabet

Pīnyīn 拼音 literally means "spelled-out sounds.

Letter	English approximation
a	father
b	bay / spit
p	pay / pit
m	may / mummy
f	fair / fun
d	day / stop
t	take / top
n	nay / nit
l	lay / love
g	gay / skill
k	kay / kill
h	hay
j	jeep / church
q	cheer / punch
x	she / push
zh	junk / choke

ch	church / chin
sh	shirt / shoe
r	leisure / reduce
z	reads
c	hats / cats
s	say / sun
y	yea / yes
w	way / water
o	saw
e	her
i	(no illustration)
i	see
u	rude
ü	French tu, German Fühlen
er	are
ai	eye
ei	eight
ao	now
ou	oh
an	can
en	turn
ang	German Gang
eng	sung
ong	German Lunge
ia	Asia
ie	yes

iao	yeowl
iu	yoke / yukon
ian	yen
in	in
iang	e + yang
ing	sing
iong	German Jünger
ua	guano
uo	wall
uai	wife
uan	one
un	went
uang	oo + ahng
üe	ü + eh
üan	ü+ an
ün	German grün
kongr	corn
wanr	w + far
dianr	d + yar

General Index

Made in the USA
Las Vegas, NV
21 March 2021